"This new and comprehensive text is an important contribution to the libraries of occupational therapy practitioners and educators alike. *Occupational Therapy and Stress: Foundations, Assessment and Interventions* first deftly and succinctly covers definitions and the history and philosophy of stress research before proceeding to explain the neurophysiology of stress responses, then assessment and treatment, finally rounding off with first person accounts. Given the many ways our OT curricula are organized, the assessment and treatment of stress and stress related disorders may be spread out over multiple courses. The logical organization of this text allows for assignment of chapters that can stand alone and also lead into a gradual integration of clinical concepts."

Juli McGruder, *Distinguished Emerita Professor of Occupational Therapy, University of Puget Sound, Tacoma, Washington, USA*

"The book, *Occupational Therapy and Stress: Foundations, Assessment and Interventions*, makes an outstanding contribution to the occupational therapy community, given that stress is not merely a mental health concern and stress management is relevant to almost all practice areas, given how disease and physical symptoms may be caused by stress, but also may precipitate a stress response. The book provides a comprehensive occupational therapy perspective on stress that is theoretically and empirically informed and offers evidenced based interventions rooted in the Person Environment Occupational model that acknowledges the biopsychosocial and interactional foundations of stress, which can lead to both positive and negative outcomes."

Ben Mortenson, *Professor and Department Head of Occupational Therapy, University of British Columbia, Vancouver, British Columbia, Canada*

"This text offers a novel synthesis of science and practice through an occupational lens, deepening understanding of how engagement in meaningful activities influences stress and resilience. Integrating evidence-based assessment tools and innovative approaches to intervention, it provides a timely and transformative resource for advancing occupational therapy education and practice in the prevention and management of stress."

Janet Njelesani, *Associate Professor of Occupational Therapy, New York University, New York, USA*

"This seminal work not only explores the historical evolution of stress research, it identifies fundamental intersections within the occupational therapy scope of practice. Stein and colleagues' integrated-pathway framework shifts the focus of occupational therapy intervention beyond learning survival skills for stress management and instead provides tools for promoting adaptation and thriving with clients; it is valuable for students, educators and practitioners."

Amy Kashiwa, *Clinical Associate Professor, School of Occupational Therapy, University of Puget Sound, Tacoma, Washington, USA*

Occupational Therapy and Stress

This is the first book aimed at occupational therapists to examine the background and impact of stress on individuals' lives, as well as providing practical interventions to address it.

Whether you work with clients coping with chronic illness, the onset of disability or a range of psychosocial challenges, stress is a hidden but often all-pervasive issue in your professional practice. This book therefore provides a comprehensive understanding of what stress means, how it can be understood and the practical tools to address it effectively. It begins by introducing the concept of stress and the neurophysiological mechanisms which underpin it. Then it deals with evaluation and assessment, including a range of clinical assessment tools, and covers topics such as lifestyle factors, cross cultural differences and the effects of technology. The final part of this book provides strategies for interventions, from mindfulness and other relaxation techniques to music, horticulture and the arts. There is also a chapter on managing group interventions, as well as addressing burnout among practitioners or students.

Emphasizing the key interplay between the individual, environment and occupation, this insightful and practical text will be essential reading for occupational therapy students and practitioners alike.

Franklin Stein is Emeritus Professor of Occupational Therapy at the University of South Dakota, former Founding Editor of *Occupational Therapy International* and life member of the American Psychological Association.

Khader A. Almhdawi is a Professor of Occupational Therapy and Rehabilitation in the Department of Rehabilitation Sciences at Jordan University of Science & Technology (JUST).

Ryan Thomure is a Clinical Assistant Professor and Academic Fieldwork Coordinator in the Department of Occupational Therapy at the University of Illinois Chicago.

Farrukh A. Chishtie is a Research Assistant in the Department of Occupational Science and Occupational Therapy, Climate Expert at the Climate Hub and Co-Lead of the Climate Migration Research Group at the Centre for Migration Studies, University of British Columbia.

George S. Tomlin is Professor Emeritus of Occupational Therapy at the University of Puget Sound, where he taught for 38 years and chaired the program for 14 years. He has authored 30 articles and 7 books/chapters and made 90+ conference presentations internationally. His professional service includes 12 years on the NBCOT Board of Directors. Current projects focus on artificial intelligence in occupational therapy and faculty research resources.

Occupational Therapy and Stress

Foundations, Assessment and Interventions

FRANKLIN STEIN, KHADER A. ALMHDAWI, RYAN THOMURE, FARRUKH A. CHISHTIE AND GEORGE S. TOMLIN

Routledge
Taylor & Francis Group
LONDON AND NEW YORK

Designed cover image: Routledge

First published 2026
by Routledge
4 Park Square, Milton Park, Abingdon, Oxon, OX14 4RN

and by Routledge
605 Third Avenue, New York, NY 10158

Routledge is an imprint of the Taylor & Francis Group, an informa business

British Library Cataloguing-in-Publication Data
A catalogue record for this book is available from the British Library

ISBN: 978-1-041-13700-9 (hbk)
ISBN: 978-1-041-13699-6 (pbk)
ISBN: 978-1-003-67108-4 (ebk)

DOI: 10.4324/9781003671084

Typeset in Vectora LT Std
by codeMantra

Access the Support Material: www.routledge.com/9781041136996

Contents

Acknowledgments

Frank Stein

My research on stress management began during my tenure as a Professor of Occupational Therapy at the University of Wisconsin-Milwaukee, from 1977 to 1989. During that time, I became interested in exploring the question: *How do people cope with stress in their everyday lives?* This question was initially posed to students through open-ended inquiries about the symptoms of stress, events that trigger stress reactions and the meaningful activities that help reduce stress. Students in the UW-Milwaukee program, especially Sharon Pape, were instrumental in collecting data from a large and diverse group of people. Later, while serving as a Professor of Occupational Therapy at the University of South Dakota, I continued my research on stress with the help of graduate students Daphne Grueshow, Melanie Hoffman, Michael Natz, Sara Taylor and Ryan Tronbak.

I am deeply grateful to my wife, Jennie, for her unwavering support, as well as to my children – Cheryl, David, Jessie and Barbara – for their encouragement throughout this journey. I would also like to thank the editors, especially Russell George, at Taylor & Francis, for the opportunity to publish this book.

Khader Almhdawi

I am deeply grateful to God, who has always guided my steps toward what is best for me. I owe a lifetime debt of gratitude to my great teacher and advisor, Dr. Virgil Mathiowetz of the University of Minnesota, USA. My first line of defense against stress has always been my beloved family – Alaa, Jude, Lujain, Ottoman and Suliman – as well as my extended family, especially Abdullah and Sawsan. I also wish to express my sincere appreciation to my generous sponsor and employer, Jordan University of Science and Technology, for funding my education and supporting my scholarly work.

Ryan Thomure

I would like to thank my family for their unending love and my colleagues for their support and generosity.

Farrukh Chistie

This textbook would not have been possible without the support and encouragement of many individuals. I am profoundly grateful to my family for their unwavering patience and understanding throughout this project and to my mentors and colleagues at the University of British Columbia for their guidance and scholarly wisdom in shaping my thinking around stress, resilience and occupational therapy practice.

I extend sincere thanks to my colleagues, including my co-authors in the rehabilitation sciences and occupational therapy communities who have generously shared their expertise, who provided thoughtful feedback and challenged me to think more deeply about the integration of positive psychology with clinical practice. To my friends and peers who listened, questioned and encouraged me along the way – your support has been invaluable.

This work is also informed by the lived experiences and insights of the many individuals who have generously contributed to research in stress management, post-traumatic growth and salutogenic approaches. It is my hope that this textbook honors their contributions and advances our collective understanding of how we can support resilience and flourishing in occupational therapy practice.

George S. Tomlin

My first encounter with stress management was during a job interview early in my occupational therapy career. My inadequate answer to the question of what my strategy was for managing stress may have been a reason I was not selected for that position. This theme has come full circle in my role as a co-author of this book, for which I am grateful. I am also thankful for Dr. Juli McGruder's explanation of family-expressed emotion and its role influencing the prognosis for individuals with mental health challenges in both developing and developed countries. Finally, I am very appreciative of the patience of my wife Sybille during the intense final month of editing the manuscript.

About the Authors

Franklin Stein has been an occupational therapist for a lifelong career. Occupational therapy has not only provided him with a profession, but it has also given him a philosophy to live by. As he learned about occupational therapy, it demonstrated to him that it is a profession based on helping individuals to cope with their disabilities and disadvantages by using purposeful and meaningful activities as interventions. For him the philosophy of occupational therapy is based on a humanistic approach where we view each individual as unique and having innate abilities and intrinsic capacities that can be positively developed to improve their lives and reach their potentials.

He is currently Emeritus Professor from the University of South Dakota, former Founding Editor of *Occupational Therapy International* and life member of the American Psychological Association. He completed his undergraduate and graduate education at Brooklyn College and New York University. He was the first recipient of a scholarship stipend from the New York State Department of Mental Hygiene to complete his certificate in occupational therapy at New York University in 1959. He worked as a psychosocial occupational therapist at the Psychiatric Institute and Director of Occupational Therapy in the Brooklyn Day Center. He received support from the New York State Scholar Incentive Program, the American Occupational Therapy Association and Vocational Rehabilitation Services to complete his master's degree in 1963 and doctoral degree from New York University in counseling psychology in 1968 with an internship at Queens College. Upon receiving his PhD in counseling psychology, he received the New York University Founder's Day Award for high scholastic performance.

He is the current author with Martin Rice and George Tomlin of the book *Stein's Research in Occupational Therapy*, 7th edition, published by Taylor and Francis (2025). He is also the author of *Occupational Therapy: A Guide for*

Students, Consumers and Advocates with Kathlyn Reed (2020), *Pocket Guide to Interventions in Occupational Therapy*, 2nd edition, with Kristine Haertl (2019), *Pocket Guide to Treatment in Occupational Therapy* (2000) with Becky Roose and over 50 articles in journals and books related to rehabilitation and psychosocial research. He has also presented more than a hundred seminars, workshops, institutes, short courses and research papers at national and international conferences.

He has taught courses as a full-time professor to undergraduate and graduate students at Boston University, the University of Wisconsin-Milwaukee, the University of Manitoba and the University of South Dakota. He also gave the keynote address at the Australian Occupational Therapy Association Conference in Perth in 1984. He has also taught in many different cultural environments. He spent sabbaticals as a Visiting Scholar at Cambridge University in England in 1974, Visiting Professor at the University of Uppsala in Sweden in 1999 and in short professorships at McGill University and the University of Alberta in Canada in 1984. He has taught short courses and workshops as a Visiting Professor at Federal University in Belo-Horizonte, Brazil, University of Texas – El Paso, Wayne State University, York College in Jamaica Queens, New York University, as well as in Mexico, Canada, Portugal, England, Australia, Sweden, Finland and Russia and in the Caribbean.

Khader Almhdawi is a Professor of Occupational Therapy and Rehabilitation in the Department of Rehabilitation Sciences at Jordan University of Science & Technology (JUST), Irbid-Jordan. Khader received his OT BSc from JUST in 2003 and an MSc from Colorado State University, USA, and a PhD in rehabilitation sciences (stroke rehabilitation) from the University of Minnesota, USA, in 2011.

Almhdawi has worked in many academic and clinical positions in Jordan and the USA including teaching and research assistant, learning disability specialist, Adjunct Faculty and Assistant/Associate/Professor of OT and rehabilitation. Khader chaired the Department of Rehabilitation Sciences (occupational therapy, physical therapy and speech/audiology) at JUST for two years and served as a member or chair for many academic-related committees. Since the start of his career, Khader has taught undergraduate and graduate courses related to adult physical dysfunctions and neurorehabilitation in addition to supervising related student research projects.

Almhdawi has published in many peer-reviewed international journals and presented at many conferences. Almhdawi and his graduate students are currently researching the field of adult physical dysfunction, particularly neurological challenges, assistive technology, occupational stress (musculoskeletal and mental health), medical education and accommodating individuals with disabilities and integrating them into the community. Almhdawi has published his work in many high-impact international peer-reviewed journals. Additionally, Khader has served as a reviewer, editorial board member and editor in many international indexed peer-reviewed journals.

Ryan Thomure is a Clinical Assistant Professor and Academic Fieldwork Coordinator in the Department of Occupational Therapy at the University of Illinois Chicago. He holds an Occupational Therapy Doctorate from Boston University and a Master of Science in Occupational Therapy from the University of Illinois Chicago (UIC), complemented by a Master of Social Work from Loyola University of Chicago.

In his current role at UIC, Thomure has provided coordination and support for fieldwork activities, ensuring that students gain meaningful and successful fieldwork experiences. He also leads several courses related to fieldwork, interpersonal communication, professional development and leadership within the occupational therapy program. His commitment to education is evident from his recognition with the 2023 Excalibur Award for Teaching Excellence, awarded by the graduating class at UIC's Department of Occupational Therapy.

Beyond his academic responsibilities, Thomure has extensive clinical experience in community settings, focusing on populations affected by homelessness, substance abuse and addiction. Since 2016 he has served as an occupational therapy supervisor at Ascension Housing and Health Alliance, providing supervision and direct clinical services.

Farrukh A. Chishtie is a Research Assistant in the Department of Occupational Science and Occupational Therapy, Climate Expert at the Climate Hub and Co-Lead of the Climate Migration Research Group at the Centre for Migration Studies, University of British Columbia. His interdisciplinary background includes two PhDs – one in applied mathematics from the University of Western Ontario and another in education with specialization in environment and sustainability. Chishtie's research focuses on occupational security and disability rehabilitation and resilience, with particular emphasis on vulnerable populations.

As president and founder of the *Peaceful Society, Science and Innovation Foundation*, he leads initiatives supporting disabled and elderly populations across Canada. His extensive experience includes developing post-disaster disability strategies following the 2005 northern Pakistan earthquake and establishing a community-based rehabilitation model specializing in spinal cord injury care delivery. Currently, he is conducting research on the lived experiences of patients with long COVID and on care management practices in British Columbia.

His contributions to rehabilitation sciences include developing frameworks for occupational security and safety, reflecting his dedication to understanding how environmental, health and societal changes impact human occupation and well-being. With over 120 peer-reviewed publications across multiple disciplines, Chishtie's background in disaster response, disability rehabilitation, resilience and emerging health challenges positions him uniquely to address contemporary issues in stress management and occupational therapy.

George S. Tomlin is Professor Emeritus of Occupational Therapy at the University of Puget Sound, where he taught for 38 years, including 14 years as Chair of the Occupational Therapy Program. His professional practice experience spans pediatric behavioral health, physical rehabilitation, injured worker programs and ergonomic assessments. He is the author of 30 articles in professional journals and 7 book chapters or books, including with Rice and Stein, *Stein's Research in Occupational Therapy* (6th and 7th editions). He has made or contributed to over 90 presentations at state, national and international conferences, including guest lectures in the Netherlands, Germany, Austria, Switzerland and the United Kingdom. From 1989 to 1999, he created five interactive video computer-based tutorials and clinical simulations covering human anatomy, biomechanics, pediatric assessment and neurological rehabilitation. His professional service has been highlighted by four years on the NBCOT clinical simulation development team and 12 years on the NBCOT Board of Directors, five years of which he served as Chair of the Qualifications and Compliance Review Committee. He has served as a reviewer/editor for many journals. Current projects include a monograph on artificial intelligence and occupational therapy with the Global Occupational Therapy Think Tank, an analysis of decision-making portrayed in published occupational therapy case studies with a mixed team of faculty researchers and practitioners and an online resource group for faculty teaching research in occupational therapy programs.

Foreword

Occupational Therapy and Stress: Foundations, Assessment and Interventions is a thoughtfully written, innovative book that fills a significant gap in the occupational therapy literature. This book addresses a pervasive challenge of the 21st century – stress. This book offers both a comprehensive review of current research and practical guidance for application in occupational therapy practice. It provides readers with a clear, evidence-informed framework for understanding, assessing and intervening in the areas of stress and coping. As the authors clearly articulate, stress is a universal experience that can manifest either as a positive, motivating force (eustress) or as a detrimental cause of illness (distress). Authored by a team of experts from occupational therapy, occupational science and environmental science, this book establishes stress management as a core life skill integral to the scope and practice of occupational therapy.

The authors' conceptual framework – the Integrated-Pathway Model – extends beyond current thinking to integrate environmental, psychological and biological perspectives while incorporating positive psychology and flow theory into a new conceptualization highly relevant to occupational therapists. This book skillfully applies current and proposed models to occupational therapy practice via the introduction of Stein's *Stress Management Questionnaire* and the inclusion of practical strategies for individual and group interventions. While many health professionals address stress management, this text fills a crucial need by offering a stress management perspective rooted specifically in occupational therapy. I highly recommend this text for faculty, students, researchers and practitioners seeking a comprehensive and practice-oriented resource on stress and occupational therapy.

Kristine Haertl, PhD, OTR/L, FAOTA
Professor
Department of Occupational Therapy, St. Catherine University
St. Paul, Minnesota, USA

Preface

Inception

This book's inception was in 2022. Having published several manuscripts on stress management and served as editor of *Occupational Therapy International*, I contacted Khader Almhdawi, whose scholarly interest in the physiology of stress I was familiar with. We began brainstorming the book's contents and soon recognized the need for an occupational therapist actively using stress management in their practice. Subsequently, we added Ryan Thomure from the University of Illinois in Chicago, whose clinical expertise with groups was a welcome addition. Farrukh Chishtie, whom I met through his involvement with the Global Occupational Therapy Think Tank, was another key contributor. As a writer and thinker of the highest caliber, Farrukh impressively navigates both the physical sciences and health professions at the University of British Columbia, with a focus on positive health and occupational therapy. The project was rounded out by George S. Tomlin, who brought his excellent research-minded approach to occupational therapy knowledge and pedagogy, who helped to edit and unify the book.

Frank Stein, October 23, 2025

PRELUDE

Why Did the Authors Select the Subject of This Book?

One of the major assumptions of this book is that stress is a pervasive experience in everyone's life. Ironically, stress can be either a positive motivating force or a cause of illness. We cannot escape stressful events in our everyday lives as human beings. Stress occurs as we pursue our goals while following the rules of life that we live under. In the 21st century, life can be competitive, for example, as we engage in sports, perform in public, complete an education, seek spouses and companions, try to get into college, apply for jobs, interact on social media and conform to the standards of acceptable behavior. There are also the hassles of everyday life as we engage with friends and relatives, co-workers and those people we encounter in stores, offices and online. Driving in heavy commuter traffic or extreme weather conditions can cause distress. There are also major events in our lives, such as the death of a loved one, a severe illness or injury, the loss of a job, financial ruin, loss of property or being in a war zone, which can produce lasting trauma. In the extreme, this can manifest itself as post-traumatic stress disorder (PTSD). In order to cope with stress, we need personal strength, perseverance, resilience and critical life skills that can help us to lessen its destructive impacts. Distress can trigger and exacerbate symptoms of and vulnerabilities to disorders. The authors' goals are to inform the reader (occupational therapy students, faculty and practitioners, as well as other health professionals) about the latest knowledge and research on stress and to present assessment tools and practical strategies and interventions that occupational therapists can use to help individuals prevent and manage stress. We present a holistic approach to stress management based on empirical research evidence.

Why Is a Book Needed on Stress Management for Occupational Therapists?

The authors are occupational therapists and health scientists representing diverse cultural and professional backgrounds. We all agree that there is a need for a textbook on stress management from an occupational therapy perspective. Stress can trigger symptoms in individuals who are vulnerable to a physical, psychological, developmental or environmental disorder. At the same time, learning stress management strategies is a critical life skill. Occupational therapists work with individuals, many of whom have chronic disabilities and are coping with distress that often is the result of loss of function and the inability to perform activities of daily living. For those living with a physical, psychological, developmental or environmental disorder, there is a need to learn how to cope with the inevitable stress. While many health professionals work on stress management with individuals, few focus specifically on the occupational therapy perspective, which emphasizes the role of occupation, adaptation, the just-right challenge and functional independence. In fact, what occupational therapy practitioners do at the core of their profession overlaps considerably with healthy stress management. That is, activity analysis and adaptation, customized instruction and therapeutic support and occupation- and client-centered intervention are at the heart of both occupational therapy and stress management approaches. Therapists have not often conceptualized their practice as one of promoting stress management, but there is in fact a strong case to be made that this is indeed true. As Courtney and Escobedo (1990) noted, "Stress is a factor in many modern illnesses. The development of coping skills to deal with stress is an occupational therapy goal for many patients" (p. 306).

This book addresses the gap between theory and practice by offering practical research-based strategies that occupational therapists can implement with their clients, helping them simultaneously meet their therapy goals and manage the inevitable stress in their lives.

How Will This Book Improve Intervention for Individuals with Chronic Disorders and Chronic Diseases?

Occupational therapists frequently see individuals with chronic disorders and diseases (arthritis, multiple sclerosis, stroke, cardiovascular disease, respiratory illness, severe mental illness, cognitive dysfunction and developmental conditions such as autism). In the USA in 2023, chronic conditions accounted for about 75% of the $4.9 trillion annual healthcare expenditure (Centers for Medicare and Medicaid Services, 2025). For example, the lifetime cost of stroke care in the USA, including inpatient treatment, rehabilitation and follow-up, has been estimated at $140,048 per patient (Rochmah et al., 2021).

Chronic illness can result in financial strain, social isolation, pain and reduced quality of life, all of which contribute to stress. Occupational therapists play a central role in helping clients regain function and social participation through activity modifications, habit formation, assistive devices, ergonomic recommendations and training in daily living skills. Stress can hinder the rehabilitation process, while stress management strategies can facilitate recovery and adaptation. This book provides occupational therapists with practical interventions to apply in aiding individuals with chronic illness.

What Are the Methods for Preventing or Reducing Distress?

In this book, we discuss practical methods and interventions within an occupational therapy framework to prevent, manage and reduce stress. We provide a standardized stress assessment that identifies symptoms, stressors and coping strategies. We emphasize the interplay among the individual, environment and occupation. We introduce everyday activities and approaches through which individuals can learn to manage their stress such as breathing exercises, meditation, meditative walking, listening to music, aerobic exercise, tai chi, yoga, arts and crafts, sleep hygiene, positive psychology and other related techniques. As occupational therapists, we consider the purpose and meaningfulness (to the individual) of each potential activity to enhance the effectiveness of the intervention. We also apply the principles of activity analysis and consider how best to incorporate stress management strategies into one's everyday schedule.

What Is the Difference in Approach between a Psychologist and an Occupational Therapist in Implementing a Stress Management Program?

Clinical and counseling psychologists are trained in psychotherapeutic techniques, including cognitive behavioral therapy and mindfulness training, which directly relate to stress management. Intervention is usually verbal and targeted at specific symptoms such as anxiety, depression and phobias that result from moderate to severe stressors and the attendant stress reactions. Occupational therapists usually intervene with individuals using a holistic (whole person) approach, emphasizing a biopsychosocial perspective within an occupation-based therapy framework. For example, an individual seeking help from a clinical psychologist will usually be seen in an office setting for verbal therapy. On the other hand, the occupational therapist will see individuals in clinical settings such as hospitals or outpatient settings, possibly in a simulated apartment, where the therapist can demonstrate specific daily life tasks that can instigate stress. The interventions by occupational therapists are coordinated with efforts by the entire rehabilitation team. In psychosocial settings, occupational therapists work in teams with social workers, nurses, psychiatrists and psychologists, using purposeful and meaningful activities with individuals diagnosed with severe mental illnesses such as schizophrenia, bipolar disorder, Alzheimer's disease or depression. Using psychoeducational techniques in group sessions, occupational therapists aim to help the individual incorporate stress management techniques into everyday living. Techniques such as aerobic exercise, meditation and relaxation therapy, arts and crafts, keeping a stress diary and music are demonstrated and encouraged by the occupational therapist. Despite the differences in professional approach, psychologists and occupational therapists share the goal of helping individuals cope with stress and alleviate anxiety and depression in their daily lives.

What Skills Does an Occupational Therapist Need to Assess Stress and Implement Stress Management Interventions?

As occupational therapists, we work directly with individuals to help them improve function and become as independent as they seek to be in activities of daily living and social participation. Occupational therapists teach healthy habits in everyday living, recommend ergonomic adaptations and motivate individuals to persevere in their rehabilitation. In interactions with the individual, the occupational therapist of course needs to first establish rapport. Specifically, in working with individuals in a stress management program, the occupational therapist should

1. have clinical knowledge of specific physical, mental and cognitive disabilities and disorders such as hypertension, chronic obstructive pulmonary disease (COPD), dementia, cancer, schizophrenia, PTSD and arthritis;
2. understand the physiology and psychology of the stress reaction;
3. understand the relationship between stress and anxiety, depression and behavioral symptoms such as insomnia, anorexia, fatigue and substance abuse and addiction;
4. be knowledgeable in administering a stress assessment tool and evaluating the results;
5. incorporate positive health factors such as nutrition, exercise, sleep hygiene, music, social connections, healthy sexuality, spirituality and meditation into a holistic stress management program;
6. be familiar with stress management techniques such as meditation, tai chi, keeping a stress diary, aerobic exercise and group activity therapy;
7. be able to plan a customized stress management program for a specific individual;
8. maintain ethical standards in implementing an intervention program;
9. have the skills to evaluate the effectiveness of the stress management intervention and document it;
10. keep current with the research on stress management;
11. recognize and respond to signs of secondary stress and burnout in oneself;
12. incorporate an occupational therapy model such as the Model of Human Occupation (MOHO) or the Person-Environment-Occupation-Performance (PEOP) into a stress management program.

Because the authors believe that every occupational therapy client may be a candidate for needing stress management help, we encourage the inclusion of a course or course unit on stress management in every entry-level program in occupational therapy.

REFERENCES

Centers for Medicare and Medicaid Services. (2025). National health expenditure fact sheet. https://www.cms.gov/data-research/statistics-trends-and-reports/national-health-expenditure-data/nhe-fact-sheet

Courtney, C., & Escobedo, B. (1990). A stress management program: Inpatient-to-outpatient continuity. *American Journal of Occupational Therapy*, *44*(4), 306–310. https://doi.org/10.5014/ajot.44.4.306

Rochmah, T. N., Rahmawati, I. T., Dahlui, M., Budiarto, W., & Bilqis, N. (2021). Economic burden of stroke disease: A systematic review. *International Journal of Environmental Research and Public Health*, *18*(14), 7552. https://doi.org/10.3390/ijerph18147552

Chapter 1
What Is Stress?

LEARNING OBJECTIVES

By the end of this chapter, the reader will be able to

1. Define the terms stressor and stress as they are used in health settings.
2. Discuss the categories of stress, including eustress and distress.
3. Identify stressors that can trigger symptoms and aggravate existing health conditions.
4. Explain how coping activities can prevent or alleviate stress.
5. Differentiate between mild, moderate and severe levels of stress.
6. Describe how stress management is one of the critical life skills as identified by the World Health Organization (WHO).
7. Identify cultural differences among people as they respond to stress.

Stress occurs in all living organisms, from plants to animals. In plants, drought, infectious diseases, insects, floods, lightning, and other events that threaten the plant's survival can cause stress that may destroy the plant. The plant can survive and continue to grow if its responses or natural coping mechanisms are resilient and enable the plant to withstand the damage.

As Bandurska (2022) explained,

> Plants' resistance to stress factors is a complex trait that is a result of changes at the molecular, metabolic, and physiological levels. The plant's resistance strategy means the ability to survive, recover, and reproduce under adverse conditions. Harmful environmental factors affect the state of stress in plant

DOI: 10.4324/9781003671084-1

> tissues, which creates a signal triggering metabolic events responsible for resistance, including avoidance and/or tolerance mechanisms.
>
> (Bandurska, 2022)

Webster (1983) in a classical study of large mammals found that stress occurs when their environment is reduced or threatened. He concluded that an adequate environment for mammals is one that meets four criteria: thermal comfort, physical comfort, disease control and behavioral satisfaction. Environmental stress, which may be direct or indirect, is anything that causes a departure from these criteria.

TYPES OF STRESS, DEFINED

In human beings, as Selye (1956) wrote, "The secret of health and happiness lies in successful adjustment to the ever-changing conditions on this globe; the penalties for failure in this great process of adaptation are disease and unhappiness" (p. vii). Stress can precipitate symptoms, as well as being a positive and motivating force. As a cause stress can be categorized (Selye, 1976) as good stress (eustress), bad stress (distress), overstress (hyperstress) and understress (hypostress). Eustress is defined as a challenge that is pleasant or motivating, such as playing a musical instrument or engaging in an amateur sport, where people are motivated to express their skills, bringing satisfaction.

On the other hand, distress can be unpleasant and contribute to the cause of a disease that may be debilitating. Distress can precipitate symptoms such as headaches, gastrointestinal pain, back pain, aggressiveness and depression. Distress can be a "trigger" to symptoms and even to relapse in individuals with existing diseases or vulnerabilities such as arthritis or clinical depression. For example, it is known that stress can trigger a relapse in individuals with a diagnosis of multiple sclerosis (Reece et al., 2024).

Hyperstress is chronic or prolonged stress and is unremitting unless resolved. It can produce damage to the internal organs such as the heart, kidney and blood vessels. Physically, the body reacts to extreme pressure or prolonged stress in a variety of ways that can precipitate a disease or an illness in an individual who is at risk. Physical damage from stress will occur if external causes are intense and long-lasting. Research has presented overwhelming evidence that severe stress over prolonged periods has a detrimental effect on physiological function (Chu et al., 2024). For example, among patients with coronary heart disease acute psychological stress has been shown to induce transient myocardial ischemia, and long-term stress can increase the risk of recurrent heart attacks and mortality (Gao et al., 2022). Chronic work stress also can increase the risk of coronary heart disease (Kivimäki & Kawachi, 2015).

Hypostress or understress can be conceptualized as a lack of motivation or hopelessness in the face of danger or challenge. In hypostress, the individual has given up and is passive to the demands of life. Frankl (1962) described this condition of hypostress in the inmates of a concentration camp during World War II when individuals gave up and no longer wanted to live.

STRESSORS AND STRESS REACTION ARE INDIVIDUALIZED

In general, stress is a complex concept that is dynamic and is derived from the everyday events in a person's life. The intensity of the stress reaction and its consequences will depend on the individual's inner ability to cope and available external resources (positive health), such as friends, and the use of coping activities like meditation, music or exercise. When a person is able to use available resources for coping, the response to distress is moderated. Some examples of stressful situations are pressure to do well on an examination, the fear of being rejected by a friend, the reaction to a loss of a job or anxious thoughts about the future. These situations are referred to as stressors that trigger a reaction in the individual. The body reacts to these stressors by a "fight or flight" mechanism that increases heart rate, blood pressure and metabolism and includes the release of certain hormones into the bloodstream. When an individual perceives that he or she is under pressure, the body mobilizes as if it is under attack. If the response is intense or prolonged, it can lead to symptoms such as headaches, heartburn, blurring of vision, anxiety or numerous other common problems (Gibbons, 2019).

Stress also refers to the everyday pressures in living that are the result of hassles that make life difficult and create discomfort. Stressors are specific to the individual. There are external stressors that are generated by the environment, including crowds, noise, poor lighting, inadequate ventilation and environmental pollutants. Internal stressors are generated by the individual and are caused by feelings of insecurity, anxiety and fear. Social stressors (Schalbroeck et al., 2024) include major life changes such as divorce, job loss, major illness, financial problems, family death, car breakdown and accidents. These stressors may negatively impact the immune system, leading to physiological disorders and a psychoneurological immune reaction (Alotiby, 2024).

PREVALENCE OF STRESS SYMPTOMS

According to the American Psychological Association (2022), symptoms of stress are widely reported among the population of the USA. Fully 76% reported having at least one symptom of stress within the last month. These symptoms included headache, fatigue, anxiety or sadness, with about one-third of respondents reporting each. Another third felt overwhelmed, had an alteration in sleep pattern or had constant worry (American Psychological Association, 2022).

MITIGATING STRESS

"Copers" are everyday activities or behavioral efforts to master, mitigate or tolerate demands created by a stressful situation. Coping refers to an individual's efforts to manage demands, regardless of the success of those efforts. When effective, copers manage or reduce stress by bringing about a feeling of relaxation, reduced anxiety and increased sense of well-being. Meng and D'Arcy (2016) found that positive coping indicated a higher level of personal well-being, whereas negative coping was associated with a lower level of personal well-being and was also related to distress.

MAGNITUDE OF STRESS, DEFINED

Everyday stress in humans can be mild, moderate or severe. A typically healthy person should be able to cope with mild or moderate stressors in daily life. Severe levels of stress, however, call for extraordinary techniques of management (see post-traumatic stress disorder, as described in Chapter 9). Mild or moderate stress as described above can also be a motivation for an individual to perform at one's best, such as in learning a new language, performing with a musical instrument or engaging in a competitive sport. On the other hand, if stress limits the individual in performing in competitions or taking an examination, it has a negative effect on the individual that could distort thinking, performance or memory. For example, Peavy et al. (2009) found that experiencing stressful life events over a period of up to three years is associated with accelerated cognitive decline in older adults with mild cognitive impairment.

Stressors are universal. Every person on the planet experiences them. How an individual responds to stressors determines whether their effects are positive (eustress) or negative (distress).

Driving a car in light traffic is a mildly stressful situation for most people who are experienced drivers. The individual has to be alert for unexpected responses from other drivers. For a new driver or someone who has a disability or physical condition such as experiencing dizziness or visual problems, even driving in light traffic can be at least moderately stressful. Driving a car in a beautiful rural area with very little traffic while enjoying the scenery can be an uplifting experience. In short, driving a car can be a positive experience or a mild, moderate or severely stressful experience depending upon the environment or context and the individual's physical and psychological states, expertise in driving a car and confidence in responding to traffic conditions such as icy roads, poor visibility, heavy traffic or having to cope with aggressive drivers.

In other instances, stress can be moderate, such as when playing in a competitive sport where the individual is driven to succeed. Severe stress can be defined as distress, such as being abused or bullied, witnessing a traumatic event, losing a family member, encountering financial ruin or living in a war zone, that is more difficult to overcome and may leave lasting health effects.

When stress is mild or moderate the individual usually feels competent in solving problems and thinks rationally. Behavior and emotions are controlled, and physiological processes, such as blood pressure and heart rate, are in equilibrium. Severe stress, on the other hand, can cause disturbances in the individual, such as difficulty in learning a new task, performing well on an examination or interacting with others. Severe stress can also contribute to an addiction to smoking, drugs or alcohol, where the individual tries to escape from the distress through behaviors that are maladaptive to long-term health. Severe distress can trigger hopelessness in the individual through a withdrawal from any attempt to resolve the stress.

Stress can also be both motivating (eustress) and simultaneously distressful, contributing to psychological and physical disorders. For example, the professional musician who performs for an audience can experience severe pressure as well as positive feelings of success. In a review of nine studies on musicians and stress, Jacukowicz (2016) found that "...musicians suffer from work-related musculoskeletal problems, they experience high work demands involving physical and mental strain and those work demands result in stress" (Section "Severe Stress May Attack the Weakest Link", Conclusion). The psychosocial stress played a role in exacerbating the repetitive physical stress on the body (Jacukowicz, 2016).

DISTRESS EFFECTS

The effects of distress can be emotional reactions such as feelings of despair or depression, cognitive problems such as difficulty making decisions, behavioral problems such as insomnia and physiological disturbances such as heightened blood pressure or stomach pains. Distress can also trigger or aggravate symptoms or episodes in individuals with existing conditions such as osteoarthritis, multiple sclerosis, clinical depression or epilepsy.

PERCEPTION OF STRESSOR AFFECTS STRESS REACTION

The stress response in an individual to the stressor is to a large degree influenced by that person's perception of the stressor. If the stressor is perceived as threatening, the autonomic nervous system will increase the heart rate, blood pressure and basal metabolism, and, by decreasing gastrointestinal digestion, shunt available blood supply to the skeletal muscles. An intense or prolonged response can lead to acute or chronic symptoms, as noted above.

How the individual then responds to the perceived stress is the key to managing stress. For example, being able to talk about a stressful event with a therapist, supportive friend or relative can ease the stress. Exercising, even walking, will help dissipate the negative buildup of "fight or flight" energy from a stressor. Listening to relaxing music, writing letters, cleaning house, doing crossword puzzles, or any number of activities can be used as stress reducers. Discovering activities that are meaningful and beneficial is a key to managing distress. Coping with stress is a unique feature of an individual. Managing stress should be a key part of everyone's daily routine, just like eating regularly and brushing teeth. Furthermore, if we accept the fact that individuals will encounter situations in their daily lives that will cause stress, then all people should be prepared to deal with stress in a health-promoting manner.

One way to help ourselves deal with stress is to toughen ourselves physically and mentally so that we can cope well with the tasks at hand. Toughening oneself means developing the resources within us and in our lives through the buildup of our physical strength and endurance and through positive personal relationships. For example, building up physical health through exercise and sports can condition the body to better handle the symptoms of stress. The process of the body responding adaptively to the stress reaction is called *hormesis*.

SEVERE STRESS MAY ATTACK THE WEAKEST LINK

When an individual is under severe stress, the weakest or most sensitive part of the body becomes most at risk. For example, if an individual is vulnerable to migraine headaches, stress will tend to precipitate this symptom. For a person with a tendency to become depressed under severe pressure, a stressful event or thought can trigger an episode of depression. Recent research has shown that major mental illnesses such as depression and schizophrenia are episodic illnesses with periods of intense symptoms and remissions. These symptoms can be triggered by an external stressor, such as the loss of a job, or an internal one, such as harboring negative thoughts about oneself. The ability of an individual to cope with these stressors before being overwhelmed is critical in preventing an episode of mental illness.

POORLY MANAGED STRESS FOSTERS DISEASE

Coping effectively with stress means accepting the fact that everyone experiences stress every day and that we are all at risk of developing symptoms that are related to common illnesses and diseases. We are best able to respond to stress when we are healthy. When we are fatigued, lack adequate sleep or nutrition or feel depressed, angry or hopeless, stress becomes an additional factor in the onset of disease. Prevention is a better alternative than cure. To prevent episodes of mental unwellness, the individual should develop an everyday strategy that promotes maximum health. Activities should be incorporated into an individual's daily life. Time should be set aside every day for talking to someone you trust, listening to relaxing music, exercising, reading, doing a craft project or engaging in other activities that you find satisfying. The key is to engage in an activity on a consistent basis so that it becomes part of your daily routine. Stress management is like a toughening regimen that prepares you for the stressors of everyday life.

Managing stress effectively starts with developing a systematic strategy by answering three questions: (1) what are the everyday hassles that trigger my stress? (2) what are the symptoms and problems that occur when I am stressed? and (3) what are the best methods or activities that have been effective in the past to cope with my stress?

Each individual will answer these questions uniquely. Symptoms of stress occur in four basic areas: (1) cognitive, such as difficulty in concentrating or learning; (2)

emotional, such as feeling anxious, angry or sad; (3) physiological, such as neck, stomach or head pain; and (4) behavioral, such as difficulty sleeping, eating or speaking. Whether and how these symptoms manifest themselves will vary from person to person.

EVIDENCE FOR STRESS INTERVENTION EFFECTIVENESS FOR THOSE WITH OR WITHOUT A MEDICAL CONDITION

An overview of example studies (see Table 1.1) demonstrates that there already is widespread evidence for the effectiveness of stress management intervention approaches for people with many different medical diagnoses and for those without a diagnosis. In Chapters 4, 8, 9 and 10, more detailed evidence will be cited.

LIFESPAN STRESS REACTION

Lupien et al. (2009) reviewed the literature on stress throughout the lifespan. They concluded:

1. Throughout the lifespan, stress causes the hypothalamic-pituitary-adrenal (HPA) axis to produce glucocorticoids. These bind to brain receptors and affect behavior.
2. Prenatal stress can increase sensitivity to stress in later life. It is associated with learning difficulties, drug abuse, and anxiety and depression in adulthood.
3. Postnatally, infant-mother separation can cause a lasting increase in glucocorticoids, while severe infant abuse decreases them, potentially affecting long-term behavior.
4. The HPA axis of adolescents is more sensitive to stress than that of adults. The impact of stress in this stage of life, however, may only manifest itself in adulthood.
5. The effects of stress in adulthood are similar to those of childhood and adolescence, except that they usually stop with the cessation of the stressor. Chronic exposure to glucocorticoids is associated with depression. In contrast, those with PTSD have lower glucocorticoid levels.
6. Stress in the elderly is associated with memory loss.
7. Exposure to stressors at different stages of life causes different effects.

STRESS MANAGEMENT – A CRITICAL LIFE SKILL

In this book, we present stress management as a critical life skill. There are three anchors for this claim. First, according to the World Health Organization (WHO), coping with stress is one of the life skills necessary for survival in the modern

Table 1.1 Sample of Empirical Support for Stress Management Approaches

Author, Year	**Activity**	**Goal**	**Diagnosis**	**Design**
Kwok et al. (2019)	Yoga, exercises	Reduce anxiety, depression	Parkinson disease	RCT
Taylor et al. (2020)	CBT	Stress management	MS	Meta-analysis of RCTs
Hinwood et al. (2023)	PP, MBSR, CBT, leisure rehab, PA, AT	Stress management	CVA	Scoping review
Chauvet-Gelinier et al. (2017)	PP, problem-focused approach	Reduce anxiety, depression	Heart disease	Literature review
Walrabenstein et al. (2023)	PA, stress management	Reduce pain, increase QoL	Arthritis	RCT
Norman et al. (2002)	Coping skills	Stress management	Schizophrenia	RCT
Mohammadi et al. (2022)	Touch, music, exercise	Chronic stress management	Alzheimer's disease	Review
Diez et al. (2022)	MBSR	Biopsychological markers	Low back pain	RCT
Mino et al. (2006)	Group CBT	Reduce depression	Workplace	Systematic review

Table 1.1 continued

Author, Year	Activity	Goal	Diagnosis	Design
Restrepo and Lemos (2021)	MBSR, AE, BT	Reduce anxiety, depression, burnout	Workplace	RCT
Chiesa and Serretti (2009)	MBSR	Stress management	Healthy people	Review & meta-analysis
Singh et al. (2023)	PA	Reduce depression, anxiety, distress	Healthy people	Systematic review
Alzahem et al. (2014)	Breathing, yoga, relaxation	Stress management	Dental students	Systematic review
van der Heijden et al. (2018)	MT	Reduce stress, pain	Children with burns	RCT
Wang et al. (2014)	TC	Reduce anxiety, depression; increase well-being	Any	Systematic review, meta-analysis

Note. Listed interventions showed a positive effect. AE- aerobic exercise, AT- aquatic therapy, BT- bibliotherapy, CBT- cognitive behavioral therapy, MBSR- mindfulness-based stress reduction, MT- music therapy, PA- physical activity, PP- positive psychology, QoL- quality of life, RCT- randomized controlled trial, TC- tai chi world (World Health Organization, 1994). Second, research on coping mechanisms has been a significant focus in psychology, emphasizing adaptive strategies to handle internal and external stressors (Folkman & Moskowitz, 2004). Third, self-perception and self-management (aspects of coping with stress) have been identified in a scoping review by Fusar-Poli et al. (2020) as two important aspects of positive mental health. In fact, they defined good mental health as "...a state of well-being that allows individuals to cope with the normal stresses of life and function productively" (p. 33). As occupational therapy practitioners are concerned with helping their clients obtain or reacquire critical life skills, it is logical that they should be prepared to help their clients adopt effective stress management programs.

CULTURAL VARIATION IN RESPONSES TO STRESS

Stress also has cultural dimensions. Below stress is discussed in relation to diverse aspects of culture.

Many definitions, both historical and contemporary, have been attempted for the concept of *culture*. One such definition is that culture comprises a consistent collection of knowledge, values, beliefs, laws, morals, habits, and other traits acquired by individuals as members of a society (Spencer-Oatey, 2012). The *Occupational Therapy Practice Framework* (OTPF) categorizes culture as a contextual personal factor, encompassing customs, beliefs, activity patterns, and societal expectations that influence an individual's activity choices and occupational performance (American Occupational Therapy Association, 2020).

Research suggests that susceptibility to various diseases and conditions varies across cultures. For example, blood pressure tends to be higher in developed nations than in less developed ones – a difference partially attributed to cultural influences on behavior and physiology (Dressler, 2004). Racial minorities tend to have higher blood pressure within societies, at least partially due to the effects of frequent discrimination. Additionally, the types of stressors individuals encounter and their responses to stress are significantly shaped by their cultural background (Aldwin, 2004). Culture may influence stress and coping in several ways:

1. Cultural context determines the types of stressors individuals encounter.
2. Cultural norms shape perceptions of stressful events and the magnitude of stress responses.
3. Coping strategies are culturally mediated.
4. Institutional mechanisms (e.g., traditions, values and habits) for managing stress vary by culture (Aldwin, 2004; Knight & Sayegh, 2010).

5. Environments high in overinvolvement and criticism, termed high expressed emotion, have been shown to predict relapse (correlated with an increase in stressors) in individuals with schizophrenia (Butzlaff & Hooley, 1998). Multiple multinational studies by the World Health Organization have consistently shown that persons diagnosed with schizophrenia recover higher function more regularly in poorer, less developed societies than in developed ones (Hopper et al., 2007). Ethnographic research provides the link between these findings, that is, that cultural beliefs and practices around the source and meaning of behavioral illness moderate criticism and control as well as support function (Jenkins, 1991, and Jenkins & Karno, 1992, as cited in McGruder, 2004).

One key stress-related factor influenced by culture is social support, a critical coping mechanism that varies across societies (Taylor et al., 2004). For instance, Asian and Asian American individuals may hesitate to seek social support during stressful situations due to fear of judgment from close others (Chen et al., 2012; Kim et al., 2008). A well-designed study comparing U.S. and Singaporean participants found significant cultural differences in perceptions of social support and stress, underscoring the need for cultural considerations in stress research (Pourmand et al., 2021). Similarly, Japanese undergraduates reported higher daily stress levels than their European Canadian counterparts, highlighting cultural variations in stress appraisal (Lee et al., 2023).

Stressors and responses differ cross-culturally. While some stressors are universal, others are culturally specific (Spradley & Phillips, 1972). Additionally, coping strategies vary by culture (Lansisalmi et al., 2000). Research has identified a positive association between stress and sociocultural adversities (e.g., discrimination, acculturative stress), while cultural resources (e.g., ethnic identity, religious support) mitigate stress (Ahmed et al., 2011).

Culture also shapes positive and negative stress responses. For example, Japanese participants reported lower personal control, higher perceived stress, and greater use of emotion-focused coping compared to British participants in one study (O'Connor & Shimizu, 2002). Negative responses, such as substance abuse, vary culturally: opioid and cocaine use is more prevalent in the USA, whereas cigarette and hookah use is higher in Middle Eastern and some Asian countries (Fouad et al., 2021; Kargar & Ansari-Moghaddam, 2023; Ritchie et al., 2022). Gambling, often another maladaptive coping behavior, is more common in Western developed nations (Calado & Griffiths, 2016). Families in an East African, Islamic nation, due to cultural beliefs that are protective of the individual with symptoms of mental illness from blame, tend to express lesser criticism of a member under mental health stress, moderating the severity of disease outcome (McGruder, 2004).

Even within societies, economic or societal upheavals – such as the COVID-19 pandemic – can alter stress levels and coping strategies (Ahmadi et al., 2023; Li et al., 2021). Thus, occupational therapists must consider cultural factors when assessing stress and designing interventions to ensure culturally sensitive, client-centered care that optimizes occupational performance (American Occupational Therapy Association, 2020; Jeong & Kim, 2025; Maitra & Erway, 2006).

Principles of occupational therapy stress management that are fundamental postulates in this book:

1. Stress can be either a positive factor (eustress) in motivating an individual to succeed or a negative factor (distress) in precipitating symptoms of illness.
2. Distress can be acute, such as having an argument with a co-worker, or chronic, such as suffering long-term pain from an illness.
3. Measuring an individual's ability to manage stress entails determining the symptoms that are precipitated by stress, identifying the stressors that an individual encounters that trigger symptoms and gaining insight into coping activities that prevent and reduce distress.
4. There is a mind-body connection between distress and the stimulation of the sympathetic nervous system and between relaxation and the stimulation of the parasympathetic nervous system.
5. Positive health emphasizes a holistic approach to promoting mental and physical health. Specifically, incorporating aerobic exercise, a Mediterranean or similar diet, restful sleep and social contact into one's daily life is a fundamental step in stress management.
6. Engaging in enjoyable activities that generate being in "flow" (Csikszentmihalyi, 1990) can prevent and mitigate stress.
7. Engaging in enjoyable activities such as sports, music, art, poetry, dance, tai chi or games can produce positive changes in dealing with distress.
8. Stress management is a critical life skill for the 21st century in dealing with the unavoidable stressors of life.
9. Occupational therapists can play an important role in helping individuals to manage their distress and promote health through satisfying activities.
10. Occupational therapy stress management entails incorporating an occupational therapy model (Model of Human Occupation or Person-Environment-Occupation-Performance) into a stress management program.

SUMMARY

Stress is a universal aspect of life. Effectively coping with stress is a critical life skill for individuals living in the 21st century. In this chapter, the authors defined the levels of stress (mild, moderate and severe), including post-traumatic stress, and differentiated between eustress and distress. A preliminary overview of some evidence for intervention effectiveness for people with a variety of diagnoses (or none at all) was presented. Cultural differences in responding to stress were also described. Including a stress management program in a comprehensive occupational therapy protocol was advocated. In the following chapters we discuss the discovery of the phenomenon of stress, the physiology of stress, assessment tools for evaluating stress and finally strategies to prevent and alleviate stress by emphasizing positive health.

DISCUSSION QUESTIONS

1. What do you see as the overlap between stress management and contemporary occupational therapy?
2. How does stress impact illness, disease and mental health?
3. Describe your understanding of eustress, distress and hormesis.
4. Identify aspects of your culture that provide resources for you to manage your own stressors in life.

REFERENCES

Ahmadi, A., Allahverdipour, H., Valiee, S., Pashazadeh, F., Ghassab-Abdollahi, N., Abdoli, F., & Matlabi, H. (2023). COVID-19 stress and coping strategies among older adults: A systematic review of qualitative evidence. *BMC Psychology, 11*(1), 333. https://doi.org/10.1186/s40359-023-01382-1

Ahmed, S. R., Kia-Keating, M., & Tsai, K. H. J. A. (2011). A structural model of racial discrimination, acculturative stress, and cultural resources among Arab American adolescents. *American Journal of Community Psychology, 48*, 181–192. https://doi.org/10.1007/s10464-011-9424-3

Aldwin, C. M. (2004). *Culture, coping, and resilience to stress*. Centre for Bhutan Studies.

Alotiby, A. (2024). Immunology of stress: A review article. *Journal of Clinical Medicine*, *13*(21), 6394. https://doi.org/10.3390/jcm13216394

Alzahem, A. M., Van der Molen, H. T., Alaujan, A. H., & De Boer, B. J. (2014). Stress management in dental students: A systematic review. *Advances in Medical Education and Practice, 5*, 167–176. https://doi.org/10.2147/AMEP.S46211

American Occupational Therapy Association. (2020). Occupational therapy practice framework: Domain and process (4th ed.). *American Journal of Occupational Therapy*, *74*(Supplement_2), 7412410010p1–7412410010p87. https://doi.org/10.5014/ajot.2020.74S2001

American Psychological Association. (2022). *More than a quarter of U.S. adults say they're so stressed they can't function*. https://www.apa.org/news/press/releases/2022/10/multiple-stressors-no-function.

Bandurska, H. (2022). Drought stress responses: Coping strategy and resistance. *Plants, 11*(7), 922. https://doi.org/10.3390/plants11070922

Butzlaff, J., & Hooley, J. M. (1998). Expressed emotion & psychiatric relapse: A meta-analysis. *Archives of General Psychiatry, 55*(6), 547–552. https://doi.org/10.1001/archpsyc.55.6.547

Calado, F., & Griffiths, M. D. (2016). Problem gambling worldwide: An update and systematic review of empirical research (2000–2015). *Journal of Behavioral Addictions, 5*(4), 592–613. https://doi.org/10.1556/2006.5.2016.073

Chauvet-Gelinier, J. C., & Bonin, B. (2017). Stress, anxiety, and depression in heart disease patients: A major challenge for cardiac rehabilitation. *Annals of Physical and Rehabilitation Medicine, 60*(1), 6–12. https://doi.org/10.1016/j.rehab.2016.09.002

Chen, J. M., Kim, H. S., Mojaverian, T., & Morling, B. (2012). Culture and social support provision: Who gives what and why. *Personality and Social Psychology Bulletin, 38*(1), 3–13. https://doi.org/10.1177/0146167211427309

Chiesa, A., & Serretti, A. (2009). Mindfulness-based stress reduction for stress management in healthy people: A review and meta-analysis. *Journal of Alternative and Complementary Medicine, 15*(5), 593–600. https://doi.org/10.1089/acm.2008.0495

Chu, B., Marwaha, K., Sanvictores, T., Awosika, A. O., & Ayers, D. (2024). Physiology, stress reaction. In *StatPearls* [Internet]. StatPearls Publishing. https://www.ncbi.nlm.nih.gov/books/NBK541120/

Csikszentmihalyi, M. (1990). *Flow: The psychology of optimal experience*. Harper & Row.

Diez, G. G., Anitua, E., Castellanos, N., Vázquez, C., Galindo-Villardón, P., & Alkhraisat, M. H. (2022). The effect of mindfulness on the inflammatory, psychological, and biomechanical domains of adult patients with low back pain: A randomized controlled clinical trial. *PLOS One, 17*(11), e0276734. https://doi.org/10.1371/journal.pone.0276734

Dressler, W. W. (2004). Culture and the risk of disease. *British Medical Bulletin, 69*, 21–31. https://doi.org/10.1093/bmb/ldh020

Folkman, S., & Moskowitz, J. T. (2004). Coping: Pitfalls and promise. *Annual Review of Psychology, 55*, 745–774. https://doi.org/10.1146/annurev.psych.55.090902.141456

Fouad, H., Commar, A., Hamadeh, R., El-Awa, F., Shen, Z., & Fraser, C. (2021). Estimated and projected prevalence of tobacco smoking in males, Eastern Mediterranean Region, 2000–2025. *Eastern Mediterranean Health Journal, 27*(1), 76–82. https://doi.org/10.26719/2021.27.1.76

Frankl, V. E. (1962). *Man's search for meaning: An introduction to logotherapy.* Beacon Press.

Fusar-Poli, P., Salazar de Pablo, G., De Micheli, A., Nieman, D. H., Correll, C. U., Kessing, L. V., Pfennig, A., Bechdolf, A., Borgwardt, S., Arango, C., & van Amelsvoort, T. (2020). What is good mental health? A scoping review. *European Neuropsychopharmacology, 31*, 33–46. https://doi.org/10.1016/j.euroneuro.2019.12.10

Gao, Y., Hu, R., Zhang, Y., Yuan, M., Xu, Y., & Ma, J. (2022). Perceived stress in Chinese patients with coronary heart disease: A cross-sectional study. *BMJ Open, 12*(3), e051419. https://doi.org/10.1136/bmjopen-2021-051419

Gibbons, C. H. (2019). Basics of autonomic nervous system function. *Handbook of Clinical Neurology*, *160*, 407–418. https://doi.org/10.1016/B978-0-444-64032-1.00027-8

Hinwood, M., Ilicic, M., Gyawali, P., Coupland, K., Kluge, M. G., Smith, A., Bowden, S., Nilsson, M., & Walker, F. R. (2023). Psychological stress management and stress reduction strategies for stroke survivors: A scoping review. *Annals of Behavioral Medicine, 57*(2), 111–130. https://doi.org/10.1093/abm/kaac002

Hopper, K., Harrison, G., Janca, A., & Sartorius, N. (Eds.). (2007). *Recovery from schizophrenia: An international perspective*. Oxford University Press.

Jacukowicz, A. (2016). Psychosocial work aspects, stress, and musculoskeletal pain among musicians: A systematic review in search of correlates and predictors of playing-related pain. *Work, 54*(3), 657–668. https://doi.org/10.3233/WOR-162323

Jenkins, J. H. (1991). Anthropology, expressed emotion and schizophrenia. *Ethos, 19*(4), 387–431. https://www.jstor.org/stable/640390

Jenkins, J. H., & Karno, M. (1992). The meaning opf expressed emotion: Theoretical issues raised by cross-cultural research. *American Journal of Psychiatry, 149*(1), 9–21. https://doi.org/10.1176/ajp.149.1.9

Jeong, H., & Kim, D. (2025). Effects of client-centered occupational therapy intervention in older adults with depression: A randomized controlled trial. *Occupational Therapy International, 2025*, 5559899. https://doi.org/10.1155/oti/5559899

Kargar, S., & Ansari-Moghaddam, A. (2023). Prevalence of cigarette and waterpipe smoking and associated cancer incidence among adults in the Middle East. *Eastern Mediterranean Health Journal, 29*(9), 749–756. https://doi.org/10.26719/emhj.23.077

Kim, H. S., Sherman, D. K., & Taylor, S. E. (2008). Culture and social support. *American Psychologist, 63*(6), 518–526. https://doi.org/10.1037/0003-066X

Kivimäki, M., & Kawachi, I. (2015). Work stress as a risk factor for cardiovascular disease. *Current Cardiology Reports*, *17*(9), 630. https://doi.org/10.1007/s11886-015-0630-8

Knight, B. G., & Sayegh, P. (2010). Cultural values and caregiving: The updated sociocultural stress and coping model. *Journals of Gerontology: Series B, 65*(1), 5–13. https://doi.org/10.1093/geronb/gbp096

Kwok, J. Y. Y., Kwan, J. C. Y., Auyeung, M., Mok, V. C. T., Lau, C. K. Y., Choi, K. C., & Chan, H. Y. L. (2019). Effects of mindfulness yoga vs stretching and resistance training exercises on anxiety and depression for people with Parkinson's disease: A randomized clinical trial. *JAMA Neurology, 76*(7), 755–763. https://doi.org/10.1001/jamaneurol.2019.0534

Lansisalmi, H., Peiró, J. M., & Kivimäki, M. (2000). Collective stress and coping in the context of organizational culture. *European Journal of Work and Organizational Psychology, 9*(4), 527–559. https://doi.org/10.1080/13594320050203120

Lee, H., Masuda, T., Ishii, K., Yasuda, Y., & Ohtsubo, Y. (2023). Cultural differences in the perception of daily stress between European Canadian and Japanese undergraduate students. *Personality and Social Psychology Bulletin, 49*(4), 571–584. https://doi.org/10.1177/01461672211070360

Li, Y., Scherer, N., Felix, L., & Kuper, H. (2021). Prevalence of depression, anxiety, and post-traumatic stress disorder in health care workers during the COVID-19 pandemic: A systematic review and meta-analysis. *PLOS One, 16*(3), e0246454. https://doi.org/10.1371/journal.pone.0246454

Lupien, S., McEwen, B., Gunnar, M., & Heim, C. (2009). Effects of stress throughout the lifespan on the brain, behavior, and cognition. *Nature Reviews Neuroscience, 10*, 434–445. https://doi.org/10.1038/nrn2639

Maitra, K. K., & Erway, F. (2006). Perception of client-centered practice in occupational therapists and their clients. *American Journal of Occupational Therapy, 60*(3), 298–310. https://doi.org/10.5014/ajot.60.3.298

McGruder, J. (2004). Disease models of mental illness and aftercare patient education: Critical observations from meta-analyses, cross-cultural practice, and anthropological study. *British Journal of Occupational Therapy, 67*(7), 310–318. https://doi.org/10.1177/030802260406700705

Meng, X., & D'Arcy, C. (2016). Coping strategies and distress reduction in psychological well-being? A structural equation modelling analysis using a national population sample. *Epidemiology and Psychiatric Sciences, 25*(4), 370–383. https://doi.org/10.1017/S2045796015000505

Mino, Y., Babazono, A., Tsuda, T., & Yasuda, N. (2006). Can stress management at the workplace prevent depression? A randomized controlled trial. *Psychotherapy and Psychosomatics, 75*(3), 177–182. https://doi.org/10.1159/000091775

Mohammadi, S., Zandi, M., Dousti Kataj, P., & Karimi Zandi, L. (2022). Chronic stress and Alzheimer's disease. *Biotechnology and Applied Biochemistry, 69*(4), 1451–1458. https://doi.org/10.1002/bab.2216

Norman, R. M., Malla, A. K., McLean, T. S., McIntosh, E. M., Neufeld, R. W., Voruganti, L. P., & Cortese, L. (2002). An evaluation of a stress management program for individuals with schizophrenia. *Schizophrenia Research, 58*(2–3), 293303. https://doi.org/10.1016/S0920-9964(01)00371-1

O'Connor, D. B., & Shimizu, M. (2002). Sense of personal control, stress, and coping style: A cross-cultural study. *International Journal of Stress Management, 18*(4), 173–183. https://doi.org/10.1002/smi.939

Peavy, G. M., Salmon, D. P., Jacobson, M. W., Hervey, A., Gamst, A. C., Wolfson, T., Patterson, T. L., Goldman, S., Mills, P. J., Khandrika, S., & Galasko, D. (2009). Effects of chronic stress on memory decline in cognitively normal and mildly impaired older adults. *American Journal of Psychiatry*, *166*(12), 1384–1391. https://doi.org/10.1176/appi.ajp.2009.09040461

Pourmand, V., Lawley, K. A., & Lehman, B. J. (2021). Cultural differences in stress and affection following social support receipt. *PLOS One, 16*(9), e0256859. https://doi.org/10.1371/journal.pone.0256859

Reece, J. C., Neate, S. L., Davenport, R. A., Milanzi, E., Nag, N., Bevens, W., Yu, M., Jelinek, G. A., & Simpson-Yap, S. (2024). Stressful life events and depression and fatigue in people with multiple sclerosis: A cross-sectional analysis of an international cohort. *Acta Neurologica Belgica, 124*(2), 457–466. https://doi.org/10.1007/s13760-023-02390-z

Restrepo, J., & Lemos, M. (2021). Addressing psychosocial work-related stress interventions: A systematic review. *Work, 70*(1), 53–62. https://doi.org/10.3233/WOR-213577

Ritchie, H., Arriagada, P., & Roser, M. (2022). Opioids, cocaine, cannabis, and other illicit drugs. *Our World in Data*. https://ourworldindata.org/drug-use

Schalbroeck, R., van Hooijdonk, C. F. M., Bos, D. P. A., Booij, J., & Selten, J. P. (2024). Chronic social stressors and striatal dopamine functioning in humans: A systematic review of SPECT and PET studies. *Molecular Psychiatry*, *29*(12), 3841–3856. https://doi.org/10.1038/s41380-024-02581-x

Selye, H. (1956). *The stress of life*. McGraw-Hill.

Selye, H. (1976). *The stress of life* (Rev. ed.). McGraw-Hill.

Singh, B., Olds, T., Curtis, R., Dumuid, D., Virgara, R., Watson, A., Szeto, K., O'Connor, E., Ferguson, T., Eglitis, E., Miatke, A., Simpson, C. E., & Maher, C. (2023). Effectiveness of physical activity interventions for improving depression, anxiety, and distress: An overview of systematic reviews. *British Journal of Sports Medicine, 57*(18), 1203–1209. https://doi.org/10.1136/bjsports-2022-106195

Spencer-Oatey, H. (2012). What is culture? A compilation of quotations. *GlobalPAD Core Concepts*. https://www2.warwick.ac.uk/fac/soc/al/globalpad/interculturalskills/

Spradley, J. P., & Phillips, M. (1972). Culture and stress: A quantitative analysis. *American Anthropologist, 74*(3), 518–529. https://www.jstor.org/stable/671532

Taylor, P., Dorstyn, D. S., & Prior, E. (2020). Stress management interventions for multiple sclerosis: A meta-analysis of randomized controlled trials. *Journal of Health Psychology, 25*(2), 266–279. https://doi.org/10.1177/1359105319860185

Taylor, S. E., Sherman, D. K., Kim, H. S., Jarcho, J., Takagi, K., & Dunagan, M. S. (2004). Culture and social support: Who seeks it and why? *Journal of Personality and Social Psychology, 87*(3), 354–362. https://doi.org/10.1037/0022-3514.87.3.354

van der Heijden, M. J. E., Jeekel, J., Rode, H., Cox, S., van Rosmalen, J., Hunink, M. G. M., & van Dijk, M. (2018). Can live music therapy reduce distress and pain in children with burns after wound care procedures? A randomized controlled trial. *Burns, 44*(4), 823–833. https://doi.org/10.1016/j.burns.2017.12.013

Walrabenstein, W., Wagenaar, C. A., van der Leeden, M., Turkstra, F., Twisk, J. W. R., Boers, M., van Middendorp, H., Weijs, P. J. M., & van Schaardenburg, D. (2023). A multidisciplinary lifestyle program for rheumatoid arthritis: The 'Plants for Joints' randomized controlled trial. *Rheumatology, 62*(8), 2683–2691. https://doi.org/10.1093/rheumatology/keac693

Wang, F., Lee, E. K., Wu, T., Benson, H., Fricchione, G., Wang, W., & Yeung, A. S. (2014). The effects of tai chi on depression, anxiety, and psychological well-being: A systematic review and meta-analysis. *International Journal of Behavioral Medicine, 21*(4), 605–617. https://doi.org/10.1007/s12529-013-9351-9

Webster, A. J. F. (1983). Environmental stress and the physiology, performance, and health of ruminants. *Journal of Animal Science, 57*(6), 1584–1593. https://doi.org/10.2527/jas1983.5761584x

World Health Organization, Division of Mental Health. (1994). *Life skills education for children and adolescents in schools* (2nd rev.). Author. https://iris.who.int/handle/10665/63552

Chapter 2

Stress, Disease, Resilience: A History of Discoveries

LEARNING OBJECTIVES

By the end of this chapter, the reader will be able to

1. Trace the historical evolution of stress research from Claude Bernard's milieu intérieur through contemporary positive health models.
2. Explain the contributions of key figures (Bernard, Cannon, Selye, Wolff, Lazarus, Antonovsky) to our understanding of stress and adaptation.
3. Understand Bernstein's constellation metaphor as a framework for integrating diverse stress theories and research traditions.
4. Compare and contrast pathogenic and salutogenic approaches to understanding stress responses and health outcomes.
5. Describe the paradigm shift from viewing stress exclusively as harmful to recognizing its potential as a catalyst for growth and resilience.
6. Analyze the integrated-pathway model of stress that demonstrates the interconnected nature of pathogenic and salutogenic responses.
7. Explain how flow theory and post-traumatic growth contribute to positive reconceptualizations of stress and adversity.
8. Apply Lazarus's cognitive appraisal theory to understand how individuals can influence their stress responses through meaning-making.
9. Evaluate the relevance of historical stress concepts to contemporary occupational therapy assessment and intervention.
10. Synthesize historical and contemporary perspectives to develop occupation-based stress management interventions that promote both resilience and flourishing.

DOI: 10.4324/9781003671084-2

11. Critically examine how power relations and social context influence stress responses and the application of stress management interventions.
12. Apply the integrated-pathway model to clinical reasoning in occupational therapy practice, recognizing that clients may simultaneously experience both challenge and threat appraisals.

INTRODUCTION: RELEVANCE TO OCCUPATIONAL THERAPY

Occupational therapists work at the intersection of mind, body and meaningful activity, making them uniquely positioned to understand and apply evolving concepts of stress within therapeutic practice. As professionals who view health through the lens of occupational engagement and participation, occupational therapists have long recognized that stress affects not merely physiological systems but the entire fabric of daily living, from self-care and productivity to leisure and social participation. This chapter traces the evolution of stress research from its physiological origins to contemporary positive health approaches, providing occupational therapists with a comprehensive framework for understanding how stress can either impede or facilitate occupational performance and well-being.

The occupational therapy profession's foundational belief in the healing power of meaningful occupation aligns naturally with emerging positive health perspectives that view stress as a potential catalyst for growth and adaptation. By understanding the historical evolution of stress concepts and their transformation toward salutogenic approaches, occupational therapists can better conceptualize interventions that not only help clients manage stress but also transform challenging experiences into opportunities for occupational adaptation and enhanced life participation.

BERNSTEIN'S CONSTELLATION METAPHOR: A FRAMEWORK FOR UNDERSTANDING

To navigate the complex evolution of stress research, this chapter employs Richard Bernstein's (1992) constellation metaphor as an organizing framework. Bernstein developed this metaphor to describe how we can bring together diverse thinkers and ideas that, while not necessarily connected in obvious ways, illuminate each other when viewed as part of a larger pattern. Like stars in a constellation, individual concepts and theories may be separated by time, discipline or philosophical orientation, yet when we draw imaginative lines between them, they form meaningful patterns that help us navigate complex intellectual terrain.

A constellation differs fundamentally from a system or hierarchy. In a system, elements have fixed relationships and predetermined functions. In a hierarchy, elements are arranged in levels of importance or causation. But in a constellation, elements maintain their individual brilliance while participating in multiple possible patterns of meaning. The constellation of stress research includes stars like Bernard's milieu intérieur, Cannon's homeostasis, Selye's adaptation syndrome, Lazarus's cognitive appraisal, Antonovsky's salutogenesis and contemporary positive psychology's focus on flourishing. Each concept retains its distinct contribution while participating in an evolving pattern of understanding.

This metaphor is particularly apt for occupational therapy, a profession that itself draws from multiple disciplines, including medicine, psychology, sociology and anthropology, to create its unique perspective on health and occupation. Just as occupational therapists synthesize knowledge from diverse sources to understand their clients holistically, this chapter brings together diverse perspectives on stress to construct a comprehensive understanding that serves therapeutic practice.

PART I: FOUNDATIONS – THE PHYSIOLOGICAL ORIGINS OF STRESS RESEARCH

Claude Bernard (1813–1878) and the Milieu Intérieur

The scientific understanding of stress finds its origins in the revolutionary work of Claude Bernard, whose concept of the milieu intérieur fundamentally transformed our understanding of physiological adaptation. Bernard's genius lay not merely in identifying the body's capacity for self-regulation but in recognizing this capacity as the foundation of what he termed "la vie libre" or free and independent life. This concept of free and independent life resonates deeply with occupational therapy's emphasis on autonomy and independent functioning.

Bernard's experimental method, grounded in the hypothetico-deductive approach, established four pillars that continue to inform stress research. First, disease represents a disruption of normal functioning rather than an entirely separate state of being. Second, therapeutic intervention requires understanding normal functioning. Third, this understanding necessitates systematic experimentation.

Fourth, such experimentation must follow rigorous scientific methodology. These principles, articulated in his 1865 work, *Introduction à l'Étude de la Médecine Expérimentale,* established the epistemological foundation for all subsequent stress research.

Bernard's concept of the internal environment maintaining constancy despite external fluctuations introduced a dynamic view of health that would later inform both homeostatic and allostatic models. His observation that excessive stimulation could exhaust the organism's capacity for maintaining equilibrium presaged later discoveries about chronic stress and allostatic load. Importantly, Bernard's framework implied that health was not merely the absence of disease but an active process of adaptation and regulation, a concept that would find full expression in later salutogenic approaches and aligns with occupational therapy's view of health as active engagement in meaningful occupation.

Walter Cannon (1871–1945) and the Wisdom of the Body

Building upon Bernard's foundation, Walter Cannon transformed our understanding of stress through his systematic investigation of the autonomic nervous system and his articulation of homeostasis. His 1932 masterwork, *The Wisdom of the Body*, introduced concepts that remain central to stress research: homeostasis, self-regulation and the fight-or-flight response. Cannon's contribution extended beyond mere description; he provided a mechanistic understanding of how the body mobilizes resources in response to threats.

Cannon's identification of the sympathetic and parasympathetic branches of the autonomic nervous system as complementary regulatory mechanisms revealed the elegant complexity of stress responses. His recognition that emotional states could trigger physiological changes comparable to physical threats established the foundation for understanding psychosomatic illness and, ultimately, the mind-body connection that underlies positive health interventions.

The concept of "emotion stress" that Cannon introduced represents a crucial bridge between purely physiological and psychological understandings of stress. By demonstrating that fear and anger could mobilize the same physiological systems activated by physical danger, Cannon laid the groundwork for understanding how cognitive appraisal and emotional regulation could influence stress responses, concepts that would become central to positive psychology interventions and occupational therapy's psychosocial approaches.

Hans Selye (1907–1982) and the General Adaptation Syndrome

Hans Selye's prodigious contributions, including over 30 books and 1,000 technical articles, established him as the architect of modern stress theory. His definition of stress as "the nonspecific response of the body to any demand" (Selye, 1976a, 1976b, p. 55) introduced a universality to stress research that transcended specific stressors. The General Adaptation Syndrome (GAS), with its three stages of Alarm, Resistance and Exhaustion, provided a temporal framework for understanding stress responses.

Selye's model, while groundbreaking, contained within it the seeds of its own transcendence. The recognition that organisms could adapt to stressors during the Resistance phase suggested that stress responses could be modified, trained, or enhanced, ideas that would later inform resilience research and stress inoculation training. Moreover, Selye's later work on "eustress" (positive stress) acknowledged that not all stress was harmful, opening the door to positive reconceptualizations of adversity that occupational therapists now use when helping clients reframe challenging occupational demands.

PART II: THE PSYCHOLOGICAL TURN – FROM MECHANISM TO MEANING

Harold Wolff (1898–1962) and the Mind-Body Connection

Harold Wolff's pioneering research on the relationship between stress and disease marked a critical transition from purely physiological to psychosomatic understandings of stress. His personal struggle with migraines informed his scientific investigations, demonstrating how lived experience can enrich scientific inquiry, a principle that resonates with occupational therapy's emphasis on understanding the client's lived experience of illness and disability.

Wolff's discovery that blood vessels could vasoconstrict and vasodilate in response to psychological stress provided concrete evidence for the mind-body connection. His recommendations that perfectionistic, driven individuals should incorporate relaxation and exercise into their lives presaged contemporary lifestyle medicine approaches and occupational therapy's focus on life balance. In this way, Wolff's work bridges the physiological tradition of Bernard, Cannon and Selye with the psychological and behavioral interventions that characterize positive health approaches.

Richard Lazarus (1922–2002) and Cognitive Appraisal

Richard Lazarus revolutionized stress research by placing cognitive appraisal at the center of stress responses. His transactional model, developed with Susan Folkman (Folkman & Lazarus, 1984), reconceptualized stress not as a simple stimulus-response phenomenon but as a dynamic interaction between person and environment mediated by cognitive evaluation and coping resources. This shift from a mechanical to meaning-centered understanding of stress opened new avenues for intervention and aligns closely with occupational therapy's Person-Environment-Occupation model.

The Hassles and Uplifts Scale (Lazarus & Folkman, 1989) represented a crucial innovation in recognizing that positive daily experiences could counteract stress, a concept that directly influenced the development of positive psychology interventions and occupational therapy's emphasis on engaging in pleasurable and meaningful activities. Lazarus's emphasis on the role of positive emotions (happiness, pride, relief, love) in modulating stress responses anticipated Fredrickson's (2001) Broaden-and-Build Theory, which demonstrates how positive emotions expand thought-action repertoires and build psychological resources.

Lazarus's statement that

> people are rarely passive in the face of what happens to them; they seek to change things if they can, and when they cannot, they use cognitive modes of coping by which they may change the meaning of the situation.
>
> (DeLongis et al., 1988, p. 248)

captures the essence of human agency in stress responses. This perspective shifts the focus from stress as something that happens to people to stress as something people actively engage with and potentially transform, a concept central to occupational therapy's emphasis on client-centered practice and empowerment.

PART III: THE SALUTOGENIC REVOLUTION – FROM PATHOGENESIS TO FLOURISHING

Aaron Antonovsky (1923–1994) and Salutogenesis

Antonovsky's introduction of salutogenesis, representing the origins (genesis) of health (saluto), marks perhaps the most fundamental paradigm shift in stress research. His work with Holocaust survivors revealed a startling finding: some individuals not only survived extreme trauma but also maintained or even enhanced their health and well-being. This observation led to his revolutionary question: "What are the origins of health?" This question parallels occupational therapy's focus on what enables occupational participation rather than what prevents it.

The Sense of Coherence (SOC) construct, with its three components of comprehensibility, manageability, and meaningfulness, provided a framework for understanding why individuals respond differently to identical stressors. These components align remarkably with occupational therapy principles: comprehensibility relates to understanding one's condition and context, manageability to identifying and utilizing resources for occupational performance and meaningfulness to engaging in occupations that provide purpose and satisfaction.

Antonovsky's insistence that health exists on a continuum from "dis-ease" to "ease" rather than as a binary state challenged the medical model's categorization of people as either healthy or ill. This perspective resonates with occupational therapy's view of function and participation as existing on continua rather than in discrete categories. His observation that "a salutogenic orientation is not likely to take over. Pathogenesis is too deeply entrenched in our thinking" (Antonovsky, 1996, p. 171) proved prescient, yet his work laid the foundation for positive psychology and positive health approaches that are increasingly influencing research and practice.

Robert Sapolsky and the Neuroscience of Stress (Contemporary)

Robert Sapolsky's integration of neuroscience, primatology and stress research provides crucial biological grounding for positive health approaches. His observation that social connection and status profoundly influence stress responses in baboons, and by extension humans, underscores the importance of relationships and community in stress management, supporting occupational therapy's emphasis on social participation as a key area of occupation.

Sapolsky's accessible writing, particularly *Why Zebras Don't Get Ulcers* (Sapolsky, 1998), has brought sophisticated stress research to public consciousness. His emphasis on the evolutionary mismatch between our stress response systems (designed for acute physical threats) and modern psychological stressors provides a framework for understanding why stress management interventions are necessary in contemporary life and why occupational adaptation is crucial for health.

PART IV: THE POSITIVE PSYCHOLOGY INTEGRATION – STRESS AS CATALYST FOR GROWTH

The Emergence of Positive Psychology

The formal establishment of positive psychology by Seligman and Csikszentmihalyi (2000) marked a decisive shift in how psychology approaches human experience, including stress. Rather than viewing stress exclusively as a problem to be eliminated, positive psychology examines how adversity can catalyze growth, build character strengths, and enhance well-being. This perspective doesn't minimize the real suffering stress can cause but recognizes that the human response to adversity is more complex and potentially transformative than previously understood.

Seligman's PERMA model consisting of Positive emotions, Engagement, Relationships, Meaning and Accomplishment provides a framework for understanding how stress management extends beyond symptom reduction to the cultivation of flourishing. Each element of PERMA can both buffer against stress and be strengthened through successfully navigating challenges. This bidirectional relationship suggests that stress, properly framed and managed, can enhance rather than diminish well-being. For occupational therapists, PERMA offers a framework for designing interventions that address multiple dimensions of well-being through occupational engagement.

FLOW AND OPTIMAL EXPERIENCE IN STRESS TRANSFORMATION

Central to positive psychology's reconceptualization of stress is Csikszentmihalyi's (1990) concept of flow, the psychological state of optimal experience characterized by complete absorption in activity, loss of self-consciousness and intrinsic motivation. Flow represents a paradigmatic example of how challenge, when properly calibrated to skill level, produces not stress but profound satisfaction and growth. This concept fundamentally challenges traditional stress models by demonstrating that demanding situations can generate positive states when specific conditions are met.

The flow model reveals that stress and engagement exist on a continuum determined by the balance between challenge and skill. When challenges exceed skills, anxiety results; when skills exceed challenges, boredom ensues. But when challenges and skills are optimally matched, individuals enter flow states characterized by:

1. **Complete concentration on the task at hand**: The focused attention required by flow states precludes rumination and worry, common features of stress responses.
2. **Clear goals and immediate feedback**: These elements provide structure and meaning that transform potential stressors into engaging challenges.
3. **Sense of control**: Despite the challenge level, individuals in flow feel capable of meeting demands, shifting appraisal from threat to opportunity.
4. **Transformation of time**: The altered temporal experience in flow states suggests fundamental changes in consciousness that protect against stress.
5. **Autotelic experience**: Activities become intrinsically rewarding, reducing dependence on external validation or outcomes.

For occupational therapists, flow theory provides crucial insights for intervention design. By carefully calibrating occupational challenges to clients' current skill levels and progressively adjusting this balance, therapists can help clients transform stressful occupations into flow-producing activities. This process, termed the "flow channel," suggests that stress management isn't about avoiding challenges but about finding the optimal challenge-skill balance that promotes engagement and growth.

Research on flow in various contexts, from work to leisure to rehabilitation, demonstrates its protective effects against stress and burnout. Individuals who regularly experience flow show enhanced well-being, increased resilience and greater life satisfaction (Nakamura & Csikszentmihalyi, 2009). Moreover, flow experiences appear to build psychological capital, creating upward spirals where successful engagement with challenges enhances confidence and skills, enabling individuals to tackle progressively greater challenges without experiencing distress.

The neurobiological correlates of flow states further illuminate their stress-protective effects. Flow is associated with transient hypofrontality, a temporary downregulation of prefrontal cortex activity that reduces self-criticism and overthinking (Dietrich, 2004). This neural signature contrasts sharply with stress states characterized by prefrontal hyperactivity and rumination. Additionally, flow states are associated with optimal arousal and the release of neurochemicals, including dopamine, norepinephrine and endorphins that enhance performance and well-being while protecting against stress-related physiological damage.

POST-TRAUMATIC GROWTH AND BENEFIT FINDING

The concept of post-traumatic growth, articulated by Tedeschi and Calhoun (2004), represents a radical reconceptualization of trauma and stress. Their research demonstrated that individuals can experience profound positive change following adversity, including enhanced appreciation for life, deeper relationships, increased personal strength, spiritual development and new life priorities. This finding challenges the assumption that trauma inevitably leads to disorder and suggests that, with appropriate support and resources, individuals can transform suffering into wisdom and strength.

Research on benefit finding and meaning-making in the context of stress (Park, 2010) reveals that individuals who can construct meaning from adverse experiences show better psychological and physical health outcomes. This aligns with Frankl's (1946) earlier observations about the importance of meaning in surviving extreme adversity and suggests that helping individuals find meaning in stressful experiences should be a central component of interventions, a principle already embedded in occupational therapy's focus on meaningful occupation.

PART V: A NEW CONCEPTUAL MODEL – THE INTEGRATED-PATHWAY FRAMEWORK

Beyond the Disease Model

The traditional model articulated by Cohen et al. (2016) viewed stress through a primarily pathogenic lens, tracing a linear progression from environmental stressors through appraisal to physiological dysregulation and disease. While this model accurately captures one potential pathway, it fails to account for the full complexity of human stress responses, particularly the potential for growth and positive adaptation that occupational therapists observe in their clients daily.

Our proposed integrated-pathway model (see Figure 2.1) recognizes that stress appraisal represents a critical bifurcation point where identical stressors can lead to divergent yet interconnected outcomes. The model emphasizes that pathogenic and salutogenic responses are not mutually exclusive but exist in dynamic interaction, with individuals potentially experiencing elements of both simultaneously or moving between pathways based on changing resources, appraisals and contexts. When stressors are appraised as threats exceeding coping resources, the pathogenic pathway is activated, potentially leading to distress, physiological dysregulation and disease. However, when stressors are appraised

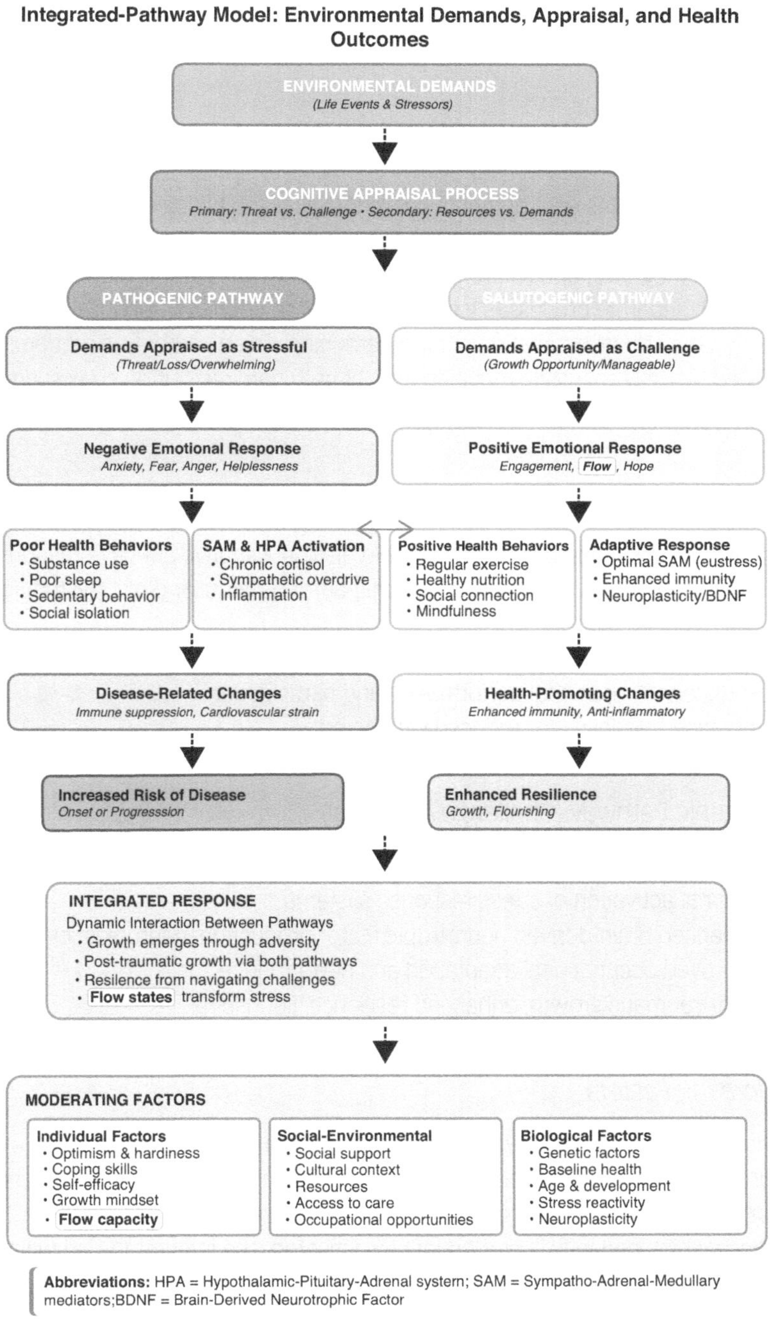

Figure 2.1 Integrated-Pathway Model: Environmental Demands, Appraisal, and Health Outcomes

as challenges that can be met with available resources, the salutogenic pathway is activated, potentially leading to eustress, growth and enhanced resilience.

The Integrated-Pathway Model Explained

This model integrates environmental, psychological and biological perspectives while incorporating positive psychology and flow theory to demonstrate both pathogenic (negative) and salutogenic (positive) pathways as interconnected rather than separate processes (see Figure 2.1). The cognitive appraisal process serves as the critical bifurcation point determining which pathway is predominantly activated, while recognizing that elements of both pathways often coexist and influence each other.

Pathogenic Pathway (Threat Appraisal)

- Environmental demands → Threat appraisal → Negative affective response
- Activation of HPA axis and sympathetic-adreno-medullar (SAM) system in dysregulated manner
- Chronic inflammation, immune suppression
- Reduced occupational performance and participation
- Increased disease risk, reduced well-being

Salutogenic Pathway (Challenge Appraisal)

- Environmental demands → Challenge appraisal → Positive affective response
- Optimal activation of stress response systems
- Enhanced brain-derived neurotropic factor production, neuroplasticity
- Improved occupational adaptation and performance
- Post-traumatic growth, enhanced resilience, flourishing

Moderating Factors

Individual factors (personality, genetics, past experiences, occupational history), social-environmental factors (support, resources, culture, occupational opportunities) and biological factors (health status, age, functional capacity) influence which pathway is predominantly activated. The integrated-pathway model recognizes that these pathways are not mutually exclusive but dynamically interconnected. Individuals may oscillate between them, experience elements of both simultaneously, and find that growth emerges through navigating difficulty. The model acknowledges that post-traumatic growth often coexists with ongoing challenges and that resilience develops not in the absence of the pathogenic pathway but through the dynamic interaction between both pathways.

This heuristic model illustrates the dynamic interaction between pathogenic and salutogenic stress responses following environmental demands and cognitive appraisal. The bidirectional arrow emphasizes that individuals often experience elements of both pathways simultaneously rather than following a single trajectory. The model integrates flow states as a key mechanism for transforming potentially stressful challenges into opportunities for engagement and growth.

Caveats: This model represents a simplified conceptual framework; actual stress responses are more complex and individualized. The pathways shown are not mutually exclusive, and individuals may move between them based on changing contexts, resources and appraisals. The model does not capture all potential moderating variables or feedback loops that influence stress responses. Cultural and contextual factors may alter the relationships depicted. The emphasis on growth through adversity should not minimize the real harm that chronic, unmanageable stress can cause, particularly when systemic inequities limit access to resources. The model is intended as a guide for understanding and intervention rather than a predictive tool for individual outcomes.

Practical Implications of the Integrated-Pathway Model for Occupational Therapy

This integrated model has profound implications for occupational therapy intervention design. Rather than focusing exclusively on stress reduction or treating pathogenic and salutogenic responses as separate phenomena, interventions should recognize their interconnected nature:

1. **Enhance Appraisal Skills**: Train individuals to differentiate between threats and challenges and to reframe stressors when appropriate through occupational experiences.
2. **Build Resources**: Develop personal (psychological capital, coping skills, occupational competence) and environmental (social support, material resources, occupational opportunities) resources.
3. **Cultivate Positive States**: Use meaningful occupations to build resilience and create upward spirals of well-being.
4. **Promote Meaning-Making**: Help individuals construct meaningful narratives about their stress experiences through occupational storytelling.
5. **Develop Stress Mindsets**: Foster beliefs about stress that emphasize its potential for growth through successful occupational challenges

PART VI: CONTEMPORARY APPLICATIONS – POSITIVE HEALTH APPROACHES

Lifestyle Medicine and Stress

The integration of lifestyle medicine with positive psychology represents a comprehensive approach to stress management that addresses both physiological and psychological dimensions. The six pillars of lifestyle medicine include nutrition, physical activity, sleep, stress management, social connections and avoiding harmful substances, providing concrete, evidence-based strategies for building resilience and managing stress. These pillars align naturally with occupational therapy's domains of practice, particularly activities of daily living, instrumental activities of daily living, health management and social participation.

Research demonstrates that individuals experiencing psychological flourishing are nine times more likely to engage in multiple health-promoting behaviors (Burke & Dunne, 2023). This suggests a positive feedback loop where well-being enhances health behaviors, which in turn support continued flourishing. This bidirectional relationship underscores the importance of addressing both psychological and behavioral factors in stress management, a principle central to occupational therapy's holistic approach.

Mindfulness and Contemplative Practices

The incorporation of mindfulness-based interventions into mainstream stress management represents a convergence of ancient wisdom traditions with contemporary neuroscience. Mindfulness-Based Stress Reduction (MBSR), developed by Kabat-Zinn (1990), demonstrates how contemplative practices can fundamentally alter stress responses by changing the relationship to thoughts, emotions and bodily sensations. Occupational therapists have successfully integrated mindfulness into occupation-based interventions, helping clients become more present and engaged in their daily activities.

Neuroimaging research reveals that mindfulness practice produces structural and functional brain changes associated with improved emotion regulation, attention and self-awareness. These changes suggest that mindfulness doesn't merely help individuals cope with stress but fundamentally alters the neural substrates of stress processing, potentially shifting the default response from threat to challenge appraisal, a shift that can enhance occupational performance across all domains.

Positive Psychology Interventions

Evidence-based positive psychology interventions (PPIs) provide practical tools for transforming stress responses that occupational therapists can readily incorporate into practice. Gratitude practices, acts of kindness, strength identification and best-possible-self exercises have been shown to improve well-being and resilience. Meta-analyses (Bolier et al., 2013; Sin & Lyubomirsky, 2009) demonstrate that PPIs can be as effective as traditional psychotherapy for improving well-being and reducing distress.

The "Three Good Things" intervention, where individuals identify and reflect on three positive events each day, exemplifies how simple practices can shift attention from stressors to resources and from problems to possibilities. For occupational therapists, this intervention can be adapted to focus on three successful occupational engagements each day. Similarly, the "Using Signature Strengths in New Ways" intervention helps individuals recognize and deploy their character strengths in facing challenges, transforming potential stressors into opportunities for growth through occupational challenges.

PART VII: INTEGRATION AND FUTURE DIRECTIONS

Occupational Stress through a Positive Lens

The workplace, often characterized as a primary source of stress in modern life, provides a compelling context for applying positive health approaches. While statistics paint a sobering picture with workplace stress causing 120,000 deaths annually in the U.S. (Goh et al., 2015), positive psychology offers transformative possibilities that occupational therapists can leverage in vocational rehabilitation and workplace wellness programs.

Organizations implementing positive health approaches report not only reduced stress-related costs but also enhanced employee engagement, creativity and performance. The concept of "thriving at work" (Spreitzer et al., 2005) demonstrates that employees can experience vitality and learning even in demanding environments when provided with appropriate resources and autonomy, principles that guide occupational therapy interventions in vocational settings.

The Neurobiology of Resilience

Recent advances in neuroscience, exemplified by research from Kalisch et al. (2024), reveal the biological substrates of stress resilience with important implications for occupational therapy practice:

1. **Neural Plasticity**: The brain's capacity for reorganization in response to stress can be enhanced through targeted occupational interventions.
2. **Positive Neuroplasticity**: Engaging in meaningful occupations that cultivate positive states produces lasting changes in neural structure and function.
3. **Gut-Brain Axis**: The bidirectional communication between gut microbiota and the brain influences stress responses and can be modulated through lifestyle interventions, including dietary occupations.
4. **Epigenetic Regulation**: Positive experiences and stress management practices can influence gene expression, potentially reversing stress-induced epigenetic changes.

These findings provide biological validation for occupation-based interventions and suggest that resilience is not a fixed trait but a dynamic capacity that can be developed through purposeful occupational engagement.

Recent Research Frontiers

Contemporary stress research increasingly recognizes the multidimensional nature of stress responses and the potential for positive adaptation, with implications for occupational therapy practice:

Stress and pregnancy. Research by Traylor et al. (2020) demonstrated that nonpharmacologic interventions, including mindfulness, exercise and expressive writing, can reduce pregnancy complications associated with stress while promoting maternal well-being, interventions that occupational therapists can adapt for perinatal practice.

Nature-based interventions. Studies on forest bathing (shinrin-yoku) and nature-based mindfulness (Menardo et al., 2022) revealed that contact with nature provides unique stress-reduction benefits while enhancing positive states, supporting occupational therapy's use of outdoor and nature-based occupations.

Creative arts and stress. Mindfulness-based art therapy (MBAT) combines creative expression with contemplative practice, engaging multiple neural networks to promote healing and growth (Beerse et al., 2020), validating occupational therapy's long-standing use of creative occupations for health promotion.

Biomarkers of positive adaptation. Research identifying biomarkers associated with flourishing rather than merely the absence of disease markers represents a fundamental shift in how we measure health (Shah et al., 2024), suggesting new outcome measures for occupational therapy that capture positive adaptation and growth.

Critical Considerations and Power Relations

Drawing from Foucault's insights, as interpreted by Flyvbjerg (2001), we must recognize that stress and its management exist within complex power relations. The individualization of stress management, making individuals responsible for managing systemic stressors, can obscure structural inequalities and social determinants of health. Occupational therapists must remain cognizant of these dynamics, advocating for environmental and systemic changes while supporting individual adaptation.

The concept of "toxic positivity," representing the pressure to maintain positive attitudes regardless of circumstances, highlights a potential shadow side of positive psychology approaches. Authentic positive health acknowledges the full spectrum of human experience, including suffering, while maintaining faith in the human capacity for growth and adaptation. Occupational therapy's commitment to meeting clients where they are provides a corrective to oversimplified positive thinking.

CONCLUSION: IMPLICATIONS FOR OCCUPATIONAL THERAPY PRACTICE

The evolution of stress research from Bernard's milieu intérieur to contemporary positive health approaches offers occupational therapists a rich theoretical foundation for practice. The integrated-pathway model proposed here recognizes the interconnected nature of pathogenic and salutogenic responses, understanding that stress can lead to breakdown, breakthrough, or most commonly, a complex interaction of both, depending on appraisal processes, available resources, and the meaning individuals construct from their experiences. These are all factors that occupational therapists can influence through carefully designed interventions that acknowledge the integrated nature of human stress responses.

For occupational therapy practice, this reconceptualization has profound implications:

1. **Assessment**: Move beyond deficit-focused evaluation to include assessment of strengths, resources and growth potential. Consider not just what occupations are impaired by stress but what occupations might transform stress into growth, while recognizing that clients may simultaneously experience both challenges and opportunities.
2. **Intervention Planning**: Design interventions that build resilience through graduated occupational challenges rather than simply reducing stressors. Use the integrated-pathway model to help clients recognize and navigate the coexistence of threat and challenge appraisals, understanding that both may be present in their experience.
3. **Therapeutic Use of Self**: Recognize that the therapeutic relationship itself can influence whether clients appraise therapeutic challenges as threats or opportunities for growth. Model resilience and positive adaptation in the therapeutic relationship while acknowledging the reality of struggle.
4. **Outcome Measurement**: Include measures of flourishing, post-traumatic growth and positive adaptation alongside traditional symptom reduction measures. Document not just the return to baseline function but the emergence of new capacities, recognizing that growth and difficulty often coexist.
5. **Program Development**: Create occupation-based stress management programs that integrate PPIs with traditional stress reduction techniques. Develop programs that help clients not just survive but thrive, while acknowledging the integrated nature of their stress experience.

The constellation of concepts explored in this chapter, including homeostasis, adaptation, coherence, hardiness, growth and flourishing, form an interconnected network that illuminates the complexity of stress responses. For occupational therapists, these concepts provide multiple entry points for intervention, recognizing that meaningful occupation can serve as both a buffer against stress and a vehicle for transforming adversity into growth.

As we move forward, the integration of positive psychology, lifestyle medicine, neuroscience and occupational science offers unprecedented opportunities for helping individuals and communities build resilience and well-being through occupation. The question for occupational therapy is no longer simply "How can we help clients manage stress?" but more fundamentally, "How can we use occupation to transform stress into a catalyst for growth and enhanced life participation?"

This shift from a deficit-based to a strength-based approach, from pathogenesis to salutogenesis, from surviving to thriving through occupation, represents not just an evolution in stress research but a reaffirmation of occupational therapy's foundational belief in the transformative power of meaningful occupation. As Mary Reilly observed, "Man, through the use of his hands, as they are energized by mind and will, can influence the state of his own health." In the context of stress, this principle suggests that through purposeful occupational engagement, individuals can not merely manage stress but transform it into a force for positive adaptation and growth.

The words of Antonovsky resonate as both a challenge and inspiration for occupational therapy practice: while pathogenic thinking remains deeply entrenched in healthcare, the growing evidence for salutogenic approaches suggests that a fundamental paradigm shift is not only possible but already underway. As occupational therapists, we are uniquely positioned to lead this transformation, using our understanding of occupation to help clients navigate the inevitable stresses of life not as passive victims but as active agents of their own growth and flourishing.

SUMMARY

The evolution of stress research represents a fundamental transformation from purely physiological models to integrated positive health approaches. This chapter synthesizes contributions spanning nearly two centuries, from Bernard's foundational work on internal environment regulation through contemporary neuroscience and positive psychology research. The integrated-pathway model presented demonstrates that stress responses are not predetermined but emerge through dynamic interactions between environmental demands, cognitive appraisal, personal resources and social context. This model challenges traditional pathogenic assumptions by illustrating how identical stressors can lead to either distress and disease or eustress and flourishing, depending on how individuals appraise and engage with challenges. For occupational therapy practice, this reconceptualization has profound implications: assessment must extend beyond deficit identification to include strengths and growth potential; interventions should build resilience through graduated occupational challenges rather than merely reducing stressors; and outcomes should capture not just symptom reduction but enhanced capacity for meaningful occupation and life participation. The chapter emphasizes occupational therapy's unique position to lead this paradigm shift, leveraging the profession's understanding of meaningful occupation to transform stress from a threat into a catalyst for positive adaptation, demonstrating that through purposeful occupational engagement, individuals can navigate life's inevitable stresses as active agents of their own growth and flourishing.

DISCUSSION QUESTIONS

1. Reflect on Bernstein's constellation metaphor as a framework for understanding stress research. How does viewing diverse theories as interconnected "stars" rather than competing paradigms change your approach to clinical reasoning in occupational therapy practice?
2. Consider Bernard's concept of the milieu intérieur and its connection to occupational therapy's view of "la vie libre" (free and independent life). How does maintaining internal equilibrium relate to your understanding of occupational adaptation and participation?
3. Selye stated that "complete freedom from stress is death." Reflect on how this challenges conventional views of stress management. What are the implications for occupational therapy interventions that aim to help clients "reduce stress"?
4. The chapter presents Lazarus's statement that "people are rarely passive in the face of what happens to them." How does this perspective of human agency align with or challenge your current approach to working with clients experiencing stress?
5. Reflect on Antonovsky's revolutionary question: "What are the origins of health?" How might asking this question instead of "What causes disease?" transform your assessment process and intervention planning with clients?
6. Consider the integrated-pathway model presented in this chapter. Can you identify a client or personal experience where you witnessed both pathogenic and salutogenic responses occurring simultaneously? How did this complexity manifest in occupational performance?
7. Csikszentmihalyi's flow theory suggests that optimal challenge-skill balance transforms potential stress into engagement. Reflect on a time when you experienced flow in your own life or practice. What conditions made that possible, and how might you intentionally create similar conditions for your clients?
8. This chapter discusses how cognitive appraisal serves as a "bifurcation point" between threat and challenge responses. What occupational

therapy strategies could help clients develop more adaptive appraisal skills, and how would you know when such intervention is appropriate?

9. Antonovsky observed that "pathogenesis is too deeply entrenched in our thinking." Reflect honestly on your own clinical practice: To what extent do you focus on deficits versus strengths? What systemic or professional barriers make salutogenic approaches challenging to implement?
10. The concept of post-traumatic growth suggests that adversity can catalyze profound positive change. How does this perspective challenge or complement your understanding of trauma-informed care in occupational therapy? What ethical considerations arise when introducing growth-oriented perspectives to clients experiencing trauma?
11. Consider the critique of "toxic positivity" and the individualization of stress management that may obscure systemic inequalities. How can occupational therapists maintain both individual empowerment approaches and advocacy for environmental and systemic changes?
12. Reflect on the statement that occupational therapists are "uniquely positioned to lead this transformation" toward positive health approaches. What unique contributions does the occupational therapy perspective offer to stress research and intervention that other disciplines may not provide?

REFERENCES

Antonovsky, A. (1996). The salutogenic model as a theory to guide health promotion. *Health Promotion International, 11*(1), 11–18. https://doi.org/10.1093/heapro/11.1.11

Beerse, M. E., Van Lith, T., Pickett, S. M., & Stanwood, G. D. (2020). Biobehavioral utility of mindfulness-based art therapy: Neurobiological underpinnings and mental health impacts. *Experimental Biology and Medicine, 245*(2), 122–130. https://doi.org/10.1177/1535370219883634

Bernard, C. (1865). *An introduction to the study of experimental medicine*. Dover Publications.

Bernstein, R. J. (1992). *The new constellation: The ethical-political horizons of modernity/post-modernity*. MIT Press.

Bolier, L., Haverman, M., Westerhof, G. J., Riper, H., Smit, F., & Bohlmeijer, E. (2013). Positive psychology interventions: A meta-analysis of randomized controlled studies. *BMC Public Health, 13*(1), 119. https://doi.org/10.1186/1471-2458-13-119

Burke, J., & Dunne, P. (2023). Lifestyle medicine pillars as predictors of psychological flourishing. *Frontiers in Psychology, 14*, 1145243. https://doi.org/10.3389/fpsyg.2022.963806

Cannon, W. B. (1932). *The wisdom of the body*. W.W. Norton.

Cohen, S., Gianaros, P. J., & Manuck, S. B. (2016). A stage model of stress and disease. *Perspectives on Psychological Science, 11*(4), 456–463. https://doi.org/10.1177/1745691616646305

Csikszentmihalyi, M. (1990). *Flow: The psychology of optimal experience*. Harper & Row.

DeLongis, A., Folkman, S., & Lazarus, R. S. (1988). The impact of daily stress on health and mood: Psychological and social resources as mediators. *Journal of Personality and Social Psychology, 54*(3), 486–495. https://doi.org/10.1037//0022-3514.54.3.486

Dietrich, A. (2004). Neurocognitive mechanisms underlying the experience of flow. *Consciousness and Cognition, 13*(4), 746–761. https://doi.org/10.1016/j.concog.2004.07.002

Flyvbjerg, B. (2001). *Making social science matter: Why social inquiry fails and how it can succeed again*. Cambridge University Press.

Folkman, S., & Lazarus, R. S. (1984). *Stress, appraisal, and coping*. Springer.

Frankl, V. E. (1946). *Man's search for meaning*. Beacon Press.

Fredrickson, B. L. (2001). The role of positive emotions in positive psychology: The broaden-and-build theory of positive emotions. *American Psychologist, 56*(3), 218–226. https://doi.org/10.1037//0003-066x.56.3.218

Goh, J., Pfeffer, J., & Zenios, S. A. (2015). The relationship between workplace stressors and mortality and health costs in the United States. *Management Science, 62*(2), 608–628. https://doi.org/10.1287/mnsc.2014.2115

Kabat-Zinn, J. (1990). *Full catastrophe living: Using the wisdom of your body and mind to face stress, pain, and illness*. Delta.

Kalisch, R., Russo, S. J., & Müller, M. B. (2024). Neurobiology and systems biology of stress resilience. *Physiological Reviews, 104*(3), 1205–1263. https://doi.org/10.1152/physrev.00042.2023

Lazarus, R. S. (1999). *Stress and emotion: A new synthesis*. Springer. https://doi.org/10.1046/j.1365-2850.1999.00227-9.x

Lazarus, R. S., & Folkman, S. (1989). *Hassles and Uplifts Scales (HSUP)*. APA PsycTests. https://doi.org/10.1037/t06473-000

Menardo, E., Di Marco, D., Ramos, S., et al. (2022). Nature and mindfulness to cope with work-related stress: A narrative review. *International Journal of Environmental Research and Public Health, 19*(10), 5948. https://doi.org/10.3390/ijerph19105948

Nakamura, J., & Csikszentmihalyi, M. (2009). Flow theory and research. In C. R. Snyder & S. J. Lopez (Eds.), *Oxford handbook of positive psychology* (pp. 195–206). Oxford University Press. https://doi.org/10.1093/oxfordhb/9780195187243.013.0018

Park, C. L. (2010). Making sense of the meaning of literature: An integrative review of meaning -making and its effects on adjustment to stressful life events. *Psychological Bulletin, 136*(2), 257–301. https://doi.org/10.1037/a0018301

Sapolsky, R. M. (1998). *Why zebras don't get ulcers* (2nd ed.). W.H. Freeman.

Seligman, M. E. P., & Csikszentmihalyi, M. (2000). Positive psychology: An introduction. *American Psychologist, 55*(1), 5–14. https://doi.org/10.1007/978-94-017-9088-8_18

Selye, H. (1956). *The stress of life*. McGraw-Hill.

Selye, H. (1976a). *The stress of life* (Rev. ed.). McGraw-Hill.

Selye, H. (1976b). Stress without distress. In G. Serban (Ed.), *Psychopathology of human adaptation* (pp. 137–146). Springer. https://doi.org/10.1007/978-1-4684-2238-2_9

Shah, K., Kumari, R., & Jain, M. (2024). Unveiling stress markers: A systematic review investigating psychological stress biomarkers. *Developmental Psychobiology, 66*(5), e22490. https://doi.org/10.1002/dev.22490

Sin, N. L., & Lyubomirsky, S. (2009). Enhancing well-being and alleviating depressive symptoms with positive psychology interventions: A practice-friendly meta-analysis. *Journal of Clinical Psychology, 65*(5), 467–487. https://doi.org/10.1002/jclp.20593

Spreitzer, G., Sutcliffe, K., Dutton, J., Sonenshein, S., & Grant, A. M. (2005). A socially embedded model of thriving at work. *Organization Science, 16*(5), 537–549. https://doi.org/10.1287/orsc.1050.0153

Tedeschi, R. G., & Calhoun, L. G. (2004). Posttraumatic growth: Conceptual foundations and empirical evidence. *Psychological Inquiry, 15*(1), 1–18. https://doi.org/10.1207/s15327965pli1501_01

Traylor, C. S., Johnson, J. D., Kimmel, M. C., & Manuck, T. A. (2020). Effects of psychological stress on adverse pregnancy outcomes and nonpharmacologic approaches for reduction: An expert review. *American Journal of Obstetrics & Gynecology MFM, 2*(4), 100229. https://doi.org/10.1016/j.ajogmf.2020.100229

Wolff, H. G. (1953). *Stress and disease*. Charles C Thomas. https://psycnet.apa.org/doi/10.1037/11785-000

Chapter 3

Stress Neurophysiology and Its Underlying Mechanisms

LEARNING OBJECTIVES

By the end of this chapter, the reader will be able to

1. Understand the etiology of stress and its normal physiological responses.
2. Recognize abnormal physiological responses to stress.
3. Understand the endocrine and immune system roles in responding to stress.
4. Appreciate the roles of various brain areas (hypothalamus, amygdala and pituitary gland) and the autonomic nervous system in stress responses.

INTRODUCTION

Stress, this complex phenomenon, can be perceived as health-promoting on some occasions and as a serious problem or pathological condition on many others. Someone might thrive on eustress during periods of productivity, hobbies or competitive games and activity. Stress, however, can become destructive, jeopardizing the individual's performance, and may even turn into a harmful condition, negatively influencing the individual's health and quality of life.

In this chapter we will explore the underlying neurophysiological mechanisms contributing to stress. The direct and indirect effects of stress on the human body will be covered as well.

DOI: 10.4324/9781003671084-3

The human body gets diverse types of environmental psychological or physical stimuli that might affect its physiological status and homeostasis. These stimuli are labeled as stressors and usually evoke behavioral and physiological changes in the human body called "stress." The World Health Organization (WHO) defines stress as "any type of change that causes physical, emotional or psychological strain." The WHO has considered stress as the health epidemic of the 21st century, as its estimated annual cost in the USA alone was about 300 billion dollars (Brulé et al., 2018).

Stress is your body's response to anything that requires attention or action. Everyone experiences stress to some degree. The way you respond to stress, however, makes a substantial difference to your overall well-being. Stress is also classically defined as any challenge facing the body's homeostasis or its sense of internal balance (Mane et al., 2011). Another simple definition of stress is being in the constant presence of physiological or psychological hazards affecting the body, which could evoke substantial pressure on neurophysiological coping mechanisms (Duric et al., 2016). Researchers claim that stress might occur when there is a lag between the current and expected perceptions or anticipation related to the individual's internal or external environments (Goldstein & McEwen, 2002).

Stress is highly prevalent among the general population as the National Health Interview Survey estimated that about 75% of the USA general population experience stress symptoms every two weeks (Balaji et al., 2019). Stress in people on a population scale usually is exacerbated during disasters and global crises. According to a recent systematic review and meta-analysis, the global prevalence of stress was 36.5% during COVID-19 (Nochaiwong et al., 2021).

It is believed that excessive stress adversely affects the immune system and thus is linked to life-threatening diagnoses, including heart disease, stroke and high blood pressure (Duric et al., 2016). Stress is also believed to be linked to many unpleasant conditions such as musculoskeletal pain. It may also lower the individuals' quality of life (Almhdawi, Alrabbaie et al., 2021; Almhdawi, Kanaan et al., 2021). Researchers have also claimed that the relationship between stress and comorbidities is bidirectional – that is, each could contribute to increasing the odds of the other (Duric et al., 2016).

Stress may take the form of acute stress disorder (ASD) if happened for a brief period or post-traumatic stress disorder (PTSD) if lasted for a long duration and had more adverse effects on the person's life, mainly related to dissociative reaction trauma (Bryant et al., 2011). Symptoms of stress can be harmful to the human body. According to the Diagnostic and Statistical Manual-V (DSM-V tr; American Psychiatric Association, 2022), ASD symptoms might last from two days to four weeks post-trauma while PTSD may get diagnosed after four weeks. Diagnostic criteria for stress include a sense of numbing or detachment, reduced awareness of surroundings, detachment from reality, personality changes and/or dissociative amnesia (Bryant et al., 2011).

Despite the well-documented negative impacts of stress on individuals' health and well-being, not all effects of stress are harmful. It has long been believed that a proper level of stress would have positive effects on an individual's productivity. Cardon and Patel (2013) found that self-employed individuals demonstrated higher levels of stress compared to employees, but self-employed individuals had better income, which could be considered a positive effect for increased stress.

The concept "fight-or-flight," the classical terminology related to the human body's molecular responses to stress, was coined by Cannon (1932). Fight-or-flight is a term used to describe the body's acute responses to stress, as the living being faces a life-threatening situation. During fight-or-flight, the living body releases the substrates of the sympathetic nervous system (SNS) – a physiological excitement in preparation for the life-preserving fight or run behavior (Cannon, 1932; Fink, 2009).

We experience stress many times in our daily life. In 2015, it was estimated that about 78% of Americans reported symptoms of stress (American Psychological Association, 2016). Stressful events might include work-related issues, professional issues, dealing with financial burdens, dealing with deadlines, dealing with academic burdens, experiencing diseases and trauma directly or through family members, life-threating events and other types of mental or physical traumas (Maslach et al., 2016; Matuska et al., 2013).

The human body automatically regulates itself in the presence of stress stimuli. The body's response to stress is operated via complex interrelated processes governed by (1) the autonomic nervous (sympathetic and parasympathetic systems), and (2) the immune and endocrine (hypothalamus, pituitary and adrenal glands) systems, as described in detail below. Repetitive and chronic exposure to internal or external stressors may introduce unhealthy levels of mental health symptoms, such as those of depression and anxiety, in addition to cognitive deficits and cardiovascular impairments (Chu et al., 2022; Ketchesin et al., 2017; Mifsud & Reul, 2018).

NERVOUS SYSTEM INVOLVEMENT IN THE STRESS REACTION MECHANISM

The nervous system and particularly the human brain are among the most complex structures of the universe. Our knowledge about the nervous system still spans only a fraction of its entire substance and underlying mechanisms. Therefore, many scientists consider the brain to be the last discovery frontier in medicine (Liebeskind et al., 2016; Restak, 1979). Basically, the nervous system consists of the central nervous system (CNS) and peripheral nervous system (PNS). The CNS consists of the spinal cord and the brain, including the medulla, pons, cerebellum, midbrain, diencephalon and the cerebral hemispheres. The PNS has a crucial role in exploring the environment and transmitting ascending sensory signals to the CNS and descending motor ones to the body through its somatic division. The autonomic division of the PNS, consisting of sympathetic and parasympathetic parts, plays a crucial role in body responses to stress (Purves et al., 2001).

The physiological mechanisms of stress encompass many interacting sets of processes triggered in response to stressors being imposed on the human body. These stressors might be of a physical, emotional or environmental nature. The body's responses to stress are organized by (1) the autonomic nervous system (ANS) and (2) the endocrine system via the hypothalamic-pituitary-adrenal (HPA) axis.

Generally speaking, the body's response to stress runs through the following stages (from Goldstein, 2006):

1. **Recognition of Stress**
   Stressors faced by people might be external (such as trauma or noise) or internal (such as physical diseases and pain, or mental health issues such as anxiety and depression). Many areas in the brain, particularly the amygdala, recognize these types of stressors. The amygdala transmits stress alerts to the hypothalamus, which is thought to be the main coordinator of the response to the stressor (Goldstein, 2006).
2. **Autonomic Nervous System (ANS) Activation**
   This activation affects the two branches of the ANS:
   Sympathetic Nervous System (SNS) – which is responsible for the fight-or-flight response. The hypothalamus sends signals through the SNS to the adrenal medulla and portions of the adrenal glands. The adrenal medulla releases catecholamines (epinephrine [adrenaline] and norepinephrine), which prepare the body to respond to the stressor. The activation of the SNS leads to increased blood pressure and heart rate, dilation of pupils, bronchodilation,

increased glucose release from the liver and inhibition of digestion and other non-essential functions (to conserve energy for immediate needs).

Parasympathetic Nervous System (PSNS) – comes into play when the stressor is removed or coped with. The PSNS activates to bring the body back to a state of rest, also called the "rest-and-digest" response (Goldstein, 2006).

3. **Activation of the HPA Axis**

   The hypothalamic-pituitary-adrenal (HPA) axis is the major component of the long-term response to stress. Upon detecting a stressor, the hypothalamus secretes corticotropin-releasing hormone (CRH). This activates the pituitary gland to secrete adrenocorticotropic hormone (ACTH) into the bloodstream. This hormone reaches the adrenal cortex (of the adrenal glands), which facilitates the secretion and release of cortisol, which is considered the primary hormone of the stress response. Cortisol increases blood sugar levels; inhibits the immune system; aids in the metabolism of fats, proteins and carbohydrates; helps maintain blood pressure; and modulates inflammatory responses. Cortisol provides energy for the body to cope with long-term stress, but chronic release of cortisol can lead to negative health effects, such as poor immunity, high blood pressure and metabolic issues (Goldstein, 2006).

4. **Feedback Mechanism**

   Once cortisol levels are sufficiently high, a negative feedback loop is initiated. Cortisol binds to receptors in the hypothalamus and pituitary gland. This helps to reduce the release of CRH and ACTH and consequently decreases the production of cortisol and ends the stress response (Goldstein, 2006).

5. **Results of Chronic Stress**

   While short-term activation of the stress response is protective, chronic stress can have detrimental effects on the body due to prolonged activation of the SNS and the HPA axis. For the cardiovascular system, chronic stress may lead to high blood pressure and increased risk of heart attack or stroke, due to continuous SNS activation. For the immune system, prolonged cortisol release can make the body more susceptible to infections and slow wound healing. For the digestive system, stress can cause irritable bowel syndrome, ulcers and acid reflux, due to reduced blood flow to the gastrointestinal tract. For the endocrine system, chronic stress affects glucose metabolism, increasing the risk of insulin resistance and type 2 diabetes. Finally, for mental and cognitive health, elevated levels of cortisol over time can impair brain function, particularly in areas involved in memory (hippocampus) and emotional regulation (prefrontal cortex). It can lead to anxiety, depression and cognitive decline (Turner et al., 2020).

6. **Adaptation to Stress**

   The body attempts to maintain homeostasis or balance during stress, but chronic exposure to stress results in an increased allostatic load, which refers to the cumulative wear and tear on the body due to constant physiological adaptation to stressors. When the allostatic load becomes too high, it can result in stress-related diseases, including cardiovascular diseases, metabolic disorders and mental health issues (Guidi et al., 2021).

7. **Stress Recovery**
   The PSNS helps return the body to a state of calm after the reaction to the stressor has passed, through mechanisms like slowing the heart rate, reducing blood pressure and promoting digestion and healing. Engaging in stress-reduction practices (like mindfulness, exercise or relaxation techniques) can help restore balance and reduce the negative impacts of chronic stress (Pascoe et al., 2017).

All processes governed by the ANS are considered to be involuntary, as they are conducted at the subconscious level. The ANS controls various processes affecting most of the body's tissues and organs, making a fundamental contribution to homeostasis. These processes include influencing blood pressure, gastrointestinal system function while digesting food, bowel and bladder operations, eye gaze and tracking responses, as well as the body's thermal regulations (Iversen et al., 2000; McCorry, 2007).

The two parts of the ANS are particularly important in the response to stress. The SNS enables the individual to fight and increases the body's alertness and readiness to withstand stressful situations. Sympathetic responses include increasing the heart rate, sweating, breathing rate and pupil diameter. The PSNS is usually associated with a relaxing state and involves the opposite processes and effects from the SNS. For example, while the SNS dilates the eye pupil, increases the heart and breathing rates and relaxes the bladder, the PSNS constricts the pupil, decreases breathing and heart rates and contracts the bladder. Processes such as food digestion, defecation, sexual alertness and slower heart and breathing rates are believed to be evoked by the PSNS (Iversen et al., 2000; McCorry, 2007; Recordati, 2003).

Neurotransmitters are also important in understanding human stress physiology. These are chemicals influencing nervous system activity that are composed in nervous system tissues and kept in cell vesicles for release upon need. The main neurotransmitters secreted by the ANS are acetylcholine (secreted by cholinergic nerve fibers) and norepinephrine (secreted by adrenergic nerve fibers). These two neurotransmitters are vital in stress management. Norepinephrine represents about 20% of the hormonal output of the adrenal medulla, while the remaining 80% consists of epinephrine hormonal output. Epinephrine is also known as adrenaline- a hormone released and significantly participating in the described PSNS responses to stress (Green & Richter, 1937; McCorry, 2007).

ENDOCRINE SYSTEM INVOLVEMENT IN THE STRESS MECHANISM

Stress physiology and underlying processes are also influenced by a complex of interrelated endocrine networks consisting of multiple glands. There is a neurohormonal interaction that mediates stress as well. The hypothalamus, pituitary and adrenal glands are the main players in these complicated hormonal-based stress mediators (Ketchesin et al., 2017). The interaction between the endocrine systems and the autonomic nervous system is referred to as the hypothalamic-pituitary-adrenocortical (HPA) axis.

The HPA action is slower than the sympathetic-adreno-medullar (SAM) network. However, the HPA network plays a fundamental role in responding to stressful situations such as injuries or invasive procedures by maintaining homeostasis, effecting allostasis and preventing further tissue damage (Fink, 2009). Scientists claimed that the pituitary gland is the autonomic governor of the adrenal cortex, as well as the thyroid and the reproductive glands. However, some researchers believe that the pituitary gland is also governed by the CNS (Fink, 2009).

The pituitary gland has connections called projections. These projections reach certain nuclei or parts in the hypothalamus that end in blood vessels, which enables neurohormones (corticotropin hormone) into bloodstream circulation. This eventually influences overall body state, including the stress reaction and its related homeostasis. These actions may eventually affect skeletal muscles, the gastrointestinal and cardiovascular systems, the subcortical brain areas, the liver and many other body tissues (Westphal & Seasholtz, 2005). The pituitary gland also activates the adrenal cortex to release its hormones, mainly cortisol, into blood circulation, which is fundamental to stress-related physiological responses (Chu et al., 2021).

The HPA axis is also believed to moderate the production of catecholamines, which are neurohormones that contribute to stress responses by increasing blood pressure, sweating, headache and anxiety. Furthermore, the HPA is involved in enhancing the role of estrogen (a hormone involved in growth, development and the reproductive system) in the stress response (Chu et al., 2022).

IMMUNE SYSTEM INVOLVEMENT IN THE STRESS MECHANISM

The immune system naturally defends the human body from any external or internal pathogens. However, this action is influenced by the HPA and the SNS during stress. In general, the stress response will inhibit the actions of the immune system, while maintaining homeostasis, to protect the body from further damage (Khoo et al., 2017).

The secretion of cortisol suppresses the immune system by releasing catecholamine, inhibiting insulin, utilizing gluconeogenesis (an alternative form of producing energy for the body via glucose) and delaying wound healing and inflammatory reactions. Stress-related hormones such as aldosterone (a sodium-retaining steroid produced by the adrenal gland) and glucocorticoid (increasing glucose levels) play vital roles in increasing blood pressure and influencing the brain, in order to preserve function (Bassett et al., 2015).

Eventually, stress and its underlying mechanisms, even under normal levels of stress, will affect many body systems, organs and tissues. These include the respiratory, cardiovascular, endocrine, nervous, reproductive and gastrointestinal systems (Vage et al., 2023). Stress influences appear in the shape of many effects, such as increasing heart rate, stronger heartbeats, larger volumes of pumped blood (dilatation of heart) and increased blood supply to skeletal muscles, which reduces the blood supply to internal muscles and viscera. To support these cardiovascular changes, stress also influences the respiratory system, constricting airways to enable faster oxygen supply and carbon dioxide extraction from cells by evoking shorter but faster breaths (Grossman, 1983). The endocrine system increases steroid hormone secretion (primarily cortisol) under stress. The gastrointestinal system's motility speed and absorption of nutrients are influenced by stress mechanisms in the short and long term. Researchers apply the term "brain of the gut" to describe this relationship (Bhatia et al., 2005). As mentioned in earlier sections, stress has a major influence in activating the SNS and launching its general effects on the body by activating adrenal glands and thus equipping the body with more energy and alertness (Cohn, 1989).

Adaptive levels of stress (eustress) are beneficial for human productivity and body protection. Stress-related changes, however, are usually counteracted or balanced by the mechanisms modulated by the PSNS, enabling recovery from stress. When physical, psychosocial or physiological stressors increase, the human body may fail to recover from stress. These effects may significantly contribute to many physical and mental diseases and health conditions, a phenomenon known as maladaptive stress level (Shen & Zipes, 2014; Tsigos et al., 2020). As a cause of cellular death, unopposed high levels of stress are strongly associated with many pathological conditions, including cardiovascular diseases, diabetes, neurological and musculoskeletal conditions, gastrointestinal conditions such as ulcers and many others (Bassett et al., 2015; Budzyński & Kłopocka, 2014; Sano & Reed, 2013).

SUMMARY

The stressors of daily life evoke a stress reaction in the human body. This reaction is moderated by elements of the nervous system and the endocrine system. The amygdala detects threats and sends signals to the hypothalamus, which orchestrates the stress response by activating the sympathetic nervous system and the hypothalamic-pituitary-adrenocortical axis. The sympathetic nervous system triggers the fight-or-flight response via adrenaline/norepinephrine, while the hypothalamic-pituitary-adrenocortical axis releases cortisol for sustained energy during prolonged stress. Cortisol, in turn, regulates metabolism and immune function and helps manage prolonged stress. The parasympathetic nervous system counterbalances the effects of the sympathetic nervous system when the crisis is perceived to be over. The sympathetic nervous system and the hypothalamic-pituitary-adrenocortical axis neurophysiological responses are crucial for survival in the face of acute threats but can become harmful if triggered too frequently or for too long, even causing serious illnesses of the cardiovascular, digestive, musculoskeletal and nervous systems.

DISCUSSION QUESTIONS

1. How does the human body react to stressors?
2. What are the main differences between the sympathetic and parasympathetic nervous system mechanisms in response to stress?
3. Describe the importance of the hypothalamic-pituitary-adrenocortical axis in the stress response.
4. What are the roles of cortisol in responding to stress?
5. Describe how the human body recovers from stress.

REFERENCES

Almhdawi, K. A., Alrabbaie, H., Kanaan, S. F., Alahmar, M. R., Oteir, A. O., Mansour, Z. M., & Obeidat, D. S. (2021). The prevalence of upper quadrant work-related musculoskeletal disorders and their predictors among registered nurses. *Work, 68*(4), 1035–1047. https://doi.org/10.3233/wor-213434

Almhdawi, K. A., Kanaan, S. F., Khader, Y., Al-Hourani, Z., Al-Jarrah, M. D., Almomani, F., & Alqhazo, M. T. (2021). Mental and physical health-related quality of life and their associated factors among students of a comprehensive allied health institution. *Work, 70*(1), 63–73. https://doi.org/10.3233/wor-205226

American Psychological Association. (2016). Stress in America: The impact of discrimination. *Stress in America survey*. https://www.apa.org/news/press/releases/stress/2015/impact

American Psychiatric Association. (2022). *Diagnostic and statistical manual of mental disorders* (5th ed., text rev; DSM-V tr.). https://doi.org/10.1176/appi.books.9780890425787

Balaji, N. K., Murthy, P. S., Kumar, D. N., & Chaudhury, S. (2019). Perceived stress, anxiety, and coping states in medical and engineering students during examinations. *Industrial Psychiatry Journal, 28*(1), 86–97. https://doi.org/10.4103/ipj.ipj_70_18

Bassett, S. M., Lupis, S. B., Gianferante, D., Rohleder, N., & Wolf, J. M. (2015). Sleep quality but not sleep quantity effects on cortisol responses to acute psychosocial stress. *Stress, 18*(6), 638–644. https://doi.org/10.3109/10253890.2015.1087503

Bhatia, V., & Tandon, R. K. (2005). Stress and the gastrointestinal tract. *Journal of Gastroenterology and Hepatology, 20,* 332–339. https://doi.org/10.1111/j.1400-1746.2004.03508.x

Brulé, G., & Morgan, R. (2018). Editorial- Working with stress: Can we turn distress into eustress? *Journal of Neuropsychology & Stress Management, 3*(4), 1–3. [no doi].

Bryant, R. A., Friedman, M. J., Spiegel, D., Ursano, R., & Strain, J. (2011). A review of acute stress disorder in DSM-5. *Depression and Anxiety, 28*(9), 802–817. https://doi.org/10.1002/da.20737

Budzyński, J., & Kłopocka, M. (2014). Brain-gut axis in the pathogenesis of Helicobacter pylori infection. *World Journal of Gastroenterology, 20*(18), 5212–5225. https://doi.org/10.3748/wjg.v20.i18.5212

Cannon, W. J. (1932). *The wisdom of the body*. W. W. Norton.

Cardon, M. S., & Patel, P. C. (2013). Is stress worth it? Stress-related health and wealth trade-offs for entrepreneurs. *Applied Psychology, 64*(2), 379–420. https://doi.org/10.1111/apps.12021

Chu, B., Marwaha, K., Sanvictores, T., & Ayers, D. (2021). Physiology, stress reaction. In *StatPearls* [Internet]. StatPearls.

Chu, B., Marwaha, K., Sanvictores, T., & Ayers, D. (2022). Physiology, stress reaction. In *StatPearls*. StatPearls.

Cohn, J. N. (1989). Sympathetic nervous system activity and the heart. *American Journal of Hypertension, 2*(12 Pt 2), 353s–356s. [no doi].

Duric, V., Clayton, S., Leong, M. L., & Yuan, L. L. (2016). Comorbidity factors and brain mechanisms linking chronic stress and systemic illness. *Neural Plasticity, 2016*, 5460732. https://doi.org/10.1155/2016/5460732

Fink, G. (2009). Stress: Definition and history. In L. R. Squire (Ed.), *Encyclopedia of Neuroscience* (pp. 549–555). Academic Press. https://doi.org/10.1016/B978-008045046-9.00076-0

Goldstein, D. S. (2006). *Adrenaline and the inner world: An introduction to scientific integrative medicine*. JHU Press.

Goldstein, D. S., & McEwen, B. (2002). Allostasis, homeostats, and the nature of stress. *Stress, 5*(1), 55–58. https://doi.org/10.1080/102538902900012345

Green, D. E., & Richter, D. (1937). Adrenaline and adrenochrome. *Biochemistry Journal, 31*(4), 596–616. https://doi.org/10.1042/bj0310596

Grossman, P. (1983). Respiration, stress, and cardiovascular function. *Psychophysiology, 20*(3), 284–300. https://doi.org/10.1111/j.1469-8986.1983.tb02156.x

Guidi, J., Lucente, M., Sonino, N., & Fava, G. A. (2021). Allostatic load and its impact on health: A systematic review. *Psychotherapy and Psychosomatics, 90*(1), 11–27. https://doi.org/10.1159/000510696

Iversen, S., Iversen, L., & Saper, C. (2000). *Principles of neural science.* McGraw-Hill.

Ketchesin, K. D., Stinnett, G. S., & Seasholtz, A. F. (2017). Corticotropin-releasing hormone-binding protein and stress: From invertebrates to humans. *Stress, 20*(5), 449–464. https://doi.org/10.1080/10253890.2017.1322575

Khoo, B., Boshier, P. R., Freethy, A., Tharakan, G., Saeed, S., Hill, N., Williams, E. L., Moorthy, K., Tolley, N., Jiao, L. R., Spaulding, D., Palazzo, F., Meeran, K., & Tan, T. (2017). Redefining the stress cortisol response to surgery. *Clinical Endocrinology, 87*(5), 451–458. https://doi.org/10.1111/cen.13439

Liebeskind, B. J., Hillis, D. M., Zakon, H. H., & Hofmann, H. A. (2016). Complex homology and the evolution of nervous systems. *Trends in Ecology & Evolution, 31*(2), 127–135. https://doi.org/10.1016/j.tree.2015.12.005

Mane Abhay, B., Krishnakumar, M. K., Niranjan Paul, C., & Hiremath Shashidhar, G. (2011). Differences in perceived stress and its correlates among students in professional courses. *Journal of Clinical and Diagnostic Research, 5*(6), 1228–1233. [no doi].

Maslach, C., & Leiter, M. P. (2016). Burnout. In G. Fink (Ed.), *Stress: Concepts, cognition, emotion, and behavior. Handbook of stress, Vol. 1* (pp. 351–358). Academic Press.

Matuska, K., Bass, J., & Schmitt, J. S. (2013). Life balance and perceived stress: Predictors and demographic profile. *Occupational Therapy Journal of Research, 33*(3), 146–158. https://doi.org/10.3928/15394492-20130614-03

McCorry, L. K. (2007). Physiology of the autonomic nervous system. *American Journal of Pharmaceutical Education, 71*(4), 78. https://doi.org/10.5688/aj710478

Mifsud, K. R., & Reul, J. (2018). Mineralocorticoid and glucocorticoid receptor-mediated control of genomic responses to stress in the brain. *Stress, 21*(5), 389–402. https://doi.org/10.1080/10253890.2018.1456526

Nochaiwong, S., Ruengorn, C., Thavorn, K., Hutton, B., Awiphan, R., Phosuya, C., Ruanta, Y., Wongpakaran, N., & Wongpakaran, T. (2021). Global prevalence of mental health issues among the general population during the coronavirus disease-2019 pandemic: A systematic review and meta-analysis. *Scientific Reports, 11*(1), 10173. https://doi.org/10.1038/s41598-021-89700-8

Pascoe, M. C., Thompson, D. R., & Ski, C. F. (2017). Yoga, mindfulness-based stress reduction, and stress-related physiological measures: A meta-analysis. *Psychoneuroendocrinology, 86*, 152–168. https://doi.org/10.1016/j.psyneuen.2017.08.008

Purves, D., Augustine, G., Fitzpatrick, D., Katz, L., LaMantia, A., McNamara, J., & Williams, S. M. (Eds.). (2001). *Neuroscience* (2nd ed.). Sinauer Associates.

Recordati, G. (2003). A thermodynamic model of the sympathetic and parasympathetic nervous systems. *Autonomic Neuroscience: Basic & Clinical, 103*(1–2), 1–12. https://doi.org/10.1016/s1566-0702(02)00260-6

Restak, R. M. (1979). *The brain: The last frontier*. Doubleday.

Sano, R., & Reed, J. C. (2013). ER stress-induced cell death mechanisms. *Biochimica Biophysica Acta, 1833*(12), 3460–3470. https://doi.org/10.1016/j.bbamcr.2013.06.028

Shen, M. J., & Zipes, D. P. (2014). Role of the autonomic nervous system in modulating cardiac arrhythmias. *Circulation Research, 114*(6), 1004–1021. https://doi.org/10.1161/circresaha.113.302549

Tsigos, C., Kyrou, I., Kassi, E., & Chrousos, G. P. (2020). Stress: Endocrine physiology and pathophysiology. In K. R. Feingold, R. A. Adler, S. F. Ahmed et al., (Eds.). *Endotext* [Internet]. MDText.com, Inc. Available from: https://www.ncbi.nlm.nih.gov/books/NBK278995/

Turner, A. I., Smyth, N., Hall, S. J., Torres, S. J., Hussein, M., Jayasinghe, S. U., Ball, K., & Clow, A. J. (2020). Psychological stress reactivity and future health and disease outcomes: A systematic review of prospective evidence. *Psychoneuroendocrinology, 114*, 104599. https://doi.org/10.1016/j.psyneuen.2020.104599

Vage, A., McCarron, E., & Hamilton, P. K. (2023). Biological testing during acute psychological stress: A hindrance or an opportunity? *Clinical Biochemistry, 114*, 11–17. https://doi.org/10.1016/j.clinbiochem.2023.01.005

Westphal, N. J., & Seasholtz, A. F. (2005). Gonadotropin-releasing hormone (GnRH) positively regulates corticotropin-releasing hormone-binding protein expression via multiple intracellular signaling pathways and a multipartite GnRH response element in alphaT3-1 cells. *Molecular Endocrinology, 19*(11), 2780–2797. https://doi.org/10.1210/me.2004-0519

Chapter 4

Technology, Stress and Participation: Harnessing Digital Tools with Intentional Boundaries

LEARNING OBJECTIVES

By the end of this chapter, readers will be able to

1. Consider the dual role of technology in stress management, identifying both its potential benefits and drawbacks.
2. Be able to develop a balanced, individualized plan for using digital tools in stress management, incorporating strategies such as digital detoxes, technology-free zones and usage tracking.

INTRODUCTION

In the last decade, the integration of technology into our daily lives has grown exponentially. From smartphones to wearable devices to the increasingly inescapable presence of artificial intelligence, technology has become an integral part of how we communicate, work and entertain ourselves (Alter, 2017; DataReportal, 2024). This rapid technological advancement has brought with it competing realities. Technology can certainly play a positive role in managing stress, but as we have often seen, it can also contribute to increased stress levels and poor mental health outcomes if not used with a degree of caution and thoughtfulness (Kuss & Griffiths, 2017).

Digital tools such as mobile apps designed to help users engage in mindfulness and meditation, wearable technology for monitoring stress and the connections and opportunities offered by online communities can be used as innovative

DOI: 10.4324/9781003671084-4

methods to help individuals manage stress effectively (Huberty et al., 2019; Mani et al., 2015). Conversely, the constant (and often unavoidable) connectivity facilitated by technology can lead to information overload, disruptions in work-life balance, sleep disturbances and even addictive behaviors, which can exacerbate stress (Bawden & Robinson, 2009; Chesley, 2005; Exelmans & Van den Bulck, 2016; Kuss & Griffiths, 2017).

This chapter aims to explore the relationship between technology and stress. It will provide an overview of how technology can both exacerbate and alleviate stress, and how for many of us, it does both (Kowalski et al., 2014; Przybylski et al., 2013; Vogel et al., 2014).

In addressing these topics, this chapter will offer readers a basic overview of technology's impact on stress – for better or for worse! The authors of this text are decidedly *not* experts on technology, but we live in the same world that you do and have seen the significant effect that technology can have on stress in both our professional and personal lives. By critically evaluating their own technology use, readers can make informed decisions to optimize their mental health and well-being and gain tools to better support the people whom they serve.

Technology and Society

Try as you might, you just can't avoid it – technology is everywhere. Despite every friend you may have who has sworn off Facebook, deleted their Instagram or proclaimed that they are only going to get their news from proper newspapers from now on, most of the world's population makes some use of technology and social media on a daily basis.

According to the Pew Research Center, as of 2021, nearly 90% of USA residents own a smartphone. Social media platforms have also seen significant user engagement, with a significant majority reporting at least some use of social media. These trends underscore how ingrained technology has become in daily life, influencing the way we live, the way we work and the way we learn about the world around us. The ubiquity of technology has made it a double-edged sword, providing convenience, efficiency and endless access to information on the one hand, while introducing new potential pitfalls on the other.

This chapter will delve into that double-edged sword, examining both technology's potential drawbacks and benefits. First, we will explore how technology can contribute to increased stress and can diminish mental health. Then, we will shift focus to the ways in which technology can be incorporated into an effective stress management routine. Technology, as with so many other things, is inherently neither good nor bad – it depends on how it is used.

PITFALLS OF TECHNOLOGY AND SOCIAL MEDIA

Social media has been linked to several high-profile cases of deteriorating mental health. One such story is that of Molly Russell, a 14-year-old girl from the United Kingdom who tragically took her own life in 2017 (BBC, 2022). Molly had become obsessed with content related to depression, self-harm and suicide on Instagram, Pinterest and other social media platforms. This case and other cases like it have sparked a debate about the role of social media in exacerbating mental health issues, especially among young people.

An investigation into her death revealed that she had viewed a significant amount of graphic and distressing material in the months leading up to her suicide. Her father has been vocal about the harmful impact of this content and has been critical of social media platforms that continually fed his daughter content that deepened her sense of despair and isolation.

This story is a sobering example of the potential dangers associated with technology use, albeit an extreme one. It underscores the need for awareness and intervention to ensure that technology serves as a tool for connection and support rather than a contributor to the mental health crisis. Technology's negative impacts on mental health are typically not so destructive, but its potential for some degree of harm is clear (Kanchan & Gaidhane, 2023; Lup et al., 2015; Seabrook et al., 2016).

This chapter cannot possibly describe all the ways that technology and social media might contribute to stress or other negative mental health outcomes. Instead, we will focus on several well-documented challenges associated with technology use, supported by evidence. Given the ever-evolving nature of this topic, the information in this chapter may become outdated soon after publication. Our goal, nonetheless, is to provide readers with an overview of well-documented pitfalls as they exist today.

Navigating a Digital Minefield

One of the primary ways that technology contributes to stress is through information overload. At any moment of every day, most of us have access to more information than someone a generation ago would have found in one of the world's great libraries. The average person is exposed to an amount of information that is roughly equivalent to 174 newspapers every day (Bawden & Robinson, 2009; Hilbert & López, 2011). Whether you're reading the *New York Times* or the *Guardian,* that's significantly more information than individuals have ever had to navigate before. This surely has its benefits – but it is not without drawbacks. This constant influx of data can make it difficult for individuals to focus and can contribute to increased stress levels and decreased productivity (Dragano & Lunau, 2020; Rosen et al., 2014).

This dynamic can create difficulties in managing work-life balance (Derks et al., 2016; Dragano & Lunau, 2020), social relationships (Kanchan & Gaidhane, 2023; Rosen et al., 2014; Seabrook et al., 2016) and general health and wellness (Chesley, 2005; Dragano & Lunau, 2020; Exelmans & Van den Bulck, 2016; Kanchan & Gaidhane, 2023; Rosen et al., 2014; Seabrook et al., 2016).

Occupational Balance

The challenge of maintaining occupational balance, including work-life balance, in a digitally connected world can be a significant contributor to stress. With the widespread adaption of smartphones and remote work, the boundaries between work, school and personal life have become increasingly blurred (Chesley, 2005). This can lead to burnout and chronic stress, as individuals struggle to find time to "unplug" from work or school, spend time with family and engage in hobbies.

Research has shown that personal use of smartphones in the workplace can contribute to occupational imbalance, increasing stress by creating pressure to be available to family, friends and work simultaneously (Derks et al., 2016; Duxbury & Smart, 2011). Moreover, the flexibility offered by mobile technology, while beneficial for some, can result in a sense of being overconnected to work and thus higher stress (Derks et al., 2016).

Challenges Associated with Social Media

Social media has received significant attention for its impact on mental health. While the popularity of particular social media platforms (e.g., MySpace, Facebook and TikTok) has ebbed and flowed over recent decades, social media as a category of product has remained a constant and is used by over half of people worldwide (DataReportal, 2024). This section will review several stress-related challenges associated with social media use, including fear of missing out, social comparison and online harassment.

One notable phenomenon stemming from social media is the fear of missing out (FOMO), which can be exacerbated by social media platforms. FOMO is characterized by a pervasive apprehension that others might be having rewarding experiences from which one is absent. Approximately 56% of social media users report experiencing FOMO, which can lead to compulsive checking of social media and increased stress and anxiety (Beyens et al., 2016; Przybylski et al., 2013).

Another challenge of note is the concept of social comparison. Platforms like Instagram and Facebook often showcase curated and idealized versions of users' lives, leading others to compare themselves to these unrealistic standards. Studies have shown that 88% of women and 65% of men compare themselves to images in the media, which can diminish self-esteem and contribute to feelings of inadequacy and stress (Vogel et al., 2014). Those of us on social media can probably relate to this – many posts are about major life events, vacations and other happy times. While those moments may make up most of our social media feeds, that does not necessarily mean that we should expect them to make up most of our lives.

Cyberbullying and forms of online harassment can also contribute to elevated levels of stress. Victims of cyberbullying, especially adolescents, often experience heightened levels of stress, anxiety and depression (Gohal et al., 2023; Maurya et al., 2022; Song et al., 2024). About 34% of school-aged individuals reported having experienced cyberbullying in their lifetime, with 17% having been cyberbullied in the past 30 days (Kowalski et al., 2014). The anonymity and reach of the internet can make cyberbullying difficult to avoid, making it a pervasive and persistent problem for many people.

While the problems described above have the potential to affect people of all ages, challenges with social media have been noted to be especially prevalent among adolescents and young adults (American Academy of Child and Adolescent Psychiatry & Children's Hospital Association, 2021). The inescapable presence of both social media and smartphones has contributed toward what has been described as a "national emergency" of mental health among young people, especially among girls and young women (American Academy of Child and Adolescent Psychiatry & Children's Hospital Association, 2021; Haidt, 2024; Nesi, 2020). This crisis has brought increased rates of anxiety, depression and suicidal ideation, among other mental health-related concerns, and it has been suggested that the ubiquitousness of technology, smartphones and social media has exacerbated the issue (Haidt, 2024).

Health and Wellness

In addition to some of the emotional and behavioral challenges stemming from technology use described above, there are potential negative physical health consequences as well. These consequences may in turn contribute to stress or make management of stress more difficult. Examples of such negative physical health consequences are described below.

Sedentary Behavior

1. Prolonged screen time often leads to sedentary lifestyles, increasing risks of cardiovascular disease, obesity, Type 2 diabetes and certain cancers (Owen et al., 2010).
2. Lack of physical activity can exacerbate stress and decrease mental well-being (Warburton & Bredin, 2017).
3. Incorporating regular movement and screen breaks is essential for maintaining both physical and mental health (Owen et al., 2010; Warburton & Bredin, 2017).

Digital Eye Strain

1. Prolonged screen use can lead to symptoms such as headaches, blurred vision and neck pain, contributing to stress in environments where screen use is constant (Anshel, 2007; Rosenfield, 2011)
2. Mitigation strategies include proper ergonomics, regular eye breaks and reducing screen time (Anshel, 2007; Rosenfield, 2011)

Tech-Induced Anxiety and Pressure to Respond

1. The expectation to be constantly available via digital communication can lead to heightened anxiety (Derks et al., 2016)
2. This "always on" mentality blurs work-life boundaries, contributing to stress and potential burnout (Derks et al., 2016)
3. Setting boundaries, such as designated "no-tech" times, can help manage this anxiety (Derks et al., 2016)

Sleep Disruptions

1. Using technology, especially screens, before bed disrupts sleep patterns due to blue light exposure, which interferes with melatonin production (Exelmans & Van den Bulck, 2016).

2. Poor sleep quality is closely linked to increased stress and a range of health issues (Exelmans & Van den Bulck, 2016).
3. Managing screen time in the evening is critical for improving sleep and reducing stress (Exelmans & Van den Bulck, 2016).

While technology and social media carry with them benefits for communication, education and entertainment, their potential pitfalls, especially related to mental and physical health, cannot be overlooked. The constant connectivity and overwhelming exposure to information, alongside the pervasive influence of social media, have led to increased stress, anxiety and negative self-perception for many individuals, particularly young people. The tragic case of Molly Russell, described earlier, underscores the need for proactive measures to ensure that digital platforms are used safely and responsibly with their potential harms in mind.

Nonetheless, it is believed that these new technologies are not inherently harmful, and it is not the intent of this chapter to "turn back the clock." Like most technologies, the "goodness" of these tools depends on how they are used. When used carefully and intentionally, they can serve as a useful tool for managing stress. The next section will explore how adopting a more intentional relationship with technology can foster balance, promote well-being and help individuals harness the positive aspects of digital tools to reduce stress and improve mental health. By using technology mindfully, we can transform it from a contributor to stress into a part of a thoughtful and holistic strategy to support mental health.

TECHNOLOGY FOR STRESS MANAGEMENT: TOOLS AND BALANCE

To this point, we have explored the numerous ways in which technology and social media can exacerbate stress and negatively impact mental health. These pitfalls underscore the complex relationship we have with our digital devices and online platforms. However, the other side of the coin reveals that when used intentionally and mindfully, technology and social media can also serve as powerful tools to support mental health and well-being. The challenge lies in striking the right balance – leveraging the benefits of technology without falling prey to its potential drawbacks. This section delves into the various digital tools available for stress management and provides strategies for integrating them into a holistic, balanced approach to maintaining mental health.

Digital Tools for Stress Management

The evolution of technology has brought about a myriad of digital tools specifically designed to help individuals manage stress. These tools leverage the power of mobile apps, wearable technology and telehealth services to provide innovative and accessible ways to enhance mental well-being. However, as with any tool, the effectiveness of these technologies depends on how they are used.

Mobile Apps for Mindfulness and Meditation

The popularity of mobile apps designed for mindfulness and meditation has surged in recent years, reflecting a growing awareness of the importance of mental well-being. Popular apps like Headspace and Calm offer guided meditation sessions, breathing exercises and mindfulness practices that are easy to access and incorporate into daily routines. These apps can help users develop a regular mindfulness practice, which has been shown to reduce stress, improve focus and enhance emotional regulation (Huberty et al., 2019; Mani et al., 2015). By making mindfulness more accessible, these apps can empower individuals to take proactive steps toward managing their stress.

Wearable Technology for Monitoring Stress Indicators

Wearable technology, such as fitness trackers and smartwatches, has evolved beyond basic activity tracking to include features that monitor physiological indicators of stress. Devices like the Apple Watch and Fitbit can track metrics such as heart rate variability, sleep patterns and even breathing rates – offering real-time feedback that helps users become more aware of their stress levels. This heightened awareness can prompt users to take immediate action, such as practicing deep breathing or taking a walk, to manage stress before it escalates.

Additionally, with features like workout tracking, wearables can encourage users to engage in movement and exercise. Wearable technology thus can serve as a valuable tool for promoting self-awareness and encouraging healthier lifestyle choices that can promote stress reduction.

Telehealth and Online Therapy

The continued growth of telehealth services, accelerated in part by the COVID-19 pandemic (McKinsey & Company, 2023; Patel et al., 2021), has made mental health services more accessible to individuals who might otherwise face barriers to receiving support. Online therapy platforms can offer convenience and flexibility, allowing individuals to engage in therapy from their homes. Research indicates that online therapy can be as effective as traditional in-person sessions for a wide range of conditions, including anxiety and depression (Barak et al., 2008; Bevan Jones et al., 2023). However, it is important to recognize that telehealth also presents barriers that can be especially impactful on marginalized communities, such as the need for reliable internet access and a device that can connect to the service being used (Barak et al., 2008; McKinsey & Company, 2023).

Balancing Technology Use for Optimal Stress Management

While technology offers numerous tools for managing stress, it is essential to use these tools mindfully. Without careful consideration, the same technologies that help us can also become new sources of stress, leading to digital overload, sleep disturbances and increased anxiety. This section explores strategies for maintaining a healthy balance in technology use, ensuring that digital tools enhance rather than detract from our well-being.

Strategies for Healthy Technology Use

Maintaining a healthy relationship with technology requires intentionality and the implementation of strategies that prevent digital tools from becoming sources of stress. By adopting practices that promote mindful technology use, individuals can enjoy the benefits of these tools without succumbing to their potential pitfalls. Below are some strategies that may be effective in achieving this balance:

1. Digital Detox and Periodic Breaks
   Engaging in regular digital detoxes – periods when one refrains from using screens and digital devices – can help reduce mental fatigue and improve focus. These breaks allow the mind to reset and recover from the constant stimulation of digital environments (Coyne & Woodruff, 2023; Derks et al., 2016).
2. Establishing Technology-Free Zones and Times
   Creating designated areas or times that are free from technology, such as during meals or in the bedroom, can help reinforce boundaries between digital and non-digital life. This practice encourages more mindful engagement with the present moment and the people around you (Alter, 2017; Coyne & Woodruff, 2023; Derks et al., 2016).

3. Mindful Usage Tracking
   Utilizing apps or built-in device features that track screen time can help users become more aware of their technology usage patterns. By monitoring how much time is spent on various apps and activities, individuals can make informed decisions about where to cut back and set limits (Alter, 2017; Bevan Jones et al., 2023; Coyne & Woodruff, 2023).
4. Practicing Digital Minimalism
   Digital minimalism involves intentionally reducing digital clutter by decluttering apps, unsubscribing from unnecessary notifications and focusing only on essential digital interactions. This approach helps minimize distractions and reduce the stress associated with information overload (Newport, 2019).
5. Leveraging "Do Not Disturb" Features
   Using "Do Not Disturb" or similar features during work hours, meetings, or personal time can minimize interruptions and help maintain focus. This strategy helps reduce the stress of constant notifications and the expectation of immediate responses (Coyne & Woodruff, 2023; Stothart et al., 2015).
6. Practicing Intentional App Use
   Prioritizing the use of apps that promote well-being and reduce stress – such as mindfulness apps, fitness trackers or educational tools – can help technology serve as a positive force in one's life. Limiting time spent on apps that contribute to stress, such as social media, can also be beneficial (Bevan Jones et al., 2023; Przybylski et al., 2013).

Integrating Technology into a Stress Management Plan

To fully leverage the potential benefits of technology for stress management, it must be thoughtfully integrated into a holistic, balanced approach (Labrique et al., 2020). While digital tools such as mindfulness apps, wearable technology and other technologies can offer innovative ways to manage stress, they are most effective when combined with more traditional stress management practices, fostering a well-rounded strategy for mental health and well-being.

A key aspect of stress management involves maintaining physical health through regular movement, proper nutrition and restful sleep. Technology can complement these strategies by serving as both a motivator and a monitor. Wearable devices, such as the Apple Watch and Fitbit, can help track physical activity levels, monitor heart rate and provide feedback on sleep quality, giving users data-driven insights into their physical well-being.

Incorporating these tools along with other activities, such as yoga, running or strength training, can contribute toward stress reduction (Fischer et al., 2022; Singh et al., 2023). Additionally, sleep-tracking apps and technologies can help users develop better sleep hygiene practices, which can play a critical role in stress management (Martire et al., 2020).

Importance of Human Connection and Social Support

One of the most important elements of any stress management plan is human connection. Technology should serve as a tool to enhance, not replace, meaningful social interactions. While online communities and social media platforms can offer some degree of support and connection, face-to-face communication often provides a deeper sense of empathy and understanding, which is essential for reducing stress (McClain et al., 2021; Stieger et al., 2023; Wickramaratne et al., 2022). The COVID-19 pandemic highlighted this fact as many people experienced increased stress during periods of prolonged isolation and lockdown (Na et al., 2022; Stieger et al., 2023).

Building strong "in real life" (offline) relationships with friends, family and colleagues can support improved mental health. Technology can help facilitate these relationships – whether through scheduling tools for family gatherings or video calls with loved ones – but cannot be used to substitute for real-world connection. Research consistently shows that having strong social support networks is one of the most powerful buffers against stress, and technology should play a supportive role in cultivating these relationships, rather than replacing them (Cohen & Janicki-Deverts, 2012; Stieger et al., 2023).

Tailoring Technology Use to Individual Needs

Just as no single stress management technique works for everyone, the use of technology in stress management should be personalized to maximize effectiveness. For client-centered healthcare providers, this will of course make sense – but it should serve as a word of caution regarding apps or services that promise to be a "cure all."

For some, daily meditation guided by an app may be a cornerstone of their routine, while others may find the idea of using apps or electronics for meditation to be inherently stressful. Some individuals might find value in regular virtual therapy sessions or connections with peers (Naslund et al., 2016), while others prefer in-person therapy or support groups (Better Help, n.d.; Talkspace, n.d.). Others may prefer to keep technology out of their lives as much as reasonably possible. Recognizing personal preferences and adapting technology use to meet those preferences is essential for creating a balanced, effective plan.

Conclusion

Technology, when used with intention and thoughtfulness, can serve as a powerful tool in managing stress. Digital tools such as mindfulness apps, wearable technology and telehealth services provide innovative ways to reduce stress and improve mental health. However, the key to successfully leveraging these tools lies in mindful usage and finding a balance that supports well-being. By setting boundaries, practicing digital minimalism and integrating these tools into a holistic stress management plan, individuals can avoid the pitfalls of overuse.

Just as we must be cautious of technology's potential to increase stress, we must also embrace its capacity to enhance mental and physical health when used with intention and moderation. Through critical evaluation of their own technology habits, readers can tailor these tools to fit their individual needs and the needs of the people they serve.

SUMMARY

This chapter mapped the double-edged role that technology can play in stress management. It described how constant connectivity, information overload, social comparison, "fear of missing out" (FOMO), cyberbullying, sleep disruption, digital eye strain and blurred work-life boundaries elevate distress and erode occupational balance. It also explored how mindful tools such as meditation apps, wearable devices that track stress indicators and telehealth platforms can support regulation and participation while acknowledging inequities in access. The chapter highlighted practical strategies, including usage tracking, digital detoxes, technology-free zones, do-not-disturb settings and digital minimalism. Through an occupational therapy lens, it emphasized the importance of balancing online and offline roles, fostering in-person connection and aligning technology use with personal values and goals. Technology itself is neither harmful nor helpful – it depends on how it is used. When used thoughtfully with intention and structure, it can move from being a source of stress to a meaningful support for well-being and participation.

DISCUSSION QUESTIONS

1. Reflect on your own technology usage. How does your use of technology contribute to both stress and stress relief? Are there specific strategies mentioned in this chapter that you could implement to create a healthier balance?
2. In healthcare settings, practitioners often face demands to be constantly available via digital tools. How might occupational therapy practitioners manage these expectations while maintaining personal well-being and professional boundaries?
3. The chapter emphasized the importance of tailoring technology use to individual preferences. How might you, as an occupational therapy practitioner, assess a client's comfort level with and interest in technology to help integrate appropriate digital tools into their stress management plans?

REFERENCES

Alter, A. (2017). *Irresistible: The rise of addictive technology and the business of keeping us hooked*. Penguin Press.

American Academy of Child and Adolescent Psychiatry, American Academy of Pediatrics & Children's Hospital Association. (2021, October). A declaration from the American Academy of Child and Adolescent Psychiatry, American Academy of Pediatrics, and the Children's Hospital Association. https://www.aacap.org/App_Themes/AACAP/Docs/press/Declaration_National_Crisis_Oct-2021.pdf

Anshel, J. R. (2007). Visual ergonomics in the workplace. *Workplace Health and Safety Journal*, *55*(10). https://doi.org/10.1177/216507990705501004

Barak, A., Hen, L., Boniel-Nissim, M., & Shapira, N. (2008). A comprehensive review and a meta-analysis of the effectiveness of internet-based psychotherapeutic interventions. *Journal of Technology in Human Services*, *26*(2–4), 109–160. https://doi.org/10.1080/15228830802094429

Bawden, D., & Robinson, L. (2009). The dark side of information: Overload, anxiety, and other paradoxes and pathologies. *Journal of Information Science*, *35*(2), 180–191. https://doi.org/10.1177/0165551508095781

BBC News. (2022). Molly Russell inquest: Online life was 'the bleakest of worlds'. https://www.bbc.com/news/uk-england-london-62981964

BetterHelp. (n.d.). You deserve to be happy. https://www.betterhelp.com

Bevan Jones, R., Hussain, F., Agha, S. S., Weavers, B., Lucassen, M., Merry, S., Stallard, P., Simpson, S. A., & Rice, F. (2023). Digital technologies to support adolescents with depression and anxiety: Review. *BJPsych Advances*, *29*(4), 239–253. https://doi.org/10.1192/bja.2022.3

Beyens, I., Frison, E., & Eggermont, S. (2016). "I don't want to miss a thing": Adolescents' fear of missing out and its relationship to adolescents' social needs, Facebook use, and Facebook-related stress. *Computers in Human Behavior*, *64*, 1–8. https://doi.org/10.1016/j.chb.2016.05.083

Chesley, N. (2005). Blurring boundaries? Linking technology use, spillover, individual distress, and family satisfaction. *Journal of Marriage and Family*, *67*(5), 1237–1248. https://doi.org/10.1111/j.1741-3737.2005.00213.x

Cohen, S., & Janicki-Deverts, D. (2012). Who's stressed? Distributions of psychological stress in the United States in probability samples from 1983, 2006, and 2009. *Journal of Applied Social Psychology*, *42*(6), 1320–1334. https://doi.org/10.1111/j.1559-1816.2012.00900.x

Coyne, P., & Woodruff, S. J. (2023). Taking a break: The effects of partaking in a two-week social media digital detox on problematic smartphone and social media use, and other health-related outcomes among young adults. *Behavioral Sciences*, *13*(12), 1004. https://doi.org/10.3390/bs13121004

DataReportal. (2024). Digital 2024: Global overview report. https://datareportal.com/reports/digital-2024-global-overview-report

Derks, D., Bakker, A. B., Peters, P., & Van Wingerden, P. (2016). Work-related smartphone use, work-family conflict and family role performance: The role of segmentation preference. *Human Relations*, *69*(5), 1045–1068. https://doi.org/10.1177/0018726715601890

Dragano, N., & Lunau, T. (2020). Technostress at work and mental health: Concepts and research results. *Current Opinion in Psychiatry*, *33*(4), 407–413. https://doi.org/10.1097/YCO.0000000000000613

Duxbury, L., & Smart, R. (2011). The "Myth of separate worlds": An exploration of how mobile technology has redefined work-life balance. In S. Kaiser, M. J. Ringlstetter, D. R. Eikhof, & M. Pina E Cunha (Eds.), *Creating balance?* (pp. 269–284). Springer. https://doi.org/10.1007/978-3-642-16199-5_15

Exelmans, L., & Van den Bulck, J. (2016). Bedtime mobile phone use and sleep in adults. *Social Science & Medicine*, *148*, 93–101. https://doi.org/10.1016/j.socscimed.2015.11.037

Fischer, J. M., Kandil, F.-I., Kessler, C. S., Nayeri, L., Zager, L. S., Rocabado Hennhöfer, T., Steckhan, N., Koppold-Liebscher, D. A., Bringmann, H. C., Schäfer, T., Michalsen, A., & Jeitler, M. (2022). Stress reduction by yoga versus mindfulness training in adults suffering from distress: A three-armed randomized controlled trial including qualitative interviews (RELAX Study). *Journal of Clinical Medicine*, *11*(19), 5680. https://doi.org/10.3390/jcm11195680

Frison, E., & Eggermont, S. (2015). The impact of daily stress on adolescents' depressed mood: The role of social support seeking through Facebook. *Computers in Human Behavior*, *44*, 315–325. https://doi.org/10.1016/j.chb.2014.11.070

Gohal, G., Alqassim, A., Eltyeb, E., Rayyani, A., Hakami, B., Al Faqih, A., Hakami, A., Qadri, A., & Mahfouz, M. (2023). Prevalence and related risks of cyberbullying and its effects on adolescent. *BMC Psychiatry*, *23*(1), 39. https://doi.org/10.1186/s12888-023-04542-0

Haidt, J. (2024). *The anxious generation: How the great rewiring of childhood is causing an epidemic of mental illness*. Random House.

Hilbert, M., & López, P. (2011). The world's technological capacity to store, communicate, and compute information. *Science*, *332*(6025), 60–65. https://doi.org/10.1126/science.1200970

Huberty, J., Green, J., Glissmann, C., Larkey, L., Puzia, M., & Lee, C. (2019). Efficacy of the mindfulness meditation mobile app "Calm" to reduce stress among college students: Randomized controlled trial. *JMIR mHealth and uHealth*, *7*(6), e14273. https://doi.org/10.2196/14273

Kanchan, S., & Gaidhane, A. (2023). Social media role and its impact on public health: A narrative review. *Cureus*, *15*(1), e33737. https://doi.org/10.7759/cureus.33737

Kowalski, R. M., Giumetti, G. W., Schroeder, A. N., & Lattanner, M. R. (2014). Bullying in the digital age: A critical review and meta-analysis of cyberbullying research among youth. *Psychological Bulletin*, *140*(4), 1073–1137. https://doi.org/10.1037/a0035618

Kuss, D. J., & Griffiths, M. D. (2017). Social networking sites and addiction: Ten lessons learned. *International Journal of Environmental Research and Public Health, 14*(3), 311. https://doi.org/10.3390/ijerph14030311

Labrique, A., Agarwal, S., Tamrat, T., & Mehl, G. (2020). WHO digital health guidelines: A milestone for global health. *npj Digital Medicine*, *3*(1), 120. https://doi.org/10.1038/s41746-020-00330-2

Lup, K., Trub, L., & Rosenthal, L. (2015). Instagram #Instasad?: Exploring associations among Instagram use, depressive symptoms, negative social comparison, and strangers followed. *Cyberpsychology, Behavior, and Social Networking*, *18*(5), 247–252. https://doi.org/10.1089/cyber.2014.0560

Mani, M., Kavanagh, D. J., Hides, L., & Stoyanov, S. R. (2015). Review and evaluation of mindfulness-based iPhone apps. *JMIR mHealth and uHealth*, *3*(3), e82. https://doi.org/10.2196/mhealth.4328

Martire, V. L., Caruso, D., Palagini, L., Zoccoli, G., & Bastianini, S. (2020). Stress & sleep: A relationship lasting a lifetime. *Neuroscience & Biobehavioral Reviews*, *117*, 65–77. https://doi.org/10.1016/j.neubiorev.2019.08.024

Maurya, C., Muhammad, T., Dhillon, P., & Maurya, P. (2022). The effects of cyberbullying victimization on depression and suicidal ideation among adolescents and young adults: A three year cohort study from India. *BMC Psychiatry*, *22*(1), 599. https://doi.org/10.1186/s12888-022-04238-x

McClain, C., Vogels, E. A., Perrin, A., Sechopoulos, S., & Rainie, L. (2021). *The internet and the pandemic*. Pew Research Center. https://www.pewresearch.org/internet/2021/09/01/the-internet-and-the-pandemic/

McKinsey & Company. (2023). Telehealth: A post-COVID-19 reality? https://www.mckinsey.com/industries/healthcare/our-insights/telehealth-a-quarter-trillion-dollar-post-covid-19-reality

Na, L., Yang, L., Mezo, P. G., & Liu, R. (2022). Age disparities in mental health during the COVID-19 pandemic: The roles of resilience and coping. *Social Science & Medicine*, *305*, 115031. https://doi.org/10.1016/j.socscimed.2022.115031

Naslund, J. A., Aschbrenner, K. A., Marsch, L. A., & Bartels, S. J. (2016). The future of mental health care: Peer-to-peer support and social media. *Epidemiology and Psychiatric Sciences*, *25*(2), 113–122. https://doi.org/10.1017/S2045796015001067

Nesi, J. (2020). The impact of social media on youth mental health: Challenges and opportunities. *North Carolina Medical Journal*, *81*(2), 116–121. https://doi.org/10.18043/ncm.81.2.116

Newport, C. (2019). *Digital minimalism: Choosing a focused life in a noisy world*. Penguin Publishing Group.

Owen, N., Healy, G. N., Matthews, C. E., & Dunstan, D. W. (2010). Too much sitting: The population health science of sedentary behavior. *Exercise and Sport Sciences Reviews*, *38*(3), 105–113. https://doi.org/10.1097/JES.0b013e3181e373a2

Patel, S. Y., Mehrotra, A., Huskamp, H. A., Uscher-Pines, L., Ganguli, I., & Barnett, M. L. (2021). Trends in outpatient care delivery and telemedicine during the COVID-19 pandemic in the US. *JAMA Internal Medicine*, *181*(3), 388–391. https://doi.org/10.1001/jamainternmed.2020.5928

Przybylski, A. K., Murayama, K., DeHaan, C. R., & Gladwell, V. (2013). Motivational, emotional, and behavioral correlates of fear of missing out. *Computers in Human Behavior*, *29*(4), 1841–1848. https://doi.org/10.1016/j.chb.2013.02.014

Rosen, L. D., Lim, A. F., Felt, J., Carrier, L. M., Cheever, N. A., Lara-Ruiz, J. M., Mendoza, J. S., & Rokkum, J. (2014). Media and technology use predicts ill-being among children, preteens and teenagers independent of the negative health impacts of exercise and eating habits. *Computers in Human Behavior*, *35*, 364–375. https://doi.org/10.1016/j.chb.2014.01.036

Rosenfield, M. (2011). Computer vision syndrome: A review of ocular causes and potential treatments. *Ophthalmic and Physiological Optics*, *31*(5), 502–515. https://doi.org/10.1111/j.1475-1313.2011.00834.x

Seabrook, E. M., Kern, M. L., & Rickard, N. S. (2016). Social networking sites, depression, and anxiety: A systematic review. *JMIR Mental Health*, *3*(4), e50. https://doi.org/10.2196/mental.5842

Singh, B., Olds, T., Curtis, R., Dumuid, D., Virgara, R., Watson, A., Szeto, K., O'Connor, E., Ferguson, T., Eglitis, E., Miatke, A., Simpson, C. E., & Maher, C. (2023). Effectiveness of physical activity interventions for improving depression, anxiety and distress: An overview of systematic reviews. *British Journal of Sports Medicine*, *57*(18), 1203–1209. https://doi.org/10.1136/bjsports-2022-106195

Song, K., Zhou, F.-J., Niu, G.-F., Fan, C.-Y., & Zhou, Z.-K. (2024). The association between cyberbullying victimization and depression among children: A moderated mediation model. *Behavioral Sciences*, *14*(5), 414. https://doi.org/10.3390/bs14050414

Stieger, S., Lewetz, D., & Willinger, D. (2023). Face-to-face more important than digital communication for mental health during the pandemic. *Scientific Reports*, *13*(1), 8022. https://doi.org/10.1038/s41598-023-34957-4

Stothart, C., Mitchum, A., & Yehnert, C. (2015). The attentional cost of receiving a cell phone notification. *Journal of Experimental Psychology: Human Perception and Performance*, *41*(4), 893–897. https://doi.org/10.1037/xhp0000100

Talkspace. (n.d.). Space to figure things out. https://www.talkspace.com

Vogel, E., Rose, J., Roberts, L., & Eckles, K. (2014). Social comparison, social media, and self-esteem. *Psychology of Popular Media Culture*, *3*, 206–222. https://doi.org/10.1037/ppm0000047

Warburton, D. E. R., & Bredin, S. S. D. (2017). Health benefits of physical activity: A systematic review of current systematic reviews. *Current Opinion in Cardiology*, *32*(5), 541–556. https://doi.org/10.1097/HCO.0000000000000437

Wickramaratne, P. J., Yangchen, T., Lepow, L., Patra, B. G., Glicksburg, B., Talati, A., Adekkanattu, P., Ryu, E., Biernacka, J. M., Charney, A., Mann, J. J., Pathak, J., Olfson, M., & Weissman, M. M. (2022). Social connectedness as a determinant of mental health: A scoping review. *PLOS One*, *17*(10), e0275004. https://doi.org/10.1371/journal.pone.0275004

Chapter 5

The Stress Management Questionnaire

LEARNING OBJECTIVES

By the end of this chapter, the reader will be able to

1. Discuss the significant factors in measuring a stress management assessment tool.
2. Administer the group version of the Stress Management Questionnaire (SMQ).
3. Identify the major symptoms triggered by stress, the stressors that trigger symptoms and the coping activities that an individual uses in managing stress.
4. Plan with an individual a stress management program based on the individual's unique profile of symptoms, stressors and coping activities.

INTRODUCTION

How can we best assess the impact of distress on an individual and the benefits of a stress management intervention program or strategy? Occupational therapists apply a pragmatic approach when working with individuals with disabilities. One of the primary goals of a stress management program is to help the individual to reduce or alleviate distress. As Cotton (1990) reported, important constructs to measure are "(1) stressors, including major life events, hassles, and appraisals: (2) the stress reaction, including cognitive, behavioral and physiological responses, and (3) personal characteristics of the client, including personal resources (strengths and weaknesses), behavior patterns, and coping styles" (p. 80). Assessment of the

DOI: 10.4324/9781003671084-5

symptoms, stressors and coping activities can help the occupational therapist to design a stress management program that is personalized to the individual's needs. In creating the Stress Management Questionnaire (SMQ), best practice for developing a reliable and valid assessment was considered (Rice et al., 2025). The following questions guided the development of and the research on the SMQ:

1. What are the purposes of the assessment?
   Can the assessment help in identifying symptoms that occur when an individual is stressed? What are the stressors in a person's life that trigger symptoms? How does the individual respond to stress? Can the assessment help in identifying positive coping strategies to effectively prevent symptoms from occurring? Does the assessment identify specific methods and strategies that the individual has used in the past to manage stress?
2. What is the reliability and validity of the assessment?
   Are there published studies to confirm that the assessment is reliable (the extent to which the test gives consistent results when administered by different testers on different occasions). Test-retest reliability is usually measured by correlation statistics. Test validity represents the ability of a test to measure what it is designed to measure, such as the type of stressors that cause discomfort (death in the family, financial crisis).
3. How is the test administered?
   Is there a standardized procedure for administering the test? Can the test be administered via pencil and paper? Can the test be taken on a computer? Is the test administered on a one-to-one basis or to a group?
4. How long will the test take for the average individual to complete?
5. Must the test be administered in a private area?
6. How can the results of the test be scored, evaluated and used in planning an intervention program or assessing the effectiveness of a stress management program?
7. What skills does the occupational therapist need for administering, scoring, evaluating and reporting test results to an individual? Reporting results to colleagues?
8. How can the test be purchased? Is it available through a publisher or free in the public domain? Was it published in a journal article?

STRESS MANAGEMENT QUESTIONNAIRE (SEE APPENDIX FOR THE PAPER AND PENCIL VERSION)

The Stress Management Questionnaire (SMQ) was developed by the first author as a tool that occupational therapists can use in helping an individual to self-regulate symptoms, identify stressors in one's everyday life and incorporate coping activities that have been beneficial in everyday living (Stein & Cutler, 2002, pp. 426–430). The SMQ is based on an occupational model where meaningful and purposeful activities are identified as coping activities used in stress management. The SMQ is the result of the first author's research on stress beginning when the author was a professor of occupational therapy at the University of Wisconsin-Milwaukee (UW-M) during the 1980s and 1990s. The author's background experience as an occupational therapist at the New York State Psychiatric Institute and the Brooklyn Day Hospital showed how distress contributed to precipitating symptoms and episodes of mental illness in individuals who had been hospitalized. At that time stress was not identified as a precipitator or "trigger" of psychiatric symptoms.

After receiving a doctorate in counseling psychology, the author used his clinical background as an occupational therapist, combining it with knowledge of psychological theory, research and statistics. Later as a professor of occupational therapy at Boston University, he was also a consultant to a residential treatment program for disadvantaged youth, where he began to gain insight on how distress can "trigger" antisocial behavior such as drug addiction and criminal activity in adolescents who came from families in crisis (father missing, mother not able to effectively parent; Stein, 1972).

The SMQ is based on the physiological principle that when an individual is under distress the body reacts by increasing cardiac and respiratory function, and when the organism is resting or relaxed, the parasympathetic branch slows down the physiological responses (Yaribeygi et al., 2017). If the stressful state is prolonged or intense, it can lead to (1) cognitive symptoms, such as impaired thinking, remembering and concentrating; (2) physiological symptoms, such as headaches, rapid heart rate and stomach pain; (3) emotional symptoms, such as anxiety, anger and panic; and (4) behavioral symptoms, such as insomnia, smoking and problems relating to people. These four construct areas were the basis for categorizing responses to the question, "what symptoms do you have when you are stressful?" The researcher found that symptoms were individual and could be mild, moderate or severe. One way for the individual to quantify the symptoms was to rank order the symptoms: 1, most severe to 10, mildest.

The next part of the SMQ was to identify the stressors in the individual's daily life. These can be considered the hassles of daily life. Holmes and Rahe (1967) initially developed the Social Readjustment Rating Scale that listed 43 life events that cause stressful reactions, starting with death of a spouse, divorce, imprisonment and health problems, to minor stresses such as holidays and vacation. Each one of the stressors was given a weighted score where death of a spouse was assigned 100 points and moving residence was assigned 20 points. Holmes and Rahe assumed that these stressors were fixed and individuals who had a high number of points would be experiencing severe stress. The limitation of the Social Readjustment Rating Scale is that stressors could affect individuals differently. A high stressor for one person may not have equal weight for another person. Holmes and Rahe did not consider that some individuals can withstand severe stress (an indication of hardiness). In contrast, the SMQ assumes that stressors are experienced individually and only the individual can weigh the impact of stressors on one's life. Dohrenwend and Dohrenwend (1981), expanding upon the work of Holmes and Rahe, also found that major life events could cause major stress reactions and prolonged physical and psychological symptoms. The debate among researchers in measuring stress regarding critical life events versus daily hassles as the major precipitators of stressful reactions was analyzed by Kanner et al. (1981). The SMQ follows in the tradition of measuring the daily stressors of life rather than examining major life events. The SMQ measures everyday events involving arguments with spouses or co-workers, driving in heavy traffic or being late for an appointment. These daily stressors were compiled by asking a large group of people what everyday situations or thoughts caused them distress.

The final version of the questionnaire has three sections, listing symptoms, stressors and coping activities. The questionnaire usually takes 20–45 minutes to complete. Individuals are asked to check yes or no to a list of symptoms and problems resulting from stress, everyday stressors that precipitate the stress response and the coping activities they use to manage or reduce stress. They are then asked to list and rank in order each symptom, stressor and coper that they have identified. The SMQ consists of 73 items describing symptoms, 37 items describing stressors and 48 items describing copers. There is also space for individuals to list other items in each of the three categories.

DEVELOPMENT OF AND RESEARCH ON THE SMQ

The first research study of the SMQ was conducted with the assistance of occupational therapy students at the University of Wisconsin-Milwaukee in 1986. Data on the SMQ was collected from 113 individuals in a first pilot study and 639 individuals in a second study.

Open-ended questions related to (1) what symptoms do you experience when you are stressful? (2) what are the stressors in your life that trigger symptoms of stress? and (3) what are the coping activities that you have used in the past to alleviate or control your stress? From the responses, the author generated lists of items that were most identified by the respondents. Further research on the SMQ was conducted (Stein, 1986, 1987, 2003, 2020; Stein et al., 1999, 2003).

The SMQ was applied in three clinical research studies: Stein and Neville (1987), Stein and Nikolic (1989) and Stein and Smith (1989). In the studies, the SMQ was used to establish the extent and nature of improved stress responses and lowered stress levels following relaxation and biofeedback therapy. The SMQ has also been used to measure stress in teachers (Austin et al., 2005). In general, the SMQ provides a personal stress profile which helps the individual to identify stressors and to reduce resultant symptoms by incorporating individual copers into one's everyday life. It is envisaged that the SMQ has wide potential for self-monitoring and regulating symptoms, stressors and "copers" as part of a holistic stress management program. It can serve as a comprehensive interactive measuring instrument for guided self-understanding and healthy lifestyle planning such as in health promotion and disease prevention programs in school and work environments. The first set of descriptor choices focuses on the feelings or problems that are a result of stress. The symptoms and problems resulting from stress were generated from four factors:

1. Physiological: such as headaches, tremors, neck/low back pain;
2. Cognitive: such as difficulty concentrating, remembering, decision-making;
3. Emotional: such as feeling angry, hopeless, tense and sad;
4. Behavioral: such as difficulty sleeping, eating and speaking.

The second set of descriptor choices on the SMQ identifies situations that cause a stress response or symptoms. These potential stressors include family arguments, criticism, encountering bureaucratic "red tape" and driving in heavy traffic. Stressors are those aspects in the environment that increase demands on the individual and tend to increase stress. The stress-inducing occurrences of daily events parallel major life changes in their potential to produce stress. The Survey of Recent Life Experiences (SLRE) is a measure that comprises a list of experiences to measure how much everyday stressors affect physical and mental health (Kohn & Macdonald, 1992). The 51-item scale of the SLRE incorporates four levels of intensity of the stress experience, from not-at-all, only slightly, moderately, to very much. The SMQ includes a range of daily hassles under the stressors heading that is related to the SLRE. Everyday stressors precipitating stress reactions were grouped under nine factors:

1. Interpersonal, such as arguments with family members;
2. Intrapersonal, such as low self-esteem;

3. Time demands, such as meeting a deadline at work;
4. Mechanical breakdown, such as dealing with a broken household appliance;
5. Performance, such as taking a test;
6. Financial pressures, such as loss of income;
7. Illness, such as having the flu;
8. Environmental disturbance, such as excessive noise;
9. Complex situations, such as raising a child alone.

The third section of the SMQ lists coping activities such as exercise, listening to music and talking to a friend. Interactional theories emphasize the mediating role of coping and adaptive mechanisms in determining the effect of stressors on the individual (Stein et al., 1999). A related scale, the Health Promotion Lifestyle Profile (Walker et al., 1987; Walker & Hill-Polerecky, 1996), incorporates six areas as indicators of positive coping: spiritual growth, interpersonal relations, nutrition, physical activity, health responsibility and stress management. The SMQ, based on an occupational therapy framework, includes eight activity "copers" that manage or reduce stress:

1. Creative, such as writing a poem;
2. Construction, such as knitting a sweater;
3. Exercise, such as walking;
4. Appreciation, such as listening to music;
5. Self-care, such as taking a bath;
6. Social, such as talking to friends;
7. Plant and animal care, such as having a pet;
8. Performance, such as singing in a choir;
9. Sports, such as swimming.

A final section of the questionnaire asks for demographic information and poses questions concerning the experience of completing the questionnaire, such as:

1. Was the questionnaire too long?
2. Were the directions clear?
3. Did the questionnaire accurately reflect your feelings?
4. Did the questionnaire help you to become more aware of the stressors in your everyday life?
5. Did you identify from the questionnaire any new methods to manage stress?
6. Do you feel you would benefit from an individualized stress management program?

The SMQ can be used clinically to help the occupational therapist in alliance with the client or patient to develop an individualized stress management program or as a qualitative outcome measure to evaluate the patient's improvement in managing stress.

SORTING OUT STRESS CARDS (SOS)

A shortened card version of the SMQ was developed by the first author and graduate students at the University of South Dakota during 1998–2002 (Stein et al., 2003). The card version is intended to be used in a clinical setting in a face-to-face interview with the client. By decreasing the time to complete the SMQ, the therapist will be able to obtain results quickly without compromising the validity or reliability of the SMQ. It takes about ten minutes to complete the card version of the SMQ, compared to 20 to 45 minutes to complete the original version. SOS Cards consist of 52 descriptor items as compared to the 158 items in the paper and pencil test. In the card version the participant is asked to sort through three packets of cards: a symptoms packet, a stressor packet and a copers packet. Participants place the individual descriptors that pertain to themselves into a yes, no or maybe pile. Participants are then asked to rank order their top five responses in the yes pile, with first place being the most troublesome.

A reliability and validity study was completed in 2001–2002 (Stein et al., 2003) and the results indicated that the card version is a highly valid and reliable instrument as compared to the long version of the SMQ. Items were selected from the symptoms, stressors and copers based on their frequency as analyzed in previous research studies and in the results from the 2001–2002 study. Eighty participants equally distributed between age categories 18–24, 22–44, 45–64 and 65+ were individually administered the SOS Cards. Twenty participants, five from each category, were then randomly selected, and each was administered a retest of the SOS Cards about two weeks following initial testing. Reliability coefficients ranged from.57 to.77 (Stein et al., 2003).

THE COMPUTERIZED VERSION OF THE SMQ

Natz (1995) developed a computerized version of the SMQ with printed reports of the test results and a client database of scores obtained. Once the software was written, the investigator compared the results of the Stress Management Questionnaire in a paper and pencil form with the computerized version. The study was conducted over a three-week period. Following screening, each subject was given a written form of the SMQ in the first test session. Eight students at the University of South Dakota participated in the study. One week later the computerized version of the questionnaire was given. A second paper and pencil version of the questionnaire was given to each subject at least one week after the computer version. In all cases the retest was taken at least one week after the previous test.

The computer version of the SMQ was administered on IBM PS/2 model 30's with color displays; a keyboard and mouse were used for input. Each mouse click was recorded with a date and time stamp. This allowed for the analysis of time spent per question and total time of the test. Individual appointments were made with subjects, and following instructions on the use of the computer, subjects were allowed to work independently in the occupational therapy department at the university.

The computerized SMQ provided subjects with a list of symptoms, stressors or coping activities and asked the subject to indicate whether items in the list apply (selection items). Upon completion of each of these sections, the subject was asked to choose and rank items from 1 to 10. If an item was selected or ranked in the first paper session and was selected again when a subject completed the computerized form, this was counted as a match.

The Stress Management Questionnaire: An Instrument for Self-regulating Stress (Stein et al., 2003) was published by Thomson Delmar Learning. This publication consisted of the paper and pencil test, SOS Cards and the computerized version on a CD-ROM. The publication is currently out of print, and an updated revision is being prepared.

STRATEGIES TO IMPLEMENT A STRESS MANAGEMENT PROGRAM BASED ON THE SMQ

The results of the SMQ can be used to develop an intervention program that uses the client's identification of symptoms, stressors and "copers."

For example, if a client lists headaches as the primary symptom of stress, then the occupational therapist can use this symptom as a baseline measure of progress. The goal would be to help the client to identify and try to eliminate or lessen those situations, which are stressors such as arguments with a spouse. The identified "copers" can be used to self-regulate the stress encountered. For example, if the client has found that classical music is calming, then the individual can schedule a time each day to listen to relaxing classical music. The occupational therapist and client can identify activities such as relaxation therapy, prescriptive exercise, tai chi, yoga, breathing, creative arts, music, meditation and visualization that can be used to self-regulate stress. The teaching of management of stress by an occupational therapist helps clients incorporate the selected stress management techniques into their everyday lives.

The general principles of stress management for a client to self-regulate stress are

1. Incorporate the "coper" into your everyday schedule as a personal habit, such as brushing your teeth.
2. Try to engage in the coping activity daily at a convenient time, such as right before breakfast, as an afternoon break or before dinner.
3. Keep a daily log of stress management activities and "copers" and how they affect your symptoms, mood, energy level and productivity.
4. Be realistic in setting up a schedule that is relevant, appropriate and attainable.
5. Do meditation and aerobic exercises in increments, starting out for five or ten minutes and working up to a half hour. For example, in walking, which is an excellent "coper" for many individuals, start out with a 15-minute relaxing walk and increase the walk to 30 minutes.
6. Monitor the impact of each "coper" in reducing stress, anxiety, depressive feelings and self-esteem.
7. Try to establish a quiet, unobtrusive environment for carrying out relaxation exercises or meditation.

SUMMARY

The Stress Management Questionnaire (SMQ) was developed as a tool for occupational therapists to help individuals self-regulate symptoms, identify stressors and select coping activities. Based on an occupational model, the SMQ emphasizes the use of meaningful and purposeful activities as strategies for managing stress.

The SMQ is a comprehensive, evidence-based assessment instrument designed to evaluate an individual's skills in managing stress. It aligns with a holistic, positive health framework by assessing stress-related responses across physical, behavioral, emotional and cognitive domains, while also considering personal characteristics and environmental influences.

Research has demonstrated that the SMQ possesses strong psychometric properties, including reliability and validity, supporting its use across diverse contexts. Occupational therapists can employ the SMQ to develop individualized intervention programs, measure pre- and post-intervention progress and conduct research on stress management.

Applicable in clinical, educational and organizational settings, the SMQ assists practitioners in evaluating stress-related issues, designing effective interventions and tracking outcomes. The SMQ integrates clinical research with practical application, offering a multidimensional approach to stress assessment and management.

DISCUSSION QUESTIONS

1. What are the components of a reliable and valid assessment instrument?
2. What are the main individual factors that are measured by the Stress Management Questionnaire?
3. How can the Stress Management Questionnaire foster hardiness in the individual's unique strategies for coping with stress?
4. How can occupational therapists incorporate the Stress Management Questionnaire in a holistic clinical practice?

REFERENCES

Austin, V., Shah, S., & Muncer, S. (2005). Teacher stress and coping strategies used to reduce stress. *Occupational Therapy International, 12*(2), 63–80. https://doi.org/10.1002/oti.16

Cotton, D. (1990). *Stress management: An integrated approach to therapy*. Brunner/Mazel.

Dohrenwend, B. P., & Dohrenwend, B. S. (1981). Socioenvironmental factors, stress, and psychopathology. *American Journal of Community Psychology*, 9(2), 128–164. https://doi.org/10.1007/BF00896364

Holmes, T. H., & Rahe, R. H. (1967). The social readjustment rating scale. *Journal of Psychosomatic Research, 11*, 213–218. https://doi.org/10.1016/0022-3999(67)90010-4

Kanner, A. D., Coyne, J. C., Schaefer, C. & Lazarus, R. S. (1981). Comparison of two modes of stress measurement: Daily hassles and uplifts versus major life events. *Journal of Behavioral Medicine, 4*, 1–39. https://doi.org/10.1007/BF00844845

Kohn, P. M., & MacDonald, J. E. (1992). The survey of recent life experiences: A decontaminated hassles scale for adults. *Journal of Behavioral Medicine, 15*, 221–236. https://doi.org/10.1007/BF00848327

Natz, M. (1995). *Comparing computer based and traditional versions of the Stress Management Questionnaire in a general population sample*. Unpublished Master's thesis, University of South Dakota at Vermillion.

Rice, M. S., Tomlin, G., & Stein, F. (2025). *Stein's research in occupational therapy* (7th ed., Chapter 11, pp. 165–188). Routledge. https://doi.org/10.4324/9781003523154

Stein, F. (1972). Community rehabilitation of disadvantaged youth. *American Journal of Occupational Therapy, 26*(6), 227–283. [no doi].

Stein, F. (1986). *Reliability and validity of the Stress Management Questionnaire*. Unpublished manuscript, University of Wisconsin-Milwaukee.

Stein, F. (1987). Stress and schizophrenia. *Alberta Psychology, 16*, 10–11. [no doi].

Stein, F. (2020). Stress Management Questionnaire. In B. J. Hemphill & C. K. Urish (Eds.), *Assessment in occupational therapy mental health: An integrative approach* (pp. 537–546). SLACK.

Stein, F., Bentley, D., & Natz, M. (1999). Computerized assessment: The Stress Management Questionnaire. In B. J. Hemphill (Ed.), *Assessment in occupational therapy mental health: An integrative approach* (pp. 301–317). SLACK.

Stein, F., & Cutler, S. (2002). *Psychosocial occupational therapy: A holistic approach* (2nd ed.). Singular Publishing Group.

Stein, F., Grueschow, D., Hoffman, M., Taylor, S., & Tronback, R. (2003). The Sorting Out Stress Cards- A version of the SMQ: A reliability study. *Occupational Therapy in Mental Health, 19*, 41–59. https://doi.org/10.1300/J004v19n01_03

Stein, F., & Neville, S. A. (1987). *Biofeedback, locus of control, and reduction of anxiety in alcohol dependent adults*. Unpublished manuscript, University of Wisconsin-Milwaukee.

Stein, F., & Nikolic, S. (1989). Teaching stress management techniques to a schizophrenic patient. *American Journal of Occupational Therapy, 43*, 162–169. https://doi.org/10.5014/ajot.43.3.162

Stein, F, & Smith, J. (1989). Short -term stress management programme with acutely depressed in-patients. *Canadian Journal of Occupational Therapy, 56*, 185–192. https://doi.org/10.1177/000841748905600407

Walker, S. N., & Hill-Polerecky, D. M. (1996). *Psychometric evaluation of the Health-Promoting Lifestyle Profile II.* Unpublished manuscript, University of Nebraska Medical Center.

Walker, S. N., Sechrist, K. R., & Pender, N. J. (1987). The health-promoting lifestyle profile: Development and psychometric characteristics. *Nursing Research, 36*(2), 76–81. [no doi].

Yaribeygi, H., Panahi, Y., Sahraei, H., Johnston, T. P., & Sahebkar, A. (2017). The impact of stress on body function: A review. *EXCLI Journal, 16*, 1057–1072. https://doi.org/10.17179/excli2017-480

Chapter 6

Other Stress Assessment Tools

LEARNING OBJECTIVES

By the end of this chapter, the reader will be able to

1. Identify and describe the major stress assessment instruments available to occupational therapists and healthcare professionals beyond the Stress Management Questionnaire (SMQ).
2. Compare and contrast the psychometric properties, administration procedures and clinical applications of various stress assessment tools.
3. Select appropriate assessment instruments based on specific clinical populations, practice settings and therapeutic objectives.
4. Integrate multiple assessment approaches to develop comprehensive stress profiles for individuals and groups.
5. Evaluate the cultural considerations and limitations of standardized stress assessment tools.
6. Apply evidence-based assessment protocols to inform stress management intervention planning and outcome measurement.

INTRODUCTION

Building upon the foundation established in Chapter 5 with the *Stress Management Questionnaire* (SMQ), this chapter expands the assessment toolkit available to occupational therapists and allied health professionals working with individuals experiencing stress-related difficulties. Over the past 50 years, numerous assessment tools have been developed to evaluate the multifaceted effects of

DOI: 10.4324/9781003671084-6

distress on psychological and physiological functioning (Frisone et al., 2021). These instruments serve as essential components in comprehensive stress assessment protocols, providing complementary perspectives that enhance clinical decision-making and intervention planning.

The assessment tools described in this chapter have been developed primarily by psychologists and health researchers to assist practitioners in gaining deeper insight into how individuals perceive, experience and respond to stressful situations (Dorsey et al., 2022). Dorsey et al. (2022) noted that it was important to use both self-reports and biomarkers to measure the three aspects of stressors, psychobiological markers, and the length of time the individual was exposed to the stressors and the stress reaction. While the SMQ provides a unique occupational therapy perspective by emphasizing the role of meaningful activities in stress management (Stein, 1986), these additional instruments offer standardized approaches to measuring specific dimensions of stress, anxiety, depression and coping responses that are crucial for evidence-based practice.

As occupational therapists increasingly work within interprofessional teams and evidence-based practice frameworks, familiarity with these widely used assessment tools becomes essential for effective communication, research participation and outcome measurement. The instruments presented in this chapter complement the holistic, occupation-focused approach of the SMQ while providing opportunities for comparison with established norms and research findings across diverse populations and clinical settings.

GENERAL STRESS ASSESSMENT INSTRUMENTS

Perceived Stress Scale (PSS)

The Perceived Stress Scale (PSS) was developed by Cohen et al. (1983) as a global measure of perceived stress that assesses the degree to which individuals appraise their lives as unpredictable, uncontrollable and overloading. The PSS represents a significant advancement in stress measurement by focusing on subjective appraisal processes rather than objective stressful events, aligning with the transactional model of stress and coping proposed by Lazarus and Folkman (1984).

Psychometric Properties. The PSS demonstrates strong psychometric properties across diverse populations. Lee (2012) conducted a comprehensive systematic review of 19 studies evaluating the PSS and found that the 10-item version (PSS-10) consistently outperformed both the 14-item and 4-item versions across all psychometric domains. Test-retest reliability coefficients typically range from 0.85 to 0.75 over short periods, with acceptable stability over longer timeframes (Cohen, 1986; Harris et al., 2023). Internal consistency has been reported as excellent across multiple cultural contexts, with Cronbach's alpha values ranging from 0.78 to 0.91 in various international samples (Andreou et al., 2011; Klein et al., 2016; Mozumder, 2022).

Recent cross-cultural validation studies have demonstrated the instrument's reliability across diverse populations. Baik et al. (2019) established measurement equivalence between English and Spanish versions among Hispanic Americans, while studies in Russian adolescents (Prokopovich et al., 2024), German adults (Klein et al., 2016) and Ethiopian university students (Ayele et al., 2019) have confirmed the instrument's cross-cultural validity. Factor analysis studies consistently support either a unidimensional structure or a two-factor model comprising perceived helplessness and perceived self-efficacy components (Prokopovich et al., 2024; Taylor, 2015).

Administration and Scoring: Available in 14-item, 10-item, and 4-item versions, the PSS uses a 5-point Likert scale ranging from 0 (never) to 4 (very often). Respondents indicate how frequently they have experienced specific thoughts and feelings during the past month. The 10-item version is most commonly used in clinical practice due to its superior psychometric properties and balance between comprehensiveness and brevity (Lee, 2012). Total scores range from 0 to 40, with higher scores indicating greater perceived stress. Normative data are available for multiple populations, including community samples from the United States (Cohen & Janicki-Deverts, 2012), Germany (Klein et al., 2016) and Bangladesh (Mozumder, 2022).

Clinical Applications: The PSS is particularly valuable for screening purposes and tracking changes in stress perception over time. Its brief administration time of three–five minutes makes it suitable for repeated assessments in intervention studies (Kechter et al., 2019). Harris et al. (2023) demonstrated that approximately half of the variance in PSS scores represents stable between-person differences, indicating the instrument captures both chronic stress patterns and acute stress responses. The scale's focus on cognitive appraisal processes makes it especially relevant for cognitive-behavioral interventions and stress management programs targeting perception and coping strategies.

Holmes and Rahe Social Readjustment Rating Scale (SRRS)

Originally developed by Holmes and Rahe in 1967, the Social Readjustment Rating Scale represents one of the earliest systematic attempts to quantify life stress through the measurement of major life events. The original scale identified 43 life events and assigned each a Life Change Unit (LCU) value based on the relative amount of adjustment required, with "death of spouse" receiving the highest rating of 100 LCU.

Contemporary Relevance. Wallace et al. (2023) recently conducted a comprehensive update and modernization of the SRRS to reflect contemporary social realities while maintaining its core theoretical foundation. The updated version addresses technological changes, evolving social structures and modern stressors that were not present in the original 1967 version. This modernization included extensive validation with contemporary samples and factor analysis confirming the continued relevance of the life events approach to stress measurement.

Strengths and Limitations. While the SRRS provides valuable information about cumulative life stress exposure and has demonstrated predictive validity for various health outcomes (Holmes & Rahe, 1967), it has important limitations that must be considered in clinical applications. The scale assumes that all individuals respond similarly to the same events and does not account for individual differences in appraisal, coping resources or cultural background (Kanner et al., 1981). Additionally, the original scale does not distinguish between positive and negative event valence, potentially overlooking the differential impact of chosen versus imposed life changes.

Clinical Utility. The SRRS remains valuable for identifying individuals who may be at elevated risk for stress-related health problems due to high levels of recent life change. Research has consistently demonstrated correlations between high SRRS scores and increased susceptibility to physical illness, psychological distress and performance decrements (Holmes & Rahe, 1967; Wallace et al., 2023). The scale provides useful context for understanding current stress responses and can inform the timing and intensity of interventions, particularly when used in conjunction with measures of current stress perception and coping resources.

Mental Health and Symptom-Specific Assessments

Hospital Anxiety and Depression Scale (HADS)

The Hospital Anxiety and Depression Scale (Zigmond & Snaith, 1983) was specifically designed to detect anxiety and depression in medical settings while avoiding somatic symptoms that might be confounded with physical illness. This design consideration makes it particularly valuable for occupational therapists working in medical settings or with individuals experiencing chronic health conditions where traditional depression scales might yield false positives due to physical symptoms.

Scale Structure and Development. The HADS consists of 14 items divided into two 7-item subscales measuring anxiety (HADS-A) and depression (HADS-D). Items are rated on a 4-point scale ranging from 0 to 3, with subscale scores ranging from 0 to 21. Cut-off scores of 8 or above on either subscale indicate probable clinical significance, while scores of 11 or above suggest definite cases requiring clinical attention (Zigmond & Snaith, 1983). The developers deliberately excluded somatic symptoms to enhance the scale's utility in medical populations where physical symptoms might confound traditional depression measures.

Psychometric Properties. Extensive international research has confirmed the HADS' robust psychometric properties across diverse populations and settings. Bjelland et al. (2002) conducted a comprehensive review of validation studies and found consistent evidence for good internal consistency, with Cronbach's alpha values typically ranging from 0.82 to 0.90 for both subscales. Factor analysis studies consistently support the two-factor structure, though some studies have identified method effects and suggested minor modifications to optimize factor structure (Helvik et al., 2017; Norton et al., 2018).

Cross-cultural validation studies have demonstrated the HADS' effectiveness across diverse populations. Recent studies have confirmed good psychometric properties in Croatian multiple sclerosis patients (Jerković et al., 2021), Colombian primary care patients (Rico-Mendoza et al., 2021), Greek hospital patients (Michopoulos et al., 2008) and Norwegian community-dwelling older adults (Sivertsen et al., 2023). Mitchell et al. (2010) conducted a comprehensive meta-analysis examining the HADS' diagnostic validity in cancer and palliative care settings, finding moderate to good sensitivity and specificity for detecting clinically significant anxiety and depression.

Clinical Applications. The HADS is particularly effective for screening and monitoring purposes in medical populations due to its non-somatic focus. Research has demonstrated its utility across diverse medical conditions, including cardiovascular disease (Stafford et al., 2007), multiple sclerosis (Watson et al., 2014), spinal cord injury (Woolrich et al., 2006) and palliative care settings (Mitchell et al., 2010). The scale's brevity and focus on psychological rather than somatic symptoms make it especially appropriate for individuals with physical health conditions where traditional depression and anxiety scales might yield false positives due to symptom overlap.

Depression, Anxiety, and Stress Scale-21 (DASS-21)

The DASS-21 (Lovibond & Lovibond, 1995) is a widely used self-report instrument that measures three related negative emotional states based on the tripartite model of depression, anxiety and stress. As a shortened version of the original 42-item DASS, the DASS-21 provides efficient assessment while maintaining strong psychometric properties and clear conceptual distinctions between the three constructs.

Theoretical Foundation. The DASS-21 is grounded in a sophisticated theoretical framework that distinguishes between depression (characterized by low positive affect and anhedonia), anxiety (characterized by autonomic arousal and specific fears) and stress (characterized by chronic non-specific arousal, negative affect and impatience). This tripartite model provides clearer conceptual distinctions compared to traditional anxiety and depression measures that often show high intercorrelations without clear discriminant validity (Watson & Clark, 1988).

Administration and Psychometric Evidence. Participants rate the extent to which they experienced each of 21 symptoms over the past week using a 4-point scale ranging from 0 (did not apply to me at all) to 3 (applied to me very much, or most of the time). Scores are doubled to provide compatibility with the full DASS, resulting in subscale scores ranging from 0 to 42. Recent systematic reviews have provided strong evidence for the instrument's psychometric properties across diverse populations and settings (de Souza et al., 2019; Lee et al., 2019).

International validation studies have consistently demonstrated the DASS-21's reliability and validity across cultural contexts. Bibi et al. (2020) established measurement invariance between Pakistani and German samples, finding good psychometric properties in both collectivistic and individualistic cultural contexts. Studies in healthcare workers from Oman (Al-Busaidi et al., 2022), Malaysian adults during COVID-19 (James et al., 2022), Bangladeshi adults (Rahman et al., 2022) and Malawian postpartum women (Udedi et al., 2022) have consistently confirmed the three-factor structure and acceptable internal consistency reliability.

Clinical Utility and Applications. The DASS-21 is freely available in the public domain and can be administered by non-clinicians, though interpretation should ideally be conducted by qualified mental health professionals to ensure appropriate clinical context (Lee et al., 2019). Its ability to discriminate between clinical and non-clinical populations makes it valuable for both screening and outcome measurement purposes. The instrument has demonstrated particular utility in healthcare settings, with studies showing its effectiveness for detecting common mental disorders in medical populations and tracking treatment response over time.

Maslach Burnout Inventory (MBI)

The Maslach Burnout Inventory (MBI; Maslach & Jackson, 1981) represents the gold standard for assessing burnout, particularly relevant for healthcare professionals and other service-oriented occupations. Burnout is conceptualized as a psychological syndrome characterized by emotional exhaustion, depersonalization and reduced personal accomplishment in response to chronic occupational stress (Maslach et al., 2018).

Three-Factor Structure and Theoretical Foundation. The MBI assesses three distinct but related dimensions of burnout that emerged from extensive empirical research with human services workers. Emotional exhaustion refers to feelings of being emotionally overextended and drained by work demands, representing the core dimension of burnout (Shirom, 2005). Depersonalization involves the development of cynical attitudes and impersonal responses toward service recipients, often serving as a coping mechanism for emotional exhaustion. Personal accomplishment (scored inversely) reflects feelings of competence and achievement in one's work, with reduced feelings indicating higher burnout levels.

Psychometric Properties and Validation. The MBI has undergone extensive psychometric evaluation across multiple versions and populations. Recent validation studies have confirmed the three-factor structure across diverse healthcare settings, including Persian medical personnel (Noroozi et al., 2022), Italian nurses (Dall'Ora et al., 2014) and international samples from the Gulf Cooperation Council Region (Hafez et al., 2020). Meta-analytic evidence demonstrates good internal consistency for emotional exhaustion ($\alpha > 0.85$), while depersonalization and personal accomplishment subscales show more variable reliability across studies (Aguayo et al., 2011).

The MBI demonstrates strong construct validity through correlations with theoretically related variables, including job stress, job satisfaction, turnover intention and mental health outcomes (Maslach et al., 2018). Recent research using both classical test theory and item response theory approaches has confirmed the instrument's psychometric adequacy across diverse healthcare populations (Noroozi et al., 2022; Wang et al., 2024).

Scoring and Clinical Applications. The MBI uses a 7-point frequency scale ranging from 0 (never) to 6 (every day) for rating the frequency of burnout-related experiences. The 2018 fourth edition of the MBI Manual removed previously published cut-off scores due to lack of diagnostic validity, instead recommending the use of burnout profiles that consider the pattern of scores across all three dimensions rather than arbitrary cut-points (Maslach et al., 2018). This approach recognizes burnout as a continuous experience rather than a categorical diagnostic condition.

For occupational therapists and healthcare workers, the MBI provides valuable insight into occupational stress levels and can inform workplace wellness initiatives, professional development programs and organizational interventions. Research has consistently demonstrated relationships between high burnout scores and various negative outcomes, including increased turnover, reduced job performance, physical health problems and compromised patient care quality (National Academy of Medicine, 2019).

Workplace-Specific Stress Assessments

Job Content Questionnaire (JCQ)

The Job Content Questionnaire (Karasek et al., 1998) is designed to measure psychosocial job characteristics based on the well-established Job Demand-Control model of occupational stress. This model proposes that job strain results from the interaction between high psychological demands and low decision latitude, with social support serving as a modifying factor that can buffer the negative effects of high-strain work conditions.

Theoretical Model and Scale Dimensions. The JCQ operationalizes Karasek's demand-control model through five primary dimensions that comprehensively assess the psychosocial work environment. Psychological demands encompass workload intensity, time pressure and conflicting demands that require sustained mental effort. Decision latitude combines two components, including skill discretion (the range of skills used and opportunities for skill development) and decision authority (control over work activities and participation in workplace decisions). Social support is assessed separately for supervisor and coworker support, recognizing the distinct roles these relationships play in buffering work stress. Additional scales assess physical demands and job insecurity, providing a comprehensive evaluation of workplace stressors.

Cross-Cultural Validity and International Applications. Extensive international research involving over 16,000 participants across four countries (United States, Sweden, Japan and Belgium) has demonstrated substantial similarity in the JCQ's psychometric properties across national boundaries (Karasek et al., 1998). This research revealed that psychological job characteristics show greater consistency across cultures than across occupations, supporting the universal applicability of the demand-control model. Reliability coefficients are generally good for most scales, with psychological job characteristics demonstrating particularly strong cross-national consistency.

The JCQ has been successfully applied across diverse occupational groups and cultural contexts, with validation studies confirming its utility for assessing psychosocial work conditions in healthcare settings, manufacturing environments, service industries, and professional occupations. Recent research has extended the model to include additional factors such as effort-reward imbalance and organizational justice, creating more comprehensive frameworks for understanding workplace stress and burnout.

Job Stress Survey (JSS)

The Job Stress Survey (Spielberger, 1994) is a comprehensive 30-item instrument designed to assess both the perceived severity and frequency of occurrence of workplace stressors commonly experienced by managerial, professional and clerical employees. The JSS represents a unique approach to job stress assessment by capturing both the intensity of stressors and their frequency of occurrence, providing a more nuanced understanding of workplace stress experiences.

Assessment Approach and Scoring. The JSS employs an innovative dual-rating system that provides comprehensive information about workplace stressor exposure. Respondents first rate the relative severity of stress associated with each item on a 9-point scale, using "assignment of disagreeable duties" as a standardized reference point assigned a value of 5. This approach allows for individual differences in stress appraisal while maintaining a common metric for comparison. Participants then indicate the frequency with which each stressor was experienced during the previous six months on a scale from 0 to 9+ days, capturing the temporal dimension of stress exposure.

The JSS yields multiple scores, including overall Severity (JSS-S) and Frequency (JSS-F) scores, as well as an overall Job Stress Index (JSS-X) based on the cross-products of severity and frequency ratings. Factor analysis has identified two primary subscales comprising Job Pressure (reflecting time pressures and workload demands) and Organizational Support (reflecting management and interpersonal relationship factors), each containing 10 items. These subscales demonstrate considerable internal consistency, with reliability coefficients exceeding 0.80 for most components (Spielberger, 1994).

Clinical Applications and Research Utility. The JSS is particularly valuable for organizational assessments and identifying specific workplace stressors that may require targeted interventions. The approximate completion time of 20 minutes makes it suitable for comprehensive workplace stress evaluations, while the detailed stressor profiles it provides can inform specific organizational change initiatives. Research has demonstrated the JSS's utility for identifying high-risk employees, evaluating the effectiveness of workplace stress management programs and understanding the relationship between specific job stressors and health outcomes.

Job Stress Scale

The Job Stress Scale (Parker & DeCotiis, 1983) was developed specifically to measure job stress dimensions in organizational settings through empirical research with managers in the restaurant industry. Based on factor analysis of stress experiences among 367 restaurant chain managers, the scale identifies two primary components of job stress that represent distinct but related aspects of workplace stress experience.

Factor Structure and Validation. The scale's development involved rigorous factor analysis procedures that identified two primary stress dimensions accounting for 77.5% of the variance in job stress experiences. Time stress represents feelings of being under substantial time pressure and excessive workload demands, reflecting the quantitative aspects of job stress related to pace and volume of work. The anxiety component encompasses job-related feelings of worry, tension and emotional distress, representing the affective response to work-related stressors.

Psychometric Properties. The Job Stress Scale demonstrates strong psychometric properties with excellent internal consistency reliability. Cronbach's alpha coefficients of 0.86 for time stress and 0.74 for anxiety indicate good to excellent internal consistency. Corrected item-total correlations range from 0.61 to 0.79 for time stress items and 0.61 to 0.75 for anxiety items, indicating that all items contribute meaningfully to their respective factors. The correlation between the two factors ($r = 0.54$) indicates substantial but not overlapping variance, supporting the discriminant validity of the two-factor structure.

The scale's development in the service industry provides particular relevance for understanding stress in fast-paced, customer-oriented work environments. However, subsequent research has confirmed its applicability across diverse occupational settings, making it a versatile tool for organizational stress assessment and research applications.

Specialized Assessment Considerations

CULTURAL ADAPTATIONS AND CROSS-CULTURAL VALIDITY

The effective use of stress assessment tools requires careful attention to cultural factors that may influence stress perception, expression and coping responses across diverse populations. Cultural considerations extend beyond simple language translation to encompass fundamental differences in how stress is conceptualized, experienced and communicated across different cultural contexts (Bibi et al., 2020; Uchida et al., 2004).

Cultural Factors Influencing Stress Assessment. Collectivistic cultures may place greater emphasis on family harmony, social obligation and interdependent well-being compared to individualistic cultures that prioritize personal achievement and autonomous functioning (Kitayama & Markus, 2000). These cultural orientations can significantly influence how individuals interpret stress assessment items and their willingness to endorse certain symptoms or experiences. For example, items related to individual achievement may be interpreted differently in cultures that emphasize collective success over personal accomplishment.

Religious and spiritual factors also play crucial roles in stress perception and coping across cultures. Research has demonstrated that spiritual coping mechanisms, social support from religious communities and meaning-making processes vary significantly across cultural groups and can influence both stress appraisal and adaptive responses (Watlington & Murphy, 2006). Assessment tools that fail to account for these cultural differences may misinterpret adaptive cultural responses as pathological or overlook significant stressors that are specific to particular cultural contexts.

Best Practices for Cross-Cultural Assessment. Contemporary research emphasizes the importance of establishing measurement invariance across cultural groups rather than simply translating existing instruments. Studies with the PSS (Baik et al., 2019; Bibi et al., 2020), DASS-21 (Bibi et al., 2020; Scholten et al., 2017) and HADS (Rico-Mendoza et al., 2021) have demonstrated that rigorous cross-cultural validation can establish whether observed differences in scores reflect true differences in stress levels or differences in how cultural groups interpret and respond to assessment items.

When validated translations are not available, practitioners should consider cultural consultation for interpretation, supplement standardized measures with culturally appropriate assessment approaches, remain aware of potential bias in normative data and consider mixed-methods approaches that include qualitative exploration of stress experiences within specific cultural contexts. These approaches help ensure that assessment results accurately reflect stress experiences rather than cultural measurement artifacts.

Integration with Occupational Therapy Practice

While standardized assessment tools provide valuable information about stress levels and related symptoms, occupational therapists must integrate these findings within their professional scope of practice and theoretical frameworks that emphasize the relationship between meaningful activity engagement and stress management outcomes (Stein & Cutler, 1998). This integration requires understanding how assessment findings relate to occupational performance, participation and well-being across diverse life contexts.

OCCUPATIONAL PERFORMANCE CONSIDERATIONS

Assessment results must be interpreted in relation to their impact on activities of daily living, instrumental activities of daily living and meaningful occupational roles. For example, elevated anxiety scores on the HADS may be most clinically significant when they interfere with work performance, social participation or self-care activities. Similarly, high burnout scores on the MBI should be understood in relation to their effects on professional role performance, work satisfaction and career sustainability.

Environmental factors that contribute to or alleviate stress represent another crucial area for integration within occupational therapy practice. The physical environment, social supports, cultural context and temporal patterns of daily occupations all influence stress experiences and coping effectiveness (Law et al., 1996). Assessment findings should inform environmental modifications, social support interventions and activity restructuring that can reduce stress exposure while enhancing coping resources.

INTERVENTION PLANNING CONSIDERATIONS

The relationship between meaningful activities and stress management outcomes suggests that intervention planning should consider how assessment findings can inform occupation-based interventions. For individuals with high perceived stress scores, interventions might focus on time management strategies, meaningful leisure engagement or stress-reducing modifications to work routines. Those with elevated depression or anxiety scores might benefit from activity scheduling, social participation enhancement or environmental modifications that support emotional regulation and well-being.

TECHNOLOGY-ENHANCED ASSESSMENT AND FUTURE DIRECTIONS

Emerging technologies offer new possibilities for stress assessment that complement traditional self-report measures by providing real-time data and objective indicators of stress responses. Smartphone-based ecological momentary assessment allows for repeated measurements of stress levels throughout daily activities, providing insights into temporal patterns and contextual factors that influence stress experiences (Shiffman et al., 2008). Wearable devices can monitor physiological indicators such as heart rate variability, cortisol levels and sleep patterns that provide objective measures of stress responses and recovery.

Virtual reality-based stress response measurement represents another promising technological advancement that allows for standardized stress exposure while monitoring both subjective and physiological responses. These approaches can provide more comprehensive understanding of individual stress reactivity and recovery patterns while offering opportunities for stress inoculation training and coping skills development within controlled environments.

Integration with Clinical Practice

Technology-enhanced assessment approaches require careful integration with traditional assessment methods and clinical judgment. While objective measures provide valuable information about physiological stress responses, they must be interpreted in conjunction with subjective experiences, functional impacts and environmental contexts that influence stress management effectiveness. The goal is to create comprehensive assessment approaches that combine the standardization and reliability of traditional measures with the ecological validity and real-time monitoring capabilities of technological innovations.

Clinical Decision-Making and Assessment Selection

EVIDENCE-BASED ASSESSMENT PROTOCOL DEVELOPMENT

The development of comprehensive stress assessment protocols requires systematic consideration of clinical questions, target populations and intended applications while balancing scientific rigor with practical feasibility. Evidence-based assessment selection involves matching assessment tools to specific clinical needs while considering psychometric properties, cultural appropriateness and resource constraints that influence implementation success.

Clinical Question Formulation. Effective assessment begins with clearly formulated clinical questions that guide instrument selection and interpretation. Questions might focus on screening for stress-related disorders, monitoring treatment progress, identifying specific stressors requiring intervention or evaluating program effectiveness across populations. Different clinical questions require different assessment approaches, with screening applications emphasizing sensitivity while diagnostic applications prioritize specificity and positive predictive value.

Assessment timing considerations also influence protocol development. Baseline assessments require comprehensive evaluation across multiple domains to establish initial status and identify intervention targets. Progress monitoring assessments should be brief enough to minimize burden while maintaining sensitivity to change. Outcome evaluations require instruments with established minimal clinically important differences and responsiveness to intervention effects.

Population-Specific Considerations. Assessment protocols must account for demographic factors, clinical characteristics and contextual variables that influence assessment validity and interpretation. Age-appropriate instruments and normative data ensure that assessment results can be meaningfully interpreted within developmental contexts. Educational level and cognitive abilities influence comprehension and response patterns, while physical limitations may affect completion methods and require accommodations.

Cultural and linguistic factors represent particularly important considerations for assessment protocol development. Instruments should have established validity within target populations, and protocols should include provisions for cultural consultation when needed. Language considerations extend beyond simple translation to encompass cultural concepts of stress, acceptable symptom expression and appropriate intervention approaches.

COMPREHENSIVE ASSESSMENT FRAMEWORK

A comprehensive stress assessment protocol typically incorporates multiple instruments selected to capture different dimensions of stress experience while avoiding excessive respondent burden. The framework should balance breadth of coverage with practical constraints, including time limitations, cost considerations and clinician training requirements.

Multi-Dimensional Assessment Approach. An optimal assessment battery might include global stress perception measures such as the Perceived Stress Scale to establish overall stress levels and temporal patterns. Specific symptom domains can be assessed using instruments like the DASS-21 or HADS that provide detailed information about anxiety, depression and related psychological symptoms. Life events and environmental stressors can be evaluated using updated versions of the Social Readjustment Rating Scale or other life event inventories that capture recent stress exposure.

Occupation-specific assessments become important for individuals whose stress is primarily related to work or specific role demands. The Maslach Burnout Inventory provides detailed assessment for healthcare workers and other human services professionals, while the Job Content Questionnaire or Job Stress Survey can assess broader workplace stress factors. The Stress Management Questionnaire described in Chapter 5 offers unique insights into occupation-based coping strategies and meaningful activity engagement.

Assessment Integration and Interpretation. Comprehensive assessment requires systematic integration of findings across multiple instruments and domains. Patterns of results provide more meaningful information than individual scale scores, with discrepancies between measures highlighting areas requiring further exploration. For example, high perceived stress combined with low specific symptom scores might suggest effective coping strategies, while the reverse pattern might indicate emerging stress-related difficulties requiring immediate attention.

Clinical interpretation should consider assessment results within broader contexts, including environmental supports, personal resources, cultural factors and intervention goals. The ultimate purpose of assessment is to inform intervention planning and outcome monitoring, requiring translation of assessment findings into actionable intervention targets and measurable outcome goals.

CONCLUSION

The assessment tools presented in this chapter provide essential components for comprehensive stress evaluation that complement the occupation-focused Stress Management Questionnaire described in Chapter 5. Each instrument offers unique perspectives on different aspects of the stress experience, from global stress perception to specific symptom domains and workplace-specific stressors. The Perceived Stress Scale provides a validated assessment of stress appraisal processes across diverse populations, while the DASS-21 and HADS offer detailed evaluations of anxiety and depression symptoms in medical and community settings.

The extensive psychometric research supporting these instruments demonstrates their reliability and validity across diverse populations and cultural contexts. Recent international validation studies have confirmed the cross-cultural applicability of major stress assessment tools while highlighting the importance of cultural considerations in assessment selection and interpretation. The Maslach Burnout Inventory continues to serve as the gold standard for occupational burnout assessment, while workplace-specific tools like the Job Content Questionnaire and Job Stress Survey provide detailed evaluations of organizational stress factors.

Effective stress assessment requires careful consideration of psychometric properties, cultural factors, and clinical applications when selecting appropriate instruments for specific populations and purposes. The integration of multiple assessment approaches provides the most comprehensive understanding of an individual's stress profile while informing evidence-based intervention planning. Technology-enhanced assessment approaches offer promising directions for real-time monitoring and ecological validity while requiring thoughtful integration with traditional assessment methods.

As the field continues to evolve toward positive psychology approaches to stress management, as explored in Chapter 7, these traditional assessment tools remain valuable for establishing baseline functioning, tracking symptom reduction and providing standardized outcome measures for research and clinical practice. The comprehensive assessment foundation established through these evidence-based instruments creates the necessary platform for implementing positive health approaches and flourishing-focused interventions that move beyond symptom reduction toward the active cultivation of human potential and resilience.

The future of stress assessment lies in the thoughtful integration of deficit-focused measures with strength-based assessments that capture the full spectrum of human stress responses and adaptive capacities. By combining rigorous assessment with culturally sensitive interpretation and technology-enhanced monitoring, practitioners can develop increasingly sophisticated understanding of stress experiences that inform more effective, personalized and meaningful interventions designed to promote not merely symptom reduction but optimal human functioning and well-being.

SUMMARY

This chapter expands the stress assessment toolkit by presenting standardized instruments that complement the occupation-focused Stress Management Questionnaire, providing occupational therapists with evidence-based tools for comprehensive stress evaluation. The Perceived Stress Scale offers a validated assessment of stress appraisal processes, while the HADS and DASS-21 provide detailed symptom evaluation for anxiety and depression in medical and community settings. The Maslach Burnout Inventory remains the gold standard for occupational burnout assessment, particularly relevant for healthcare professionals. Workplace-specific instruments, including the Job Content Questionnaire and Job Stress Survey, enable detailed evaluation of organizational stress factors based on established theoretical models. Extensive psychometric research confirms the reliability and validity of these instruments across diverse populations and cultural contexts, though careful attention to cultural adaptation and measurement invariance remains essential. The chapter emphasizes developing comprehensive assessment protocols that integrate multiple instruments while balancing scientific rigor with practical feasibility. Technology-enhanced approaches offer promising directions for real-time monitoring and ecological validity. Effective stress assessment requires thoughtful instrument selection based on clinical questions, population characteristics and intended applications, with findings interpreted within broader contexts including environmental supports, personal resources and intervention goals that inform occupation-based practice.

DISCUSSION QUESTIONS

1. Reflect on the distinction between the occupation-focused Stress Management Questionnaire (SMQ) and the standardized instruments presented in this chapter. What unique insights does each approach offer, and how might you integrate both perspectives in a comprehensive stress assessment?
2. The chapter emphasizes that the Perceived Stress Scale (PSS) focuses on subjective appraisal processes rather than objective stressful events. How does this align with Lazarus and Folkman's transactional model of stress? What are the clinical implications of assessing perceived stress versus life events exposure?
3. Consider the Hospital Anxiety and Depression Scale's (HADS) deliberate exclusion of somatic symptoms. In your experience, how might physical symptoms be misinterpreted as psychological distress in medical populations? What ethical considerations arise when distinguishing between physical and psychological symptom presentations?
4. The Maslach Burnout Inventory's 2018 edition removed fixed cut-off scores in favor of burnout profiles. Reflect on the implications of viewing burnout as a continuous experience rather than a categorical diagnosis. How does this approach align with or challenge your understanding of occupational wellness?
5. This chapter discusses extensive cross-cultural validation research for various instruments. Reflect on a time when you worked with clients from cultural backgrounds different from your own. How might cultural factors influence stress perception, symptom expression and willingness to disclose difficulties on standardized assessments?
6. Consider the Job Content Questionnaire's finding that "psychological job characteristics show greater consistency across cultures than across occupations." What does this reveal about the nature of workplace stress? How might this inform organizational-level versus individual-level interventions?
7. Reflect on the balance between assessment comprehensiveness and respondent burden. How do you decide how many assessment instruments are appropriate for a given client or situation? What factors influence this clinical decision?

8. This chapter presents various workplace stress measures (JCQ, JSS, Job Stress Scale). As an occupational therapist, how might you use workplace assessment findings to advocate for environmental modifications or systemic changes rather than focusing solely on individual coping strategies?
9. Consider the concept of measurement invariance discussed in the cross-cultural validity section. Why is it important to establish that score differences reflect true stress level differences rather than cultural interpretation differences? How might you address situations where validated translations are unavailable?
10. Reflect on the integration of standardized assessment findings with occupational therapy's focus on meaningful activity and functional performance. How do you translate a high score on the DASS-21 or PSS into occupation-based intervention targets that are meaningful to clients?
11. This chapter discusses technology-enhanced assessment approaches, including ecological momentary assessment and wearable devices. What are the potential benefits and limitations of real-time stress monitoring? How might continuous monitoring change the client-therapist relationship or client self-awareness?
12. This chapter emphasizes that comprehensive assessment protocols should capture different dimensions while avoiding excessive burden. Design a realistic assessment protocol for a specific population (e.g., healthcare workers, college students, chronic pain patients). How did you balance comprehensiveness with feasibility, and what guided your instrument selection?

REFERENCES

Aguayo, R., Vargas, C., de la Fuente, E. I., & Lozano, L. M. (2011). A meta-analytic reliability generalization study of the Maslach Burnout Inventory. *International Journal of Clinical and Health Psychology*, *11*(2), 343–361.

Al-Busaidi, Z. Q., Bhargava, K., Al-Ismaily, A., Al-Lawati, H., Al-Kindi, R., Al-Shafaee, M., & Al-Maniri, A. (2022). Psychometric properties of the depression, anxiety, stress scales-21 (DASS-21) in a sample of health care workers in Oman. *BMC Nursing*, *21*(1), 317. https://doi.org/10.1186/s12912-022-01094-z

Andreou, E., Alexopoulos, E. C., Lionis, C., Varvogli, L., Gnardellis, C., Chrousos, G. P., & Darviri, C. (2011). Perceived stress scale: Reliability and validity study in Greece. *International Journal of Environmental Research and Public Health*, *8*(8), 3287–3298. https://doi.org/10.3390/ijerph8083287

Ayele, B. A., Dhingra, S., & Mullins, C. D. (2019). Psychometric properties of the perceived stress scale in Ethiopian university students. *BMC Public Health*, *19*(1), 41. https://doi.org/10.1186/s12889-018-6310-z

Baik, S. H., Fox, R. S., Mills, S. D., Roesch, S. C., Sadler, G. R., Klonoff, E. A., & Malcarne, V. L. (2019). Reliability and validity of the Perceived Stress Scale-10 in Hispanic Americans with English or Spanish language preference. *Journal of Health Psychology*, *24*(5), 628–639. https://doi.org/10.1177/1359105316684938

Bibi, A., Lin, M., Zhang, X. C., & Margraf, J. (2020). Psychometric properties and measurement invariance of Depression, Anxiety and Stress Scales (DASS-21) across cultures. *International Journal of Psychology*, *55*(6), 916–925. https://doi.org/10.1002/ijop.12671

Bjelland, I., Dahl, A. A., Haug, T. T., & Neckelmann, D. (2002). The validity of the Hospital Anxiety and Depression Scale: An updated literature review. *Journal of Psychosomatic Research*, *52*(2), 69–77. https://doi.org/10.1016/s0022-3999(01)00296-3

Cohen, S. (1986). Contrasting the hassle scale and the perceived stress scale. *American Psychologist*, *41*(7), 716–719. https://doi.org/10.1037/0003-066X.41.7.716

Cohen, S., & Janicki-Deverts, D. (2012). Who's stressed? Distributions of psychological stress in the United States in probability samples from 1983, 2006, and 2009. *Journal of Applied Social Psychology*, *42*(6), 1320–1334. https://doi.org/10.1111/j.1559-1816.2012.00900.x

Cohen, S., Kamarck, T., & Mermelstein, R. (1983). A global measure of perceived stress. *Journal of Health and Social Behavior*, *24*(4), 385–396. https://doi.org/10.2307/2136404

Dall'Ora, C., Griffiths, P., Ball, J., Simon, M., & Aiken, L. H. (2014). Association of 12 h shifts and nurses' job satisfaction, burnout, and intention to leave: Findings from a cross-sectional study of 12 European countries. *BMJ Open*, *5*(9), e008331. https://doi.org/10.1136/bmjopen-2015-008331

de Souza, L. A. S., Lopes, C. S., Barbosa, M. T. S., Caldas, C. P., & Veras, R. P. (2019). Systematic review of the measurement properties of the Depression Anxiety Stress Scales-21 by applying updated COSMIN methodology. *Quality of Life Research*, *28*(9), 2325–2339. https://doi.org/10.1007/s11136-019-02198-0

Dorsey, A., Scherer, E., Eckhoff, R., Furberg, R., Harmon, B., Holden, K., Khan, S., Kim, Y., Kolodka, O., Lipperman-Kreda, S., Maddock, J., McLaughlin, I., Mumford, E., Patel, S., Pearson, J., Rao, P., Richardson, L., Sapp, L., Schwarz, M., & Sullivan, P. (2022). *Measurement of human stress: A multidimensional approach*. RTI Press. https://doi.org/10.3768/rtipress.2022.op.0073.2206

Frisone, F., Sicari, F., Settineri, S., & Merlo, E. M. (2021). Clinical psychological assessment of stress: A narrative review of the last 5 years. *Clinical Neuropsychiatry*, *18*(2), 91–100. https://doi.org/10.36131/cnfioritieditore20210203

Hafez, D., Al-Rashdan, W., Al-Sharman, A., Rababah, J., Al-Mistarehi, A. H., Aldalaykeh, M., & Al-Zayyat, A. S. (2020). Examining and adapting the psychometric properties of the Maslach Burnout Inventory-Health Services Survey (MBI-HSS) among healthcare professionals. *Applied Sciences*, *10*(5), 1890. https://doi.org/10.3390/app10051890

Harris, K. M., Gaffey, A. E., Schwartz, J. E., Krantz, D. S., & Burg, M. M. (2023). The Perceived Stress Scale as a measure of stress: Decomposing score variance in longitudinal behavioral medicine studies. *Annals of Behavioral Medicine*, *57*(10), 846–854. https://doi.org/10.1093/abm/kaad015

Helvik, A. S., Engedal, K., Skancke, R. H., & Selbæk, G. (2017). A psychometric evaluation of the Hospital Anxiety and Depression Scale for the medically hospitalized elderly. *Nordic Journal of Psychiatry*, *71*(6), 458–465. https://doi.org/10.1080/08039488.2017.1321948

Holmes, T. H., & Rahe, R. H. (1967). The Social Readjustment Rating Scale. *Journal of Psychosomatic Research*, *11*(2), 213–218. https://doi.org/10.1016/0022-3999(67)90010-4

James, T. G., Cheah, J. H., Chai, J. H., Sim, M. S., Mohd Shahwan, M. K., Thurasamy, R., Yeap, B. Y., Rajah, S. S., Liew, L. S., & Kwan, Y. H. (2022). Psychometric properties of the 21-item Depression, Anxiety, and Stress Scale (DASS-21) among Malaysians during COVID-19: A methodological study. *Humanities and Social Sciences Communications*, *9*(1), 220. https://doi.org/10.1057/s41599-022-01229-x

Jerković, A., Proroković, A., Matijaca, M., Vuko, J., Poljičanin, A., Mastelić, A., Ćurković Katić, A., Košta, V., Kustura, L., Dolić, K., Đogaš, Z., & Rogić Vidaković, M. (2021). Psychometric properties of the HADS measure of anxiety and depression among multiple sclerosis patients in Croatia. *Frontiers in Psychology*, *12*, 794353. https://doi.org/10.3389/fpsyg.2021.794353

Kanner, A. D., Coyne, J. C., Schaefer, C., & Lazarus, R. S. (1981). Comparison of two modes of stress measurement: daily hassles and uplifts versus major life events. *Journal of Behavioral Medicine*, *4*(1), 1–39. https://doi.org/10.1007/bf00844845

Karasek, R., Brisson, C., Kawakami, N., Houtman, I., Bongers, P., & Amick, B. (1998). The Job Content Questionnaire (JCQ): An instrument for internationally comparative assessments of psychosocial job characteristics. *Journal of Occupational Health Psychology*, *3*(4), 322–355. https://doi.org/10.1037/1076-8998.3.4.322

Kechter, A., Black, D. S., Riggs, N. R., Warren, C. M., Ritt-Olson, A., Chou, C. P., & Pentz, M. A. (2019). Factors in the perceived stress scale differentially associate with mindfulness disposition and executive function among early adolescents. *Journal of Child and Family Studies*, *28*(3), 814–821. https://doi.org/10.1007/s10826-018-01313-4

Kitayama, S., & Markus, H. R. (2000). The pursuit of happiness and the realization of sympathy: Cultural patterns of self, social relations, and well-being. In E. Diener & E. M. Suh (Eds.), *Culture and subjective well-being* (pp. 113–161). MIT Press.

Klein, E. M., Brähler, E., Dreier, M., Reinecke, L., Müller, K. W., Schmutzer, G., Wölfling, K., & Beutel, M. E. (2016). The German version of the Perceived Stress Scale – psychometric characteristics in a representative German community sample. *BMC Psychiatry*, *16*(1), 159. https://doi.org/10.1186/s12888-016-0875-9

Law, M., Cooper, B., Strong, S., Stewart, D., Rigby, P., & Letts, L. (1996). The Person-Environment-Occupation Model: A transactive approach to occupational performance. *Canadian Journal of Occupational Therapy*, *63*(1), 9–23. https://doi.org/10.1177/000841749606300103

Lazarus, R. S., & Folkman, S. (1984). *Stress, appraisal, and coping*. Springer.

Lee, E. H. (2012). Review of the psychometric evidence of the perceived stress scale. *Asian Nursing Research*, *6*(4), 121–127. https://doi.org/10.1016/j.anr.2012.08.004

Lee, J., Lee, E. H., & Moon, S. H. (2019). Systematic review of the measurement properties of the Depression Anxiety Stress Scales–21 by applying updated COSMIN methodology. *Quality of Life Research*, *28*(9), 2325–2339. https://doi.org/10.1007/s11136-019-02177-x

Lovibond, P. F., & Lovibond, S. H. (1995). The structure of negative emotional states: Comparison of the Depression Anxiety Stress Scales (DASS) with the Beck Depression and Anxiety Inventories. *Behaviour Research and Therapy*, *33*(3), 335–343. https://doi.org/10.1016/0005-7967(94)00075-u

Maslach, C., & Jackson, S. E. (1981). The measurement of experienced burnout. *Journal of Organizational Behavior*, *2*(2), 99–113. https://doi.org/10.1002/job.4030020205

Maslach, C., Jackson, S. E., & Leiter, M. P. (2018). *Maslach Burnout Inventory Manual* (4th ed.). Mind Garden.

Michopoulos, I., Douzenis, A., Kalkavoura, C., Christodoulou, C., Michalopoulou, P., Kalemi, G., Fineti, K., Patapis, P., Protopapas, K., & Lykouras, L. (2008). Hospital Anxiety and Depression Scale (HADS): Validation in a Greek general hospital sample. *Annals of General Psychiatry*, *7*(1), 4. https://doi.org/10.1186/1744-859X-7-4

Mitchell, A. J., Meader, N., & Symonds, P. (2010). Diagnostic validity of the Hospital Anxiety and Depression Scale (HADS) in cancer and palliative settings: A meta-analysis. *Journal of Affective Disorders*, *126*(3), 335–348. https://doi.org/10.1016/j.jad.2010.01.067

Mozumder, M. K. (2022). Reliability and validity of the Perceived Stress Scale in Bangladesh. *PLoS One*, *17*(10), e0276837. https://doi.org/10.1371/journal.pone.0276837

National Academy of Medicine. (2019). *Valid and reliable survey instruments to measure burnout, well-being, and other work-related dimensions*. https://nam.edu/product/valid-and-reliable-survey-instruments-to-measure-burnout-well-being-and-other-work-related-dimensions/

Noroozi, M., Kouzekanani, K., Eslami, A. A., Tahmasebi, R., & Hashemiparast, M. (2022). Psychometric properties of the Maslach Burnout Inventory for Medical Personnel (MBI-HSS-MP). *Heliyon*, *8*(2), e08832. https://doi.org/10.1016/j.heliyon.2022.e08832\

Norton, S., Cosco, T., Doyle, F., Done, J., & Sacker, A. (2018). The Hospital Anxiety and Depression Scale: A meta confirmatory factor analysis. *Journal of Psychosomatic Research*, *74*(1), 74–81. https://doi.org/10.1016/j.jpsychores.2012.10.010

Parker, D. F., & DeCotiis, T. A. (1983). Organizational determinants of job stress. *Organizational Behavior and Human Performance*, *32*(2), 160–177. https://doi.org/10.1016/0030-5073(83)90145-9

Prokopovich, D. S., Petrova, N. N., Morozova, T. I., Rakhmanina, A. A., Iosifescu, D. V., & Gayanova, V. V. (2024). Factor structure and psychometric properties of the Perceived Stress Scale in Russian adolescents. *Scientific Reports*, *14*(1), 778. https://doi.org/10.1038/s41598-023-51104-1

Rahman, M. A., Hoque, N., Alif, S. M., Salehin, M., Islam, S. M. S., Banik, B., Sharif, A., Nazim, N. B., Sultana, F., & Cross, W. (2022). The psychometric properties of the Depression, Anxiety, and Stress Scale-21 (DASS-21) Bangla version. *Acta Psychologica*, *223*, 103498. https://doi.org/10.1016/j.actpsy.2022.103509

Rico-Mendoza, A., Borrero, A., Molina, D., López-Jaramillo, C., & Torres, M. (2021). Validity of the Hospital Anxiety and Depression Scale (HADS) for depression and anxiety screening in primary care patients in Colombia. *General Hospital Psychiatry*, *69*, 110–117. https://doi.org/10.1016/j.genhosppsych.2021.01.014

Scholten, S., Velten, J., Bieda, A., Zhang, X. C., & Margraf, J. (2017). Testing measurement invariance of the Depression, Anxiety, and Stress Scales-21 across four countries. *Psychological Assessment*, *29*(11), 1376–1390. https://doi.org/10.1037/pas0000440

Shiffman, S., Stone, A. A., & Hufford, M. R. (2008). Ecological momentary assessment. *Annual Review of Clinical Psychology*, *4*, 1–32. https://doi.org/10.1146/annurev.clinpsy.3.022806.091415

Shirom, A. (2005). Reflections on the study of burnout. *Work & Stress*, *19*(3), 263–270. https://doi.org/10.1080/02678370500376649

Sivertsen, H. E., Helvik, A. S., Gjøra, L., & Haugan, G. (2023). Psychometric validation of the Hospital Anxiety and Depression Scale (HADS) in community-dwelling older adults. *BMC psychiatry*, *23*(1), 903. https://doi.org/10.1186/s12888-023-05407-2

Spielberger, C. D. (1994). *Job Stress Survey: Professional manual*. Psychological Assessment Resources.

Stafford, L., Berk, M., & Jackson, H. J. (2007). Validity of the hospital anxiety and depression scale and patient health questionnaire-9 to screen for depression in patients with coronary artery disease. *General Hospital Psychiatry*, *29*(5), 417–424. https://doi.org/10.1016/j.genhosppsych.2007.06.005

Stein, F. (1986). *The Stress Management Questionnaire (SMQ)*. University of Wisconsin-Milwaukee.

Stein, F., & Cutler, S. (1998). *Psychosocial occupational therapy: A holistic approach*. Singular.

Taylor, J. M. (2015). Psychometric analysis of the ten-item Perceived Stress Scale. *Psychological Assessment*, *27*(1), 90–101. https://doi.org/10.1037/a0038100

Uchida, Y., Norasakkunkit, V., & Kitayama, S. (2004). Cultural constructions of happiness: Theory and empirical evidence. *Journal of Happiness Studies*, *5*(3), 223–239. https://doi.org/10.1007/s10902-004-8785-9

Udedi, M., Stockton, M. A., Kulisewa, K., Hosseinipour, M. C., Gaynes, B. N., Mphonda, S. M., Go, V. F., & Miller, W. C. (2022). Reliability and validity of depression anxiety stress scale (DASS)-21 in screening for common mental disorders among postpartum women in Malawi. *BMC Psychiatry*, *22*(1), 352. https://doi.org/10.1186/s12888-022-03994-0

Wallace, D., Cooper, N. R., Sel, A., & Russo, R. (2023). The social readjustment rating scale: Updated and modernised. *PLoS One*, *18*(12), e0295943. https://doi.org/10.1371/journal.pone.0295943

Wang, A., Duan, Y., Norton, P. G., Leiter, M. P., & Estabrooks, C. A. (2024). Validation of the Maslach Burnout Inventory-General Survey 9-item short version: Psychometric properties and measurement invariance across age, gender, and continent. *Frontiers in Psychology*, *15*, 1439470. https://doi.org/10.3389/fpsyg.2024.1439470

Watlington, C. G., & Murphy, C. M. (2006). The roles of religion and spirituality among African American survivors of domestic violence. *Journal of Clinical Psychology*, *62*(7), 837–857. https://doi.org/10.1002/jclp.20268

Watson, D., & Clark, L. A. (1988). Development and validation of brief measures of positive and negative affect: The PANAS scales. *Journal of Personality and Social Psychology*, *54*(6), 1063–1070. https://doi.org/10.1037/0022-3514.54.6.1063

Watson, S., Turk, D., Mure, J., & Padfield, N. (2014). Validation of mood measures for people with multiple sclerosis. *International Journal of MS Care*, *16*(2), 105–109. https://doi.org/10.7224/1537-2073.2013-013

Woolrich, R. A., Kennedy, P., & Tasiemski, T. (2006). A preliminary psychometric evaluation of the Hospital Anxiety and Depression Scale (HADS) in 963 people living with a spinal cord injury. *Psychology, Health & Medicine*, *11*(1), 80–90. https://doi.org/10.1080/13548500500294211

Zigmond, A. S., & Snaith, R. P. (1983). The Hospital Anxiety and Depression Scale. *Acta Psychiatrica Scandinavica*, *67*(6), 361–370. https://doi.org/10.1111/j.1600-0447.1983.tb09716.x

Chapter 7

Positive Health Approaches to Stress: Flourishing through Adversity

LEARNING OBJECTIVES

By the end of this chapter, the reader will be able to

1. Define positive psychology and explain its core theoretical foundations, including the PERMA framework (Positive Emotion, Engagement, Relationships, Meaning and Accomplishment).
2. Describe the concept of flow states and explain how optimal challenge-skill balance can transform stress responses into opportunities for growth and engagement.
3. Understand stress mindset theory and apply Crum's three-phase intervention (acknowledge, welcome and use stress) to help clients develop stress-is-enhancing perspectives.
4. Differentiate between post-traumatic stress disorder (PTSD) and post-traumatic growth (PTG), identifying the five domains of growth that can emerge following adversity.
5. Explain corporeal post-traumatic growth and its relevance to occupational therapy practice with clients experiencing physical trauma, illness or disability.
6. Integrate the Stress Management Questionnaire (SMQ) with standardized anxiety/depression measures and positive psychology assessments to create comprehensive evaluation frameworks.
7. Design and implement evidence-based positive psychology interventions, including gratitude practices, acts of kindness, mindfulness meditation, benefit-finding and flow cultivation techniques.

DOI: 10.4324/9781003671084-7

8. Apply cultural considerations when adapting positive psychology interventions for diverse populations, recognizing variations in individualistic versus collectivistic values.
9. Develop personalized positive psychology intervention protocols that match individual strengths, preferences and specific stress-related challenges.
10. Evaluate the effectiveness of positive psychology stress management programs through longitudinal tracking of both distress reduction and well-being enhancement measures.

INTRODUCTION

The landscape of stress research has undergone a fundamental paradigm shift from a deficit-focused pathology model to a comprehensive positive health approach that recognizes stress as a potential catalyst for human flourishing (Keyes, 2007; Seligman, 2008). While stress has traditionally been conceptualized primarily through its negative impacts on psychological and physiological functioning, emerging positive psychology research reveals that adversity can serve as a springboard for growth, resilience and the development of character strengths (Peterson & Seligman, 2004; Tedeschi & Calhoun, 2004). This chapter explores how lifestyle responses to stress can be transformed through evidence-based positive psychology interventions (PPIs) that not only mitigate distress but also actively cultivate well-being, meaning and human thriving.

Seligman's (2008) positive health framework moves beyond traditional pathology-focused models by emphasizing five core elements that contribute to human flourishing: experiencing positive affect, achieving deep engagement in activities, maintaining meaningful relationships, pursuing purpose and accomplishing valued goals, which are components that together form the foundation for comprehensive well-being. This framework, termed PERMA (Positive Emotion, Engagement, Relationships, Meaning and Accomplishment), provides a robust foundation for understanding how individuals can not only cope with stress but also leverage challenging experiences to develop greater psychological capital and life satisfaction (Fredrickson, 2001; Ryan & Deci, 2001). Rather than viewing stress as an inherently pathological force, positive psychology recognizes that optimal stress levels can enhance performance, foster creativity and flow and promote personal growth when properly channeled through evidence-based interventions (Csikszentmihalyi, 1990; Dweck, 2006).

The integration of positive psychology interventions with traditional stress management approaches represents a revolutionary advancement in promoting comprehensive well-being. Research consistently demonstrates that individuals who engage in structured gratitude practices, acts of kindness, mindfulness-based interventions and character strength identification show significant improvements not only in mood and life satisfaction but also in their capacity to navigate stressful circumstances with greater resilience and adaptive coping strategies (Bolier et al., 2013; Lyubomirsky et al., 2005; Sin & Lyubomirsky, 2009). These findings challenge the conventional wisdom that stress management should focus primarily on reduction and avoidance, instead suggesting that growth-oriented interventions can transform stress into a vehicle for enhanced psychological functioning.

FLOW STATES AND OPTIMAL STRESS ENGAGEMENT

Central to understanding how stress can be leveraged for human flourishing is Csikszentmihalyi's concept of flow, which is a psychological state characterized by complete immersion in an activity with effortless concentration and intrinsic motivation (Csikszentmihalyi, 1990). Optimal experience occurs when people become completely immersed in their activities with deep concentration and intrinsic motivation. During these states, individuals experience intense focus that often obscures their awareness of time and surroundings, with full appreciation of the experience emerging upon reflection (Nakamura & Csikszentmihalyi, 2014).

Flow states emerge when there is a precise balance between the perceived challenges of a situation and an individual's perceived skills to meet those challenges. This balance creates what Csikszentmihalyi described as the "golden ratio" of experience – when challenge levels are too low relative to skills, boredom ensues; when challenges exceed skills, anxiety results; but when challenges and skills are optimally matched, flow occurs (Csikszentmihalyi, 1990; Engeser & Rheinberg, 2008). This dynamic relationship between challenge and skill reveals how stress, when properly calibrated, can become a gateway to optimal experience rather than a source of distress.

The connection between flow and stress management is profound yet often overlooked in traditional therapeutic approaches. Research demonstrates that individuals who regularly experience flow states show enhanced psychological resilience, improved emotional regulation and greater capacity to transform challenging situations into opportunities for growth and engagement (Bakker, 2008; Jackson & Marsh, 1996). In the context of positive psychology interventions, cultivating flow experiences provides a powerful mechanism for reframing stress from a threat to be avoided into a challenge to be embraced and optimized.

Overall, with the abovementioned considerations, this chapter presents an innovative framework that combines the Stress Management Questionnaire (SMQ; Stein, 1986) with standardized anxiety and depression measures and evidence-based positive psychology interventions to create a comprehensive approach to stress that emphasizes human potential and flourishing. Specifically designed for occupational therapists and allied health professionals, this integrated model draws upon psychosocial occupational therapy principles (Stein & Cutler, 1998) and incorporates cutting-edge research on stress mindset (Crum et al., 2013, 2017) and post-traumatic growth (Hefferon, 2013; Tedeschi & Calhoun, 2004) to move beyond symptom reduction and actively cultivate the conditions necessary for sustained well-being and personal growth (Keyes, 2002; Seligman, 2011).

POSITIVE PSYCHOLOGY: THEORETICAL FOUNDATIONS AND STRESS APPLICATIONS

The Science of Well-Being and Stress Resilience

Positive psychology emerged as a scientific discipline dedicated to understanding what makes life worth living, shifting psychology's focus from merely repairing damage to building positive qualities and fostering human flourishing (Seligman & Csikszentmihalyi, 2000). This movement represented a fundamental reconceptualization of human nature, moving from a disease model that viewed people as passive victims of negative forces to a strengths-based model that recognizes humans as active agents capable of growth, resilience and self-actualization (Hart, 2021; Peterson & Park, 2003).

The theoretical foundations of positive psychology rest on extensive empirical research demonstrating that positive emotions, character strengths and meaningful relationships serve as powerful protective factors against stress and psychological distress (Boehm & Lyubomirsky, 2008; Fredrickson, 2001). The Broaden-and-Build Theory of Positive Emotions (Fredrickson, 2001) provides particularly compelling evidence for how positive emotional experiences expand individuals' thought-action repertoires and build enduring psychological resources that enhance stress resilience. When individuals experience positive emotions such as joy, gratitude, serenity and love, their awareness broadens, their creativity increases and their capacity to cope with adversity strengthens (Fredrickson & Joiner, 2002; Kok et al., 2013).

The classification system developed by Peterson and Seligman (2004) identifies fundamental positive attributes that promote optimal functioning across diverse cultural settings. Empirical evidence demonstrates that when individuals recognize and deliberately apply their most prominent strengths, they report elevated satisfaction with life, enhanced occupational involvement and superior stress regulation abilities (Proctor et al., 2011; Seligman et al., 2005). The VIA (Virtue in Action) Survey of Character Strengths has become a cornerstone assessment tool in positive psychology interventions, enabling individuals to recognize their unique constellation of strengths and leverage them in challenging situations (Peterson & Park, 2009).

Evidence-Based Positive Psychology Interventions for Stress

The empirical foundation for positive psychology interventions has grown exponentially, with meta-analytic studies demonstrating significant effects on well-being, life satisfaction and stress reduction across diverse populations (Bolier et al., 2013; Sin & Lyubomirsky, 2009; White et al., 2019). These interventions are designed not merely to alleviate negative symptoms but to actively cultivate positive emotions, meaningful relationships and purposeful engagement with life challenges.

Stress Mindset Interventions

One of the most significant advances in positive psychology approaches to stress management has emerged from the groundbreaking research of Alia Crum and colleagues at Stanford University's Mind and Body Lab. Their work on "stress mindset" demonstrates that how individuals think about stress fundamentally alters its impact on their psychological and physiological functioning (Crum et al., 2013, 2017). This research revealed that people generally hold one of two mindsets about stress: stress-is-enhancing or stress-is-debilitating, and these mindsets profoundly influence stress outcomes.

According to research by Crum and colleagues (2013, 2017), individuals who perceive stress as potentially beneficial tend to experience improved outcomes. This adaptive perspective frames stress responses as mechanisms that activate personal resources and facilitate skill development, contrasting sharply with views that characterize stress as purely detrimental. In contrast, the stress-is-debilitating mindset sees stress as inherently harmful, depleting and something to be avoided at all costs. Research consistently demonstrates that individuals with a stress-is-enhancing mindset show superior psychological and physiological responses to stressors, including increased anabolic hormone production, improved cognitive flexibility and better emotional regulation (Crum et al., 2017; Park et al., 2018).

Crum's three-phase intervention for developing a positive stress mindset provides occupational therapists with a practical framework for helping clients transform their relationship with stress (Crum et al., 2022). The first phase involves acknowledging stress by identifying current stressors and typical mental, physical and behavioral reactions. The second phase welcomes stress by recognizing that stress only occurs when we care about something meaningful, thereby identifying the underlying values and purposes that make situations stressful. The third phase uses stress by leveraging this understanding to transform typical stress reactions in ways that enhance rather than hinder personal values and goals.

Clinical applications of stress mindset interventions show remarkable promise for professional practice in occupational therapy. Research demonstrates that educational interventions on the positive effects of stress can alter brain wave patterns measured by EEG, confirming neurological changes that reduce stress's adverse effects (Park et al., 2018). Furthermore, stress mindset interventions have been successfully adapted for various populations, including healthcare workers experiencing pandemic-related stress (Emirza & Yılmaz Kozcu, 2023), individuals with chronic pain conditions (Heathcote et al., 2018) and employees facing workplace challenges (Hammond et al., 2021).

FLOW COMPONENTS AND STRESS TRANSFORMATION

The Nine Components of Flow and Their Role in Stress Leverage

Csikszentmihalyi's research identified nine core components of flow experiences that directly relate to how individuals can transform their relationship with stress (Csikszentmihalyi, 1990; Jackson & Marsh, 1996).

Clarity of objectives and progress monitoring. Activities conducive to optimal experience feature explicit aims with real-time performance indicators. When applied to stress management, practitioners help clients establish concrete, attainable targets for navigating challenging circumstances while implementing systems to evaluate their coping effectiveness (Csikszentmihalyi, 1990; Jackson & Marsh, 1996).

Balance between task demands and personal competence. Optimal experience requires careful alignment of environmental challenges with individual abilities. Applied to stress management, this principle involves progressively expanding clients' capacity for managing difficult circumstances while concurrently building requisite competencies. Through this method, stressors become opportunities for skill acquisition rather than overwhelming barriers (Csikszentmihalyi, 1990; Engeser & Rheinberg, 2008).

Focused awareness in the present. Achieving optimal states demands undivided attention and focus on current engagement. Within stress management contexts, cultivating moment-to-moment consciousness through mindfulness practices enables clients to direct their cognitive resources toward controllable aspects of their situation, thereby reducing preoccupation with anticipated difficulties or historical regrets (Garland et al., 2010; Kabat-Zinn, 2003).

Self-consciousness disappears. During flow, the critical inner voice quiets, and self-doubt diminishes. This component is particularly relevant for stress management, as it addresses the rumination and negative self-talk that often amplify stress responses. Positive psychology interventions that cultivate flow experiences help individuals move beyond self-critical thought patterns that exacerbate stress.

Time transformation. Flow experiences alter temporal perception, with time either speeding up or slowing down depending on the activity. This time distortion can be therapeutically valuable in stress management, as it provides relief from the time pressure and urgency that often characterize stressful experiences (Csikszentmihalyi, 1990).

The integration of flow principles with stress management interventions creates a paradigm where stress becomes a signal for potential growth and optimal experience rather than a threat to be eliminated. Research in occupational settings demonstrates that employees who approach workplace stressors with a flow-oriented mindset show improved performance, reduced burnout and greater job satisfaction compared to those using traditional stress reduction approaches (Bakker, 2008; Demerouti, 2006).

GRATITUDE INTERVENTIONS AND STRESS RESILIENCE

Gratitude interventions represent one of the most extensively researched categories of positive psychology practices. Empirical evidence demonstrates that systematic gratitude practices, including journaling exercises focused on appreciation, yield measurable benefits across multiple well-being domains, encompassing enhanced contentment, better physiological functioning, improved rest patterns and decreased stress indicators (Emmons & McCullough, 2003;

Seligman et al., 2005). More sophisticated gratitude interventions, such as gratitude letters and gratitude visits, demonstrate even stronger effects on well-being and relationship quality (Kumar & Epley, 2018; Toepfer et al., 2012). Recent research has revealed that gratitude practices work by shifting attention away from negative rumination and toward positive aspects of experience, creating upward spirals of positive emotion and improved coping (Fuller et al., 2025; Watkins et al., 2003).

Acts of kindness and interventions centered on prosocial behavior have proven especially effective for improving personal wellness and interpersonal bonds. Empirical findings indicate that engaging in benevolent actions toward others stimulates neural reward pathways, triggers beneficial neurochemical responses and produces sustained enhancements in affective states and overall contentment (Curry et al., 2018; Rowland & Curry, 2019). The psychological benefits of kindness extend beyond immediate mood enhancement to include reduced stress reactivity, improved immune function and greater sense of life purpose (Nelson et al., 2016; Post, 2005). Structured kindness interventions that encourage variety and social connection show particularly strong and sustained effects on well-being measures (Lyubomirsky et al., 2005; Sheldon & Lyubomirsky, 2006).

Mindfulness-based positive psychology interventions combine traditional mindfulness meditation practices with specific focus on cultivating positive mental states such as loving-kindness, appreciation and self-compassion. Research indicates that these integrated approaches produce superior outcomes compared to either mindfulness or positive psychology interventions alone, with participants showing significant improvements in stress management, emotional regulation and overall psychological well-being (Garland et al., 2010; Goldberg et al., 2018; Malouff & Schutte, 2020). The integration of mindfulness with positive psychology practices appears to create synergistic effects that enhance both present-moment awareness and future-oriented optimism.

AN INTEGRATED POSITIVE HEALTH MODEL FOR STRESS MANAGEMENT

Comprehensive Assessment through a Positive Lens: Occupational Therapy Applications

The integration of the Stress Management Questionnaire (SMQ; Stein, 1986) with standardized anxiety and depression measures within a positive psychology framework creates a comprehensive assessment approach that captures both areas of concern and existing strengths, perfectly aligned with occupational therapy's holistic approach to client care. This dual-focus assessment strategy, grounded in psychosocial occupational therapy principles (Stein & Cutler, 1998), recognizes that effective intervention must address not only what is wrong but also what is right with individuals experiencing stress (Clifton & Harter, 2003; Seligman, 2002).

Originally designed for clinical applications within occupational therapy contexts, the SMQ offers practitioners a structured approach to understanding clients' cognitive appraisals and behavioral reactions to everyday stressors, encompassing multiple dimensions of stress experience and coping patterns. The questionnaire's strength lies in its ability to capture the multidimensional nature of stress responses, including physical symptoms (headaches, sleep disruptions), interpersonal dynamics (conflicts, family tensions), environmental factors (work pressures, financial concerns) and coping strategies (both adaptive and maladaptive) that clients employ in their daily occupational performance.

When viewed through a positive psychology lens, SMQ responses can be understood not merely as adaptive or maladaptive coping strategies but as indicators of underlying character strengths and growth opportunities. For example, individuals who report using problem-solving approaches to stress may be demonstrating the character strength of prudence or perseverance, while those who seek social support may be exhibiting the strengths of social intelligence or love (Peterson & Seligman, 2004). This strengths-based interpretation of stress responses aligns with occupational therapy's commitment to client-centered practice and the recognition of individual capabilities and resources.

The clinical applications of the SMQ in occupational therapy settings have been well-documented through case studies and intervention research. Stein and Nikolic (1989) demonstrated the effectiveness of systematic stress management approaches with individuals experiencing severe mental illness, while Stein and Smith (1989) showed positive outcomes when implementing structured stress management programs with acutely depressed inpatients. These studies highlight the SMQ's utility in both assessment and intervention planning within occupational therapy practice.

Anxiety and depression measures, such as the Hospital Anxiety and Depression Scale (HADS; Zigmond & Snaith, 1983) or the Kessler Psychological Distress Scale (K10; Kessler et al., 2002), provide essential information about symptom severity and functional impairment that directly impacts occupational performance. However, within a positive health framework, these measures also serve as baseline indicators for tracking improvements in well-being and flourishing that extend beyond mere symptom reduction. Research demonstrates that individuals can experience significant reductions in anxiety and depression while simultaneously developing greater life satisfaction, meaning and positive emotion through targeted positive psychology interventions (Chakhssi et al., 2018; Fava et al., 2005).

The integration of traditional stress and mental health assessments with positive psychology measures creates a comprehensive evaluation framework that captures both areas of concern and existing strengths and resources. This dual-focus approach recognizes that effective intervention requires understanding not only what challenges individuals face but also what capacities they possess for addressing those challenges (Lopez & Snyder, 2009; Peterson & Park, 2003). For occupational therapists, this comprehensive assessment approach provides the foundation for developing intervention plans that address both symptom reduction and capacity building, consistent with the profession's focus on promoting health, well-being and participation in life through engagement in occupation.

Tailored Positive Psychology Intervention Protocols

The development of personalized positive psychology intervention protocols requires careful consideration of individual strengths, preferences, cultural background and specific stress-related challenges. Research indicates that intervention effectiveness is significantly enhanced when activities are matched to individual characteristics and delivered in culturally sensitive ways (Hendriks et al., 2019; Parks & Boucher, 2020). This personalization process begins with comprehensive strength identification using validated assessments such as the VIA Survey of Character Strengths, followed by collaborative selection of interventions that align with individual strengths and values.

For individuals whose stress primarily manifests through worry and rumination, interventions that cultivate present-moment awareness and optimistic thinking show particular effectiveness. The Best Possible Self intervention, which involves writing about and visualizing an optimal future, has demonstrated significant effects on reducing anxiety and increasing hope and positive expectations (King, 2001; Meevissen et al., 2011).

Individuals experiencing stress-related social withdrawal and isolation benefit particularly from relationship-focused positive psychology interventions. Active-constructive responding training teaches individuals to respond to others' good news in ways that strengthen relationships and build social resources (Gable et al., 2004; Reis & Gable, 2015). Loving-kindness meditation practices expand compassion and social connection while reducing stress-related inflammation and improving immune function (Klimecki et al., 2013; Pace et al., 2009). These interventions work synergistically to rebuild social support networks that serve as powerful buffers against future stress exposure.

Cultivating Flow Experiences as Stress Management Interventions

The systematic cultivation of flow experiences provides a unique avenue for transforming stress responses within professional practice in occupational therapy. Unlike traditional stress management approaches that focus primarily on relaxation and stress reduction, flow-based interventions actively engage individuals with challenging situations in ways that promote growth, mastery and intrinsic satisfaction (Csikszentmihalyi, 1997; Nakamura & Csikszentmihalyi, 2014).

Progressive challenge mapping. This intervention involves systematically identifying activities or situations that match an individual's current skill level while providing optimal challenge. Clients work with therapists to create "challenge ladders" that progressively increase in difficulty while ensuring that each step remains within the individual's zone of proximal development. For example, someone experiencing social anxiety might begin with brief, structured social interactions before progressing to more complex social situations. The key is maintaining the delicate balance between challenge and skill that characterizes flow states (Stavrou et al., 2015).

Skill development protocols. Flow theory emphasizes that optimal experience requires not just appropriate challenges but also the continuous development of relevant skills. Flow-based stress management interventions include systematic skill-building components that prepare individuals to meet increasing challenges with confidence and competence. This might involve teaching specific coping techniques, communication skills, problem-solving strategies or emotional regulation methods that directly address the types of stressors individuals encounter (Engeser & Rheinberg, 2008).

Attention training exercises. Since flow requires complete concentration on the task at hand, interventions often include mindfulness and attention training components. These exercises help individuals develop the capacity to maintain focus on relevant aspects of challenging situations while filtering out distracting thoughts or environmental factors. Research demonstrates that attention training not only facilitates flow experiences but also reduces stress reactivity and improves emotional regulation (Lutz et al., 2008; Moore & Malinowski, 2009).

Intrinsic motivation enhancement. Flow experiences are characterized by intrinsic rather than extrinsic motivation – individuals engage in activities for their inherent satisfaction rather than external rewards. Flow-based stress management interventions help clients identify the intrinsic values and meanings within challenging situations. For instance, a healthcare worker experiencing burnout might reconnect with the inherent satisfaction of helping others, transforming workplace stress into meaningful engagement (Bakker & van Wingerden, 2021; Ryan & Deci, 2000).

Environmental optimization. Flow research emphasizes the importance of environmental factors in facilitating optimal experience. Interventions include strategies for modifying physical, social, and organizational environments to support flow states. This might involve eliminating unnecessary distractions, creating clear boundaries around focused work time or establishing social support systems that encourage risk-taking and growth (Csikszentmihalyi, 1990).

The integration of flow-based interventions with SMQ assessment data provides a powerful framework for personalized stress management. Individuals whose SMQ profiles indicate avoidance-based coping strategies may benefit particularly from progressive challenge mapping that gradually increases their confidence in facing difficult situations. Those showing patterns of overwhelm and anxiety might benefit most from attention training and environmental optimization interventions that help them focus on manageable aspects of stressful situations.

Implementation and Integration Strategies

Successful implementation of integrated positive psychology approaches to stress management requires systematic attention to intervention delivery, progress monitoring and sustainable behavior change. Research indicates that positive psychology interventions are most effective when delivered through structured programs that combine initial assessment, psychoeducation, skill-building exercises, practice opportunities and ongoing support (Seligman et al., 2005; Sin & Lyubomirsky, 2009).

The timing and sequencing of interventions appear crucial for maximizing effectiveness and preventing intervention fatigue. Meta-analytic research suggests that interventions delivered over periods of one to three months with regular practice requirements show superior long-term outcomes compared to single-session interventions or extended programs that exceed participants' motivation and capacity (Bolier et al., 2013; White et al., 2019). Progressive intervention models that begin with simple, easily implemented practices and gradually introduce more complex activities demonstrate enhanced participant engagement and sustained behavior change.

Technology-enhanced delivery platforms have emerged as particularly promising vehicles for positive psychology intervention implementation. Online and mobile applications allow for real-time practice reminders, progress tracking, social sharing capabilities and personalized feedback that enhance intervention adherence and effectiveness (Gander et al., 2018; Parks & Boucher, 2020). Research indicates that technology-delivered positive psychology interventions can achieve effect sizes comparable to face-to-face delivery while offering enhanced accessibility and scalability.

POST-TRAUMATIC STRESS AND GROWTH: TRANSFORMING ADVERSITY IN OCCUPATIONAL THERAPY PRACTICE

Understanding Post-Traumatic Stress Disorder (PTSD) through a Positive Health Lens

Post-traumatic stress disorder (PTSD) represents one of the most challenging mental health conditions that occupational therapists encounter in practice. PTSD is a complex condition that arises following exposure to or witnessing deeply distressing events, manifesting through symptoms including flashbacks, nightmares, intense anxiety, intrusive thoughts and significant functional impairments that disrupt daily activities and overall well-being. Traditional approaches to PTSD have focused primarily on symptom reduction and trauma processing, but the positive health framework offers additional pathways for promoting recovery and growth beyond the trauma experience.

The integration of positive psychology principles with PTSD treatment represents a paradigm shift that acknowledges both the devastating impact of trauma and the potential for profound growth and transformation. This approach does not minimize the severity of PTSD symptoms or suggest that positive thinking alone can resolve trauma-related difficulties. Rather, it recognizes that individuals possess inherent capacities for resilience, meaning-making and post-traumatic growth that can be systematically cultivated alongside traditional trauma-focused interventions.

Research demonstrates that lifestyle medicine interventions show particular promise for PTSD treatment. Exercise interventions have emerged as especially effective treatments for individuals with PTSD, offering both physiological and psychological benefits that complement traditional therapeutic approaches (Rosenbaum et al., 2015). Given the increased cardiovascular risks associated with PTSD, comprehensive lifestyle medicine programs that address sleep, exercise, nutrition and stress management provide holistic approaches that target both trauma symptoms and overall health outcomes (Kibler et al., 2023).

Post-Traumatic Growth: The Science of Thriving After Adversity

Post-traumatic growth (PTG) represents one of the most compelling areas of positive psychology research, challenging the assumption that trauma inevitably leads to lasting psychological damage. This form of growth describes transformative psychological developments that may follow intense struggle with difficult life circumstances. Rather than simply returning to baseline functioning, individuals experiencing PTG often report substantive shifts in their worldview, relationships and sense of purpose that extend beyond pre-trauma levels (Tedeschi & Calhoun, 2004).

The concept of PTG encompasses five key domains that the majority of trauma survivors experience to varying degrees. The domains of post-traumatic growth include:

Expanded life trajectories. Trauma survivors often identify previously unrecognized opportunities, prompting major lifestyle modifications, including professional shifts or engagement in novel pursuits.

Enhanced interpersonal connections. Many individuals report stronger empathetic capacity, more robust social networks and heightened motivation to support others facing comparable adversities (Tedeschi et al., 1998).

Personal strength. Survivors experience recognition and development of inner resilience, courage and self-efficacy, often accompanied by increased confidence in facing future challenges.

Spiritual change. Trauma survivors reevaluate beliefs and values to find meaning and purpose within suffering, frequently leading to deeper spiritual or existential understanding.

Appreciation of life. This involves increased awareness and gratitude for life's beauty and simple pleasures, fostering enhanced mindfulness and meaning-finding in everyday experiences.

It is crucial to understand that PTG does not necessarily eliminate distress or guarantee increased happiness; significant growth often coexists with substantial subjective distress (Tedeschi et al., 1998). The objective of PTG is not to restore individuals to their pre-trauma state but to facilitate transformation that enriches their lives with greater purpose, meaning and fulfillment. Research indicates that PTG is a natural adjustment process experienced by the majority of trauma survivors, suggesting that growth represents a fundamental human response to adversity rather than an exceptional outcome.

Flow States as Catalysts for Post-Traumatic Growth

The intersection of flow theory and post-traumatic growth reveals how individuals can transform traumatic experiences into opportunities for optimal functioning and enhanced well-being. Research demonstrates that the capacity to experience flow states plays a crucial role in determining whether individuals develop PTSD symptoms or experience post-traumatic growth following adverse events (Joseph, 2011; Tedeschi & Calhoun, 2004).

Flow and meaning-making. One of the core mechanisms through which flow facilitates post-traumatic growth is through enhanced meaning-making processes. A primary pathway through which immersive engagement promotes growth following trauma involves strengthened capacity for constructing personal significance. When experiencing optimal states, individuals frequently describe heightened awareness of transcendent connections and greater clarity regarding their core values and priorities (Csikszentmihalyi, 1990). For trauma survivors, cultivating flow experiences provides a pathway for reconstructing meaning and purpose in the aftermath of adverse events. Activities that promote flow, whether creative pursuits, physical challenges or service to others, create opportunities for individuals to discover new meanings and purposes that may not have emerged without the catalyst of traumatic experience (Hefferon et al., 2009).

Skill development through challenge. Post-traumatic growth often involves the development of new coping skills, enhanced relationships and increased appreciation for life. Flow theory's emphasis on the progressive matching of challenges to skills provides a framework for systematic growth following trauma. Rather than avoiding reminders of traumatic events, flow-based approaches help individuals gradually re-engage with challenging situations in ways that build confidence and mastery. This progressive exposure occurs within the safety of flow states, where individuals feel capable and in control rather than overwhelmed and helpless (Kilmer, 2006).

Embodied recovery and corporeal flow. For individuals experiencing corporeal post-traumatic growth, namely transformative changes in their relationship with their bodies following trauma, flow experiences offer particularly powerful healing opportunities. Physical activities that promote flow states, such as yoga, martial arts, dance or outdoor adventures, help trauma survivors reconnect with their bodies as sources of strength and pleasure rather than vulnerability and pain. Research demonstrates that embodied flow experiences can restore a sense of agency and competence in individuals whose trauma involved physical injury or violation (Hefferon, 2012; van der Kolk, 2014).

Social flow and relationship enhancement. Many flow experiences occur in social contexts, and the cultivation of "social flow" can be particularly valuable for trauma survivors whose ability to trust and connect with others has been compromised. Collaborative activities that promote flow – team sports, group music-making, community service projects – provide safe contexts for rebuilding social connections and developing the enhanced empathy and compassion that characterize post-traumatic growth (Csikszentmihalyi, 1997; Walker, 2010).

Corporeal Post-Traumatic Growth in Occupational Therapy

A particularly relevant concept for occupational therapists is corporeal post-traumatic growth, which refers to transformative changes within an individual's physical being following trauma that affects their relationship with their body (Hefferon, 2012). This concept is especially pertinent for individuals who have experienced medical trauma, accidents, chronic illness diagnoses or other physical health challenges that fundamentally alter their embodied experience. Embodied or corporeal PTG manifests through multiple dimensions that correspond directly to occupational therapy's emphasis on functional performance and life quality. These transformations include:

Reconceptualized body-self connection. Individuals often develop heightened self-kindness, acknowledge corporeal constraints without judgment and adopt more deliberate approaches to physical engagement.

Amplified health consciousness. Increased awareness of bodily needs commonly prompts intentional modifications in health behaviors, including nutritional improvements, addiction cessation and enhanced self-maintenance routines (Hefferon, 2012; van der Kolk, 2014).

For occupational therapists, corporeal PTG provides a framework for understanding how clients can transform their relationship with their bodies following illness, injury or disability. Rather than focusing solely on restoration of previous function, this approach emphasizes the potential for developing new ways of being in and with the body that may ultimately prove more sustainable, meaningful and health-promoting than pre-trauma patterns.

Facilitating Post-Traumatic Growth in Practice

Several evidence-based factors contribute to the promotion of PTG that occupational therapists can incorporate into their practice approaches. Individuals who engage in adaptive emotional processing, including the sharing of both positive and negative emotions about their trauma experience, tend to demonstrate higher levels of growth. The use of positive coping strategies such as benefit finding, meaning-making, and positive reappraisal facilitates PTG development, as does the cultivation of social support networks and the maintenance of realistic optimism about the future.

Benefit-Finding Interventions

One of the most practical interventions for facilitating PTG is benefit finding, which involves the systematic exploration of positive changes, insights or developments that have emerged from traumatic experiences. This intervention can be adapted for use with individuals experiencing various forms of adversity, including chronic illness, acute medical events, accidents or other life-disrupting circumstances.

The benefit-finding process involves structured reflection on how traumatic or adverse experiences have contributed to personal development, enhanced coping capabilities or created new opportunities for growth and meaning. Practitioners guide clients through structured reflection using prompts such as, "In what ways has navigating this difficulty contributed to your personal development?" and "What new capabilities for managing adversity have emerged from this experience?" This exploration is conducted with careful attention to timing, client readiness and the integration of both the difficulties and the growth that may have emerged from the experience.

Research has demonstrated that benefit-finding interventions can be effectively implemented across diverse populations and settings, showing particular promise for individuals dealing with medical trauma, chronic pain conditions and other health-related adversities that frequently present in professional practice in occupational therapy (King & Miner, 2000; Tennen & Affleck, 2005).

Integrating PTG with Occupational Therapy Practice

The integration of post-traumatic growth principles with occupational therapy practice requires careful attention to timing, client readiness and the therapeutic relationship. PTG interventions are most effective when implemented after initial stabilization and when clients demonstrate readiness to explore growth-oriented perspectives on their experiences. These interventions complement rather than replace trauma-focused treatments and should be integrated within comprehensive care approaches that address both symptoms and growth potential.

For occupational therapists, PTG provides a valuable framework for understanding client resilience and for designing interventions that promote not just functional recovery but meaningful transformation. This approach recognizes that the goal of therapy extends beyond returning clients to their previous level of functioning to include the possibility of discovering new capacities, meanings and ways of engaging with life that may ultimately prove more fulfilling and sustainable than pre-trauma patterns.

LIFESTYLE TRANSFORMATION THROUGH POSITIVE PSYCHOLOGY

Daily Practices and Sustainable Change

The transformation of lifestyle responses to stress through positive psychology requires systematic attention to daily practices that gradually shift automatic patterns of thinking, feeling and behaving. Research has demonstrated that sustainable change occurs through the accumulation of small, consistent actions rather than dramatic interventions, making daily positive psychology practices particularly well-suited for stress management applications (Lyubomirsky et al., 2005; Sheldon & Lyubomirsky, 2006).

Morning gratitude practices have shown remarkable effectiveness in setting a positive trajectory for daily stress management. Research indicates that beginning each day with gratitude reflection or journaling primes the cognitive system to notice and appreciate positive aspects of experience throughout the day, creating natural stress-buffering effects (Emmons & McCullough, 2003; Watkins et al., 2003). These practices work by activating positive emotion networks in the brain that broaden attention and enhance creative problem-solving capacities when stressful situations arise (Fredrickson, 2001; Isen, 2000).

Evening reflection practices that focus on identifying daily strengths usage, meaningful moments and acts of kindness create powerful consolidation effects that transform stress experiences into opportunities for growth and learning. The "Three Good Things" intervention, which involves writing about positive events and one's role in creating them, has demonstrated significant effects on reducing depression and increasing life satisfaction that persist for months after initial implementation (Mongrain & Anselmo-Matthews, 2012; Seligman et al., 2005). When integrated with stress management goals, these reflection practices help individuals recognize their agency in creating positive experiences even within challenging circumstances.

Physical Health and Positive Psychology Integration

Combining positive psychology principles with health-promoting behaviors generates complementary benefits that simultaneously strengthen stress resistance and holistic wellness. Empirical investigations reveal that constructive emotional states and hopeful cognitive orientations support enhanced immune system functioning, decreased inflammatory responses, superior cardiac health and extended lifespan (Boehm & Lyubomirsky, 2008; Chida & Steptoe, 2008; Diener & Chan, 2011).

Physical activity programs infused with positive psychology components demonstrate amplified efficacy relative to conventional exercise regimens. Interventions such as appreciation-focused walking, where participants consciously acknowledge environmental beauty and bodily capabilities during movement yield heightened benefits for emotional states, stress mitigation and sustained participation (Emmons & Mishra, 2011; Nezlek, 2001). Group exercise programs that emphasize social connection, shared accomplishment and mutual encouragement create positive feedback loops that sustain both physical activity and psychological well-being over time.

Nutrition practices guided by positive psychology principles focus on appreciation, mindful consumption and the social aspects of eating rather than restriction and deprivation. Research indicates that individuals who approach healthy eating from a self-compassionate, strengths-based perspective show greater long-term success in maintaining nutritional goals and lower levels of food-related stress and anxiety (Bacon & Aphramor, 2011; Tylka & Homan, 2015). Mindful eating practices that emphasize gratitude for food, awareness of hunger and satiety cues and appreciation for the social connections created through shared meals demonstrate significant effects on both physical health and psychological well-being.

Social Connection and Community Building

Developing supportive interpersonal bonds constitutes a fundamental element of evidence-based stress management within positive psychology frameworks. Converging research findings confirm that people maintaining robust social networks display superior stress resistance, accelerated recovery trajectories following difficulties and elevated wellness and contentment indicators (Holt-Lunstad et al., 2010; Umberson & Montez, 2010). Positive psychology interventions that focus on building and strengthening relationships create powerful protective factors against stress-related mental health challenges.

Active listening and empathy training programs teach individuals to engage with others in ways that build connection and mutual support. Research indicates that individuals who develop strong active listening skills experience reduced interpersonal stress, greater relationship satisfaction and enhanced sense of meaning and purpose (Gable & Reis, 2010; Reis & Gable, 2015). These skills become particularly valuable during times of stress when social support serves as a critical resource for coping and recovery.

Civic participation and service-oriented activities serve as potent positive psychology strategies that concurrently diminish stress responses while strengthening interpersonal networks. Evidence indicates that those consistently involved in charitable work exhibit decreased stress sensitivity, enhanced psychological functioning and more pronounced sense of existential meaning relative to individuals not engaged in such activities (Jenkinson et al., 2013; Thoits & Hewitt, 2001). The psychological benefits of helping others appear to arise through multiple pathways, including enhanced self-efficacy, expanded social networks, increased meaning and purpose and the activation of reward centers in the brain associated with positive emotions.

ASSESSMENT INTEGRATION AND PROGRESS MONITORING

Comprehensive Evaluation Frameworks

The integration of traditional stress and mental health assessments with positive psychology measures creates a comprehensive evaluation framework that captures both areas of concern and existing strengths and resources. This dual-focus approach recognizes that effective intervention requires understanding not only what challenges individuals face but also what capacities they possess for addressing those challenges (Lopez & Snyder, 2009; Peterson & Park, 2003).

Traditional measures such as the Stress Management Questionnaire (SMQ; Stein, 1986), Hospital Anxiety and Depression Scale (HADS; Zigmond & Snaith, 1983) and Perceived Stress Scale (PSS; Cohen et al., 1983) provide essential information about symptom severity, functional impairment, and stress perception. These measures serve as important baseline indicators and progress monitoring tools that track reductions in distress over time. However, within a positive psychology framework, these assessments are complemented by measures that capture growth in positive functioning and well-being.

Kern and colleagues' (2015) PERMA assessment instrument offers systematic evaluation across the five well-being dimensions central to Seligman's theoretical framework: affective positivity, absorption in activities, interpersonal connections, purposeful living and achievement. Empirical work confirms that enhancements across these areas may emerge separate from symptom amelioration, rendering positive functioning metrics crucial for documenting comprehensive intervention outcomes (Keyes, 2005; Westerhof & Keyes, 2010). The VIA Survey of Character Strengths (Peterson & Seligman, 2004) identifies individuals' signature strengths and provides a foundation for strengths-based intervention planning and progress monitoring.

Longitudinal Tracking and Outcome Measurement

Successful implementation of positive psychology stress management necessitates methodical monitoring of both distress decrease and wellness augmentation across extended timeframes. Scientific evidence suggests that positive psychology interventions frequently demonstrate temporal lag effects, with benefits materializing and intensifying during subsequent weeks or months post-initiation, thus rendering extended assessment periods vital for documenting authentic intervention impact (Seligman et al., 2005; Sin & Lyubomirsky, 2009).

Weekly brief assessments using validated measures such as the PANAS (Watson & Clark, 1988) for positive and negative affect, single-item life satisfaction scales and brief stress ratings provide efficient tracking of intervention effects without creating assessment burden. These frequent measurements allow for real-time intervention adjustments and help maintain participant motivation by providing visible evidence of progress over time.

Monthly comprehensive assessments using the full battery of stress, anxiety, depression and well-being measures provide more detailed information about intervention effects and guide long-term treatment planning. Research demonstrates that individuals who engage in regular self-monitoring show enhanced intervention effects and greater sustained behavior change compared to those who receive interventions without systematic progress tracking (Harkin et al., 2016; Korotitsch & Nelson-Gray, 1999).

Flow Assessment Integration with SMQ and Well-being Measures

The systematic assessment of flow experiences provides a valuable complement to traditional stress and mental health measures in professional practice in occupational therapy. The Flow Short Scale (FSS; Rheinberg et al., 2003) and the Dispositional Flow Scale-2 (DFS-2; Jackson & Eklund, 2002) offer validated instruments for measuring both state and trait aspects of flow that can be integrated with SMQ and anxiety/depression assessments to create comprehensive evaluation profiles.

Flow assessment components. The FSS measures the nine components of flow during specific activities, providing insights into which aspects of optimal experience individuals access readily and which require development. When combined with SMQ data, flow assessments reveal whether individuals have identified activities that provide optimal challenge-skill balance or whether their current coping strategies consistently under-challenge or overwhelm their capabilities (Engeser & Rheinberg, 2008).

Longitudinal flow tracking. Regular assessment of flow experiences throughout intervention provides valuable feedback about the effectiveness of stress management approaches. Individuals who show increases in flow frequency and intensity typically demonstrate corresponding improvements in stress resilience and well-being measures. This tracking can be accomplished through brief daily flow ratings combined with periodic comprehensive assessments (Csikszentmihalyi & Larson, 1987).

Flow obstacles assessment. Understanding barriers to flow provides crucial information for intervention planning. Common flow obstacles include perfectionism, external pressure, unclear goals, inadequate feedback and mismatched challenge-skill ratios. Assessment protocols that identify these barriers enable targeted interventions that remove obstacles to optimal experience while building conditions that support flow states (Jackson et al., 2001).

The integration of flow assessment with positive psychology measures creates opportunities for strength-based intervention planning that builds upon individuals' existing capacities for optimal experience while addressing areas where flow is blocked or limited.

CULTURAL CONSIDERATIONS AND ADAPTATION

Cross-Cultural Validity and Adaptation

The implementation of positive psychology approaches to stress management requires careful attention to cultural context, values and meaning systems that influence how individuals experience and express both distress and well-being. Research demonstrates significant cultural variation in the conceptualization of positive emotions, social relationships and life satisfaction, necessitating thoughtful adaptation of interventions to align with diverse cultural perspectives (Diener et al., 2003; Kitayama & Markus, 2000).

Cultural contexts emphasizing collective values typically prioritize familial cohesion, communal responsibilities and interdependent flourishing, contrasting with individualistic societies that elevate personal accomplishment and independent satisfaction. When tailoring positive psychology approaches for collectivist populations, practitioners emphasize relational enhancement, household-level appreciation exercises and communal contributions rather than self-focused interventions (Kitayama & Park, 2007; Uchida et al., 2004).

Religious and spiritual frameworks also provide important context for understanding how individuals conceptualize meaning, purpose and transcendence within positive psychology approaches. Interventions that incorporate prayer, meditation, spiritual gratitude and service to others aligned with religious teachings show enhanced effectiveness for individuals with strong spiritual commitments (McCullough & Willoughby, 2009; Watlington & Murphy, 2006). The integration of positive psychology with existing spiritual practices creates natural bridges that enhance intervention acceptance and long-term adherence.

COMMUNITY-BASED IMPLEMENTATION MODELS

The translation of positive psychology approaches from research settings to community applications requires attention to accessibility, cultural relevance and sustainable delivery systems. Community-based implementation models that train local leaders, integrate with existing social service systems and adapt to community resources and constraints show enhanced reach and sustainability compared to researcher-delivered interventions (Glasgow et al., 2019; Proctor et al., 2011).

School-based positive psychology programs represent particularly promising models for community implementation due to their ability to reach large numbers of individuals during formative developmental periods. Research demonstrates that school-based positive psychology curricula that focus on character strength development, gratitude practices and social-emotional learning show significant effects on student well-being, academic performance and stress resilience (Adler, 2017; Seligman et al., 2009; White & Waters, 2015). These programs create positive ripple effects that extend to families and communities as students share practices and perspectives learned through school-based interventions.

Workplace positive psychology programs offer another valuable community implementation model that can reach adults during peak stress periods of their lives. Research indicates that workplace interventions focusing on character strengths, gratitude and meaningful work show significant effects on employee well-being, job satisfaction and stress management while also benefiting organizational outcomes such as productivity and retention (Cameron et al., 2003; Peterson et al., 2010; Seligman & Schulman, 1986). The integration of positive psychology with existing employee wellness programs creates comprehensive approaches that address both stress reduction and well-being enhancement.

FUTURE DIRECTIONS AND EMERGING RESEARCH

Technology-Enhanced Interventions

The rapid advancement of digital technology platforms has created unprecedented opportunities for delivering personalized, accessible and scalable positive psychology interventions for stress management. Mobile applications that provide real-time intervention delivery, progress tracking, social connection and adaptive feedback represent the cutting edge of positive psychology implementation research (Lyubomirsky & Layous, 2013; Parks & Boucher, 2020).

Computational intelligence technologies and algorithmic learning systems demonstrate potential for generating customized intervention prescriptions derived from individual trait profiles, preference patterns and response histories. Emerging research suggests that algorithmically driven positive psychology platforms may produce therapeutic effects approximating those of clinician-administered programs while simultaneously improving availability and decreasing implementation expenses (Gander et al., 2018; Mohr et al., 2017).

Virtual and augmented reality technologies offer exciting possibilities for creating immersive positive psychology experiences that enhance traditional intervention approaches. Preliminary research suggests that VR-delivered gratitude experiences, virtual nature exposures and immersive loving-kindness practices may produce stronger and more sustained effects compared to traditional delivery methods (Anderson et al., 2017; Riva et al., 2019). The ability to create controlled, engaging and repeatable positive experiences through virtual environments represents a significant advancement in positive psychology intervention technology.

Precision Medicine Approaches

The emerging field of precision medicine offers promising directions for personalizing positive psychology interventions based on genetic, neurobiological and individual difference factors that influence intervention response. Research is beginning to identify genetic polymorphisms and neural markers that predict differential response to various positive psychology practices, creating possibilities for truly personalized intervention prescription (Fredrickson et al., 2013; Haas et al., 2016).

Neuroimaging research has revealed distinct brain activation patterns associated with different positive psychology interventions, providing insights into mechanisms of action and individual variation in response. Studies using fMRI and EEG demonstrate that gratitude practices, loving-kindness meditation and character strengths interventions activate different neural networks and produce distinct patterns of brain change over time (Fox et al., 2016; Kini et al., 2016). This neurobiological research creates opportunities for matching interventions to individual neural profiles and optimizing intervention effectiveness through precision targeting.

Pharmacogenomic research is exploring how genetic variations in neurotransmitter systems may influence response to positive psychology interventions either alone or in combination with psychotropic medications. Preliminary findings suggest that individuals with certain genetic profiles may show enhanced responses to specific positive psychology practices, while others may benefit more from combined approaches that integrate medication with positive psychology interventions (Geschwind et al., 2019; Khazanov & Ruscio, 2016).

SUMMARY

The integration of positive psychology approaches with traditional stress management represents a fundamental paradigm shift that moves beyond symptom reduction toward the active cultivation of human flourishing and resilience. This comprehensive approach recognizes that individuals possess inherent capacities for growth, meaning-making and positive adaptation that can be systematically developed through evidence-based interventions. The combination of the Stress Management Questionnaire, standardized anxiety and depression measures and carefully selected positive psychology interventions creates a robust framework for assessment, intervention and progress monitoring that addresses both areas of concern and existing strengths. Research consistently demonstrates that positive psychology interventions produce significant and sustained improvements in well-being, life satisfaction, and stress resilience across diverse populations and settings. The cultivation of positive emotions, character strengths, meaningful relationships and purposeful engagement creates upward spirals of positive functioning that enhance quality of life and protect against future stress-related difficulties. By combining rigorous assessment with evidence-based positive psychology interventions, occupational therapists can help individuals not only cope with stress but also transform challenging experiences into opportunities for growth, connection and deeper life satisfaction. This paradigm shift from pathology to potential represents a fundamental advancement in understanding human resilience and promoting flourishing in the face of adversity.

DISCUSSION QUESTIONS

1. How does the positive psychology approach to stress management differ from traditional deficit-focused models, and what are the implications of this paradigm shift for occupational therapy practice?
2. Reflect on a time when you experienced a flow state. What conditions enabled that experience, and how might you intentionally cultivate similar conditions for clients dealing with stress?
3. Consider Alia Crum's stress mindset theory (stress-is-enhancing versus stress-is-debilitating). How might your own beliefs about stress influence the way you assess and intervene with clients experiencing stress-related challenges?
4. How can occupational therapists balance (1) acknowledging the reality of clients' distress while simultaneously (2) recognizing and building upon their existing strengths and capacities for growth?

5. Reflect on the concept of post-traumatic growth. How might you recognize when a client is ready to explore growth-oriented perspectives following trauma, and what ethical considerations should guide this process?
6. How does corporeal post-traumatic growth align with occupational therapy's emphasis on embodied experience and functional performance? What implications does this have for clients recovering from physical illness or injury?
7. Consider the nine components of flow experiences described in the chapter. How might you systematically assess and remove obstacles to flow in your clients' daily occupations?
8. What cultural considerations should occupational therapists reflect upon when implementing positive psychology interventions, particularly when working with clients from collectivistic versus individualistic cultural backgrounds?
9. How can occupational therapists integrate positive psychology interventions into their practice without minimizing or invalidating clients' legitimate struggles with mental health symptoms or life adversities?

REFERENCES

Adler, A. (2017). Teaching well-being increases academic performance: Evidence from Bhutan, Mexico, and Peru. *Dissertation Abstracts International Section A: Humanities and Social Sciences*, 78(4–A(E)), 1–89.

American Psychological Association. (2017). *Ethical principles of psychologists and code of conduct.* Retrieved from https://www.apa.org

Anderson, A. P., Mayer, M. D., Fellows, A. M., Cowan, D. R., Hegel, M. T., & Buckey, J. C. (2017). Relaxation with immersive natural scenes presented using virtual reality. *Aerospace Medicine and Human Performance*, *88*(6), 520–526. https://doi.org/10.3357/amhp.4747.2017

Bacon, L., & Aphramor, L. (2011). Weight science: Evaluating the evidence for a paradigm shift. *Nutrition Journal*, *10*(1), 9–13. https://doi.org/10.1201/b16308-26

Bakker, A. B. (2008). The work-related flow inventory: Construction and initial validation of the WOLF. *Journal of Vocational Behavior*, *72*(3), 400–414. https://doi.org/10.1016/j.jvb.2007.11.007

Bakker, A. B., & van Wingerden, J. (2021). Do personal resources and strengths use increase work engagement? The effects of a training intervention. *Journal of Occupational Health Psychology*, *26*(1), 20–30. https://doi.org/10.1037/ocp0000266

Boehm, J. K., & Lyubomirsky, S. (2008). Does happiness promote career success? *Journal of Career Assessment*, *16*(1), 101–116. https://doi.org/10.1177/1069072707308140

Bolier, L., Haverman, M., Westerhof, G. J., Riper, H., Smit, F., & Bohlmeijer, E. (2013). Positive psychology interventions: A meta-analysis of randomized controlled studies. *BMC Public Health*, *13*(1), 119. https://doi.org/10.1186/1471-2458-13-119

Cameron, K. S., Dutton, J. E., & Quinn, R. E. (Eds.). (2003). *Positive organizational scholarship: Foundations of a new discipline*. Berrett-Koehler Publishers.

Chakhssi, F., Kraiss, J. T., Sommers-Spijkerman, M., & Bohlmeijer, E. T. (2018). The effect of positive psychology interventions on well-being and distress in clinical samples with psychiatric or somatic disorders: A systematic review and meta-analysis. *BMC Psychiatry*, *18*(1), 211. https://doi.org/10.1186/s12888-018-1739-2

Chida, Y., & Steptoe, A. (2008). Positive psychological well-being and mortality: A quantitative review of prospective observational studies. *Psychosomatic Medicine*, *70*(7), 741–756. https://doi.org/10.1097/psy.0b013e31818105ba

Clifton, D. O., & Harter, J. K. (2003). Investing in strengths. In K. S. Cameron, J. E. Dutton, & R. E. Quinn (Eds.), *Positive organizational scholarship* (pp. 111–121). Berrett-Koehler Publishers.

Cohen, S., Kamarck, T., & Mermelstein, R. (1983). A global measure of perceived stress. *Journal of Health and Social Behavior*, *24*(4), 385–396. https://doi.org/10.2307/2136404

Csikszentmihalyi, M. (1990). *Flow: The psychology of optimal experience*. Harper & Row.

Csikszentmihalyi, M. (1997). *Finding flow: The psychology of engagement with everyday life*. Basic Books.

Csikszentmihalyi, M., & Larson, R. (1987). Validity and reliability of the experience-sampling method. *Journal of Nervous and Mental Disease*, *175*(9), 526–536. https://doi.org/10.1097/00005053-198709000-00004

Crum, A. J., Akinola, M., Martin, A., & Fath, S. (2017). The role of stress mindset in shaping cognitive, emotional, and physiological responses to challenging and threatening stress. *Anxiety, Stress, & Coping*, *30*(4), 379–395. https://doi.org/10.1080/10615806.2016.1275585

Crum, A. J., Salovey, P., & Achor, S. (2013). Rethinking stress: The role of mindsets in determining the stress response. *Journal of Personality and Social Psychology*, *104*(4), 716–733. https://doi.org/10.1037/a0031201

Crum, A. J., Santoro, E., Handley-Miner, I., Smith, E. N., Evans, K., Moraveji, N., … & Salovey, P. (2022). Evaluation of the "rethink stress" mindset intervention: A metacognitive approach to changing mindsets. *Journal of Experimental Psychology: General*, *152*(9), 2603–2622. https://doi.org/10.1037/xge0001396

Curry, O. S., Rowland, L. A., Van Lissa, C. J., Zlotowitz, S., McAlaney, J., & Whitehouse, H. (2018). Happy to help? A systematic review and meta-analysis of the effects of performing acts of kindness on the well-being of the actor. *Journal of Experimental Social Psychology*, *76*, 320–329. https://doi.org/10.1016/j.jesp.2018.02.014

Demerouti, E. (2006). Job characteristics, flow, and performance: The moderating role of conscientiousness. *Journal of Occupational Health Psychology*, *11*(3), 266–280. https://doi.org/10.1037/1076-8998.11.3.266

Diener, E., & Chan, M. Y. (2011). Happy people live longer: Subjective well-being contributes to health and longevity. *Applied Psychology: Health and Well-Being*, *3*(1), 1–43. https://doi.org/10.1037/e675972011-001

Diener, E., Oishi, S., & Lucas, R. E. (2003). Personality, culture, and subjective well-being: Emotional and cognitive evaluations of life. *Annual Review of Psychology*, *54*(1), 403–425. https://doi.org/10.1146/annurev.psych.54.101601.145056

Dweck, C. S. (2006). *Mindset: The new psychology of success*. Random House.

Emirza, S., & Yılmaz Kozcu, G. (2023). Protecting healthcare workers' mental health against COVID-19-related stress: The effects of stress mindset and psychological resilience. *Nursing & Health Sciences*, *25*(2), 216–230. https://doi.org/10.1111/nhs.13018

Emmons, R. A., & McCullough, M. E. (2003). Counting blessings versus burdens: An experimental investigation of gratitude and subjective well-being in daily life. *Journal of Personality and Social Psychology*, *84*(2), 377–389. https://doi.org/10.1037/0022-3514.84.2.377

Emmons, R. A., & Mishra, A. (2011). Why gratitude enhances well-being: What we know, what we need to know. In K. M. Sheldon, T. B. Kashdan, & M. F. Steger (Eds.), *Designing positive psychology* (pp. 248–262). Oxford University Press. https://psycnet.apa.org/doi/10.1093/acprof:oso/9780195373585.003.0016

Engeser, S., & Rheinberg, F. (2008). Flow, performance and moderators of challenge-skill balance. *Motivation and Emotion*, *32*(3), 158–172. https://doi.org/10.1007/s11031-008-9102-4

Fava, G. A., Ruini, C., & Belaise, C. (2005). The concept of recovery in major depression. *Psychological Medicine*, *37*(3), 307–317. https://doi.org/10.1017/s0033291706008981

Fox, K. C., Nijeboer, S., Dixon, M. L., Floman, J. L., Ellamil, M., Rumak, S. P., … & Christoff, K. (2016). Is meditation associated with altered brain structure? A systematic review and meta-analysis of morphometric neuroimaging in meditation practitioners. *Neuroscience & Biobehavioral Reviews*, *68*, 649–658. https://doi.org/10.1016/j.neubiorev.2014.03.016

Fredrickson, B. L. (2001). The role of positive emotions in positive psychology: The broaden-and-build Theory of positive emotions. *American Psychologist*, *56*(3), 218–226. https://doi.org/10.1037//0003-066x.56.3.218

Fredrickson, B. L., & Joiner, T. (2002). Positive emotions trigger upward spirals toward emotional well-being. *Psychological Science*, *13*(2), 172–175. https://doi.org/10.1111/1467-9280.00431

Fredrickson, B. L., Grewen, K. M., Coffey, K. A., Algoe, S. B., Firestine, A. M., Arevalo, J. M., … & Cole, S. W. (2013). A functional genomic perspective on human well-being. *Proceedings of the National Academy of Sciences*, *110*(33), 13684–13689. https://doi.org/10.1073/pnas.1305419110

Fuller, C., Marin-Dragu, S., Iyer, R. S., & Meier, S. M. (2025). A mobile app–based gratitude intervention's effect on mental well-being in university students: Randomized controlled trial. *JMIR mHealth and uHealth*, *13*, e53850. https://doi.org/10.2196/53850

Gable, S. L., & Reis, H. T. (2010). Good news! Capitalizing on positive events in an interpersonal context. *Advances in Experimental Social Psychology*, *42*, 195–257. https://doi.org/10.1016/s0065-2601(10)42004-3

Gable, S. L., Reis, H. T., Impett, E. A., & Asher, E. R. (2004). What do you do when things go right? The intrapersonal and interpersonal benefits of sharing positive events. *Journal of Personality and Social Psychology*, *87*(2), 228–245. https://doi.org/10.4324/9780203732496-6

Gander, F., Proyer, R. T., & Ruch, W. (2018). A placebo-controlled online study on potential mediators of a pleasure-based positive psychology intervention: The role of emotional and cognitive components. *Journal of Happiness Studies*, *19*(7), 2035–2048. https://doi.org/10.1007/s10902-017-9909-3

Garland, E. L., Fredrickson, B., Kring, A. M., Johnson, D. P., Meyer, P. S., & Penn, D. L. (2010). Upward spirals of positive emotions counter downward spirals of negativity: Insights from the broaden-and-build theory and affective neuroscience on the treatment of emotion dysfunctions and deficits in psychopathology. *Clinical Psychology Review*, *30*(7), 849–864. https://doi.org/10.1016/j.cpr.2010.03.002

Geschwind, N., Arntz, A., Bannink, F., & Peeters, F. (2019). Positive cognitive behavior therapy in the treatment of depression: A randomized order within-subject comparison with traditional cognitive behavior therapy. *Behaviour Research and Therapy*, *116*, 119–130. https://doi.org/10.1016/j.brat.2019.03.005

Glasgow, R. E., Harden, S. M., Gaglio, B., Rabin, B., Smith, M. L., Porter, G. C., … & Estabrooks, P. A. (2019). RE-AIM planning and evaluation framework: Adapting to new science and practice with a 20-year review. *Frontiers in Public Health*, *7*, 64. https://doi.org/10.3389/fpubh.2019.00064

Goldberg, S. B., Tucker, R. P., Greene, P. A., Davidson, R. J., Wampold, B. E., Kearney, D. J., & Simpson, T. L. (2018). Mindfulness-based interventions for psychiatric disorders: A systematic review and meta-analysis. *Clinical Psychology Review*, *59*, 52–60. https://doi.org/10.1016/j.cpr.2017.10.011

Haas, B. W., Ishak, A., Anderson, I. W., & Filkowski, M. M. (2016). The tendency to trust is reflected in human brain structure. *NeuroImage*, *107*, 175–181. https://doi.org/10.1016/j.neuroimage.2014.11.060

Hammond, M. M., Murphy, C., & Demsky, C. A. (2021). Stress mindset and the work-family interface. *International Journal of Manpower*, *42*(1), 150–166. https://doi.org/10.1108/ijm-05-2018-0161

Harkin, B., Webb, T. L., Chang, B. P., Prestwich, A., Conner, M., Kellar, I., Benn, Y., & Sheeran, P. (2016). Does monitoring goal progress promote goal attainment? A meta-analysis of the experimental evidence. *Psychological Bulletin*, *142*(2), 198–229. https://doi.org/10.1037/bul0000025

Hart, R. (2021). *Positive psychology:The basics*. Routledge. https://doi.org/10.4324/9781315147857

Heathcote, L., Hernandez, J., Kronman, C., Mahmud, F., Crum, A., & Simons, L. (2018). 'Stress helps me learn and grow': Does stress mindset matter for children and young adults with chronic pain? *Journal of Pain*, *19*, S56. https://doi.org/10.1016/j.jpain.2017.12.137

Hefferon, K. (2012). Bringing back the body into positive psychology: The theory of corporeal posttraumatic growth in breast cancer survivorship. *Psychology*, *3*(12A), 1238–1242. https://doi.org/10.4236/psych.2012.312a183

Hefferon, K., Grealy, M., & Mutrie, N. (2009). Post-traumatic growth and life threatening physical illness: A systematic review of the qualitative literature. *British Journal of Health Psychology*, *14*(2), 343–378. https://doi.org/10.1348/135910708x332936

Hendriks, T., Warren, M. A., Schotanus-Dijkstra, M., Hassankhan, A., Graafsma, T., Bohlmeijer, E., & de Jong, J. (2019). How WEIRD are positive psychology interventions? A bibliometric analysis of randomized controlled trials on the science of well-being. *Journal of Positive Psychology*, *14*(4), 489–501. https://doi.org/10.1080/17439760.2018.1484941

Holt-Lunstad, J., Smith, T. B., & Layton, J. B. (2010). Social relationships and mortality risk: A meta-analytic review. *PLoS Medicine*, *7*(7), e1000316. https://doi.org/10.4016/19911.01

Isen, A. M. (2000). Positive affect and decision making. In M. Lewis & J. M. Haviland-Jones (Eds.), *Handbook of emotions* (2nd ed., pp. 417–435). Guilford Press.

Jackson, S. A., & Eklund, R. C. (2002). Assessing flow in physical activity: The Flow State Scale-2 and Dispositional Flow Scale-2. *Journal of Sport and Exercise Psychology*, *24*(2), 133–150. https://doi.org/10.1123/jsep.24.2.133

Jackson, S. A., & Marsh, H. W. (1996). Development and validation of a scale to measure optimal experience: The Flow State Scale. *Journal of Sport and Exercise Psychology*, *18*(1), 17–35. https://doi.org/10.1123/jsep.18.1.17

Jackson, S. A., Thomas, P. R., Marsh, H. W., & Smethurst, C. J. (2001). Relationships between flow, self-concept, psychological skills, and performance. *Journal of Applied Sport Psychology*, *13*(2), 129–153. https://doi.org/10.1080/104132001753149865

Jenkinson, C. E., Dickens, A. P., Jones, K., Thompson-Coon, J., Taylor, R. S., Rogers, M., … & Richards, S. H. (2013). Is volunteering a public health intervention? A systematic review and meta-analysis of the health and survival of volunteers. *BMC Public Health*, *13*(1), 773. https://doi.org/10.1186/1471-2458-13-773

Joseph, S. (2011). *What doesn't kill us: The new psychology of posttraumatic growth*. Basic Books.

Kabat-Zinn, J. (2003). Mindfulness-based interventions in context: Past, present, and future. *Clinical Psychology: Science and Practice*, *10*(2), 144–156. https://doi.org/10.1093/clipsy/bpg016

Kern, M. L., Waters, L. E., Adler, A., & White, M. A. (2015). A multidimensional approach to measuring well-being in students: Application of the PERMA framework. *Journal of Positive Psychology*, *10*(3), 262–271. https://doi.org/10.1080/17439760.2014.936962

Kessler, R. C., Andrews, G., & Colpe, L. J. (2002). Short screening scales to monitor population prevalences and trends in non-specific psychological distress. *Psychological Medicine*, *32*(6), 959–976. https://doi.org/10.1017/s0033291702006074

Keyes, C. L. M. (2002). The mental health continuum: From languishing to flourishing in life. *Journal of Health and Social Behavior*, *43*(2), 207–222. https://doi.org/10.2307/3090197

Keyes, C. L. M. (2005). Mental illness and/or mental health? Investigating axioms of the complete state model of health. *Journal of Consulting and Clinical Psychology*, *73*(3), 539–548. https://doi.org/10.1037/0022-006x.73.3.539

Keyes, C. L. M. (2007). Promoting and protecting mental health as flourishing: A complementary strategy for improving national mental health. *American Psychologist*, *62*(2), 95–108. https://doi.org/10.1037/0003-066x.62.2.95

Khazanov, G. K., & Ruscio, A. M. (2016). Is low positive emotionality a specific risk factor for depression? A meta-analysis of longitudinal studies. *Psychological Bulletin*, *142*(9), 991–1015. https://doi.org/10.1037/bul0000059

Kilmer, R. P. (2006). Resilience and posttraumatic growth in children. In L. G. Calhoun & R. G. Tedeschi (Eds.), *Handbook of posttraumatic growth: Research and practice* (pp. 264–288). Lawrence Erlbaum Associates.

Kini, P., Wong, J., McInnis, S., Gabana, N., & Brown, J. W. (2016). The effects of gratitude expression on neural activity. *NeuroImage*, *128*, 1–10. https://doi.org/10.1016/j.neuroimage.2015.12.040

Kibler, J., Ma, M., Hrzich, J., & Choe, J. (2023). Pilot findings indicate a cognitive behavioral healthy lifestyle intervention for PTSD improves sleep and physical activity. *Brain Sciences*, *13*(11), 1565. https://doi.org/10.3390/brainsci13111565

King, L. A. (2001). The health benefits of writing about life goals. *Personality and Social Psychology Bulletin*, *27*(7), 798–807. https://doi.org/10.1177/0146167201277003

King, L. A., & Miner, K. N. (2000). Writing about the perceived benefits of traumatic events: Implications for physical health. *Personality and Social Psychology Bulletin*, *26*(2), 220–230. https://doi.org/10.1177/0146167200264008

Kitayama, S., & Markus, H. R. (2000). The pursuit of happiness and the realization of sympathy: Cultural patterns of self, social relations, and well-being. In E. Diener & E. M. Suh (Eds.), *Culture and subjective well-being* (pp. 113–161). MIT Press.

Kitayama, S., & Park, J. (2007). Cultural shaping of self, emotion, and well-being: How does it work? *Social and Personality Psychology Compass*, *1*(1), 202–222. https://doi.org/10.1111/j.1751-9004.2007.00016.x

Klimecki, O. M., Leiberg, S., Lamm, C., & Singer, T. (2013). Functional neural plasticity and associated changes in positive affect after compassion training. *Cerebral Cortex*, *23*(7), 1552–1561. https://doi.org/10.1093/cercor/bhs142

Kok, B. E., Coffey, K. A., Cohn, M. A., Catalino, L. I., Vacharkulksemsuk, T., Algoe, S. B., Brantley, M., & Fredrickson, B. L. (2013). How positive emotions build physical health: Perceived positive social connections account for the upward spiral between positive emotions and vagal tone. *Psychological Science*, *24*(7), 1123–1132. https://psycnet.apa.org/doi/10.1177/0956797612470827

Korotitsch, W. J., & Nelson-Gray, R. O. (1999). An overview of self-monitoring research in assessment and treatment. *Psychological Assessment*, *11*(4), 415–425. https://doi.org/10.1037//1040-3590.11.4.415

Kumar, A., & Epley, N. (2018). Undervaluing gratitude: Expressers misunderstand the consequences of showing appreciation. *Psychological Science*, *29*(9), 1423–1435. https://doi.org/10.1177/0956797618772506

Lopez, S. J., & Snyder, C. R. (Eds.). (2009). *Oxford handbook of positive psychology*. Oxford University Press.

Lutz, A., Slagter, H. A., Dunne, J. D., & Davidson, R. J. (2008). Attention regulation and monitoring in meditation. *Trends in Cognitive Sciences*, *12*(4), 163–169. https://doi.org/10.1016/j.tics.2008.01.005

Lyubomirsky, S., & Layous, K. (2013). How do simple positive activities increase well-being? *Current Directions in Psychological Science*, *22*(1), 57–62. https://doi.org/10.1177/0963721412469809

Lyubomirsky, S., Sheldon, K. M., & Schkade, D. (2005). Pursuing happiness: The architecture of sustainable change. *Review of General Psychology*, *9*(2), 111–131. https://doi.org/10.1037/1089-2680.9.2.111

Malouff, J. M., & Schutte, N. S. (2020). The efficacy of interventions aimed at reducing procrastination: A meta-analysis of randomized controlled trials. *Journal of Counseling & Development*, *98*(3), 319–326. https://doi.org/10.1002/jcad.12243

McCullough, M. E., & Willoughby, B. L. (2009). Religion, self-regulation, and self-control: Associations, explanations, and implications. *Psychological Bulletin*, *135*(1), 69–93. https://doi.org/10.1037/a0014213

Meevissen, Y. M., Peters, M. L., & Alberts, H. J. (2011). Become more optimistic by imagining a best possible self: Effects of a two week intervention. *Journal of Behavior Therapy and Experimental Psychiatry*, *42*(3), 371–378. https://doi.org/10.1016/j.jbtep.2011.02.012

Mohr, D. C., Burns, M. N., Schueller, S. M., Clarke, G., & Klinkman, M. (2017). Behavioral intervention technologies: Evidence review and recommendations for future research in mental health. *General Hospital Psychiatry*, *32*(4), 332–338. https://doi.org/10.1016/j.genhosppsych.2013.03.008

Mongrain, M., & Anselmo-Matthews, T. (2012). Do positive psychology exercises work? A replication of Seligman et al. (2005). *Journal of Clinical Psychology*, *68*(4), 382–389. https://doi.org/10.1002/jclp.21839

Moore, A., & Malinowski, P. (2009). Meditation, mindfulness and cognitive flexibility. *Consciousness and Cognition*, *18*(1), 176–186. https://doi.org/10.1016/j.concog.2008.12.008

Nakamura, J., & Csikszentmihalyi, M. (2014). The concept of flow. In M. Csikszentmihalyi (Ed.), *Flow and the foundations of positive psychology* (pp. 239–263). Springer.

Nelson, S. K., Layous, K., Cole, S. W., & Lyubomirsky, S. (2016). Do unto others or treat yourself? The effects of prosocial and self-focused behavior on psychological flourishing. *Emotion*, *16*(6), 850–861. https://doi.org/10.1037/emo0000178

Nezlek, J. B. (2001). Daily psychological adjustment and the planfulness of day-to-day behavior. *Journal of Social and Clinical Psychology*, *20*(4), 452–475. https://doi.org/10.1521/jscp.20.4.452.22398

Pace, T. W., Negi, L. T., Adame, D. D., Cole, S. P., Sivilli, T. I., Brown, T. D., Issa, M. J., & Raison, C. L. (2009). Effect of compassion meditation on neuroendocrine, innate immune and behavioral responses to psychosocial stress. *Psychoneuroendocrinology*, *34*(1), 87–98. https://doi.org/10.1016/j.psyneuen.2008.08.011

Park, D., Yu, A., Metz, S. E., Tsukayama, E., Crum, A. J., & Duckworth, A. L. (2018). Beliefs about stress attenuate the relation among adverse life events, perceived distress, and self-control. *Child Development*, *89*(6), 2059–2069. https://doi.org/10.1111/cdev.12946

Parks, A. C., & Boucher, E. M. (2020). Positive psychological interventions (PPIs) in the age of COVID-19: On the potential impact of digital PPIs on loneliness. *Journal of Positive Psychology*, *15*(5), 569–571. https://doi.org/10.1080/17439760.2020.1789715

Peterson, C., & Park, N. (2003). Positive psychology as the evenhanded positive psychologist views it. *Psychological Inquiry*, *14*(2), 143–147. https://www.jstor.org/stable/1449822

Peterson, C., & Park, N. (2009). Classifying and measuring strengths of character. In S. J. Lopez & C. R. Snyder (Eds.), *Oxford handbook of positive psychology* (pp. 25–33). Oxford University Press.

Peterson, C., & Seligman, M. E. P. (2004). *Character strengths and virtues: A handbook and classification*. Oxford University Press.

Peterson, C., Stephens, J. P., Park, N., Lee, F., & Seligman, M. E. P. (2010). Strengths of character and work. In P. A. Linley, S. Harrington, & N. Garcea (Eds.), *Oxford handbook of positive psychology and work* (pp. 221–231). Oxford University Press.

Post, S. G. (2005). Altruism, happiness, and health: It's good to be good. *International Journal of Behavioral Medicine*, *12*(2), 66–77. https://doi.org/10.1207/s15327558ijbm1202_4

Proctor, C., Maltby, J., & Linley, P. A. (2011). Strengths use as a predictor of well-being and health-related quality of life. *Journal of Happiness Studies*, *12*(1), 153–169. https://doi.org/10.1007/s10902-009-9181-2

Reis, H. T., & Gable, S. L. (2015). Responsiveness. *Current Opinion in Psychology*, *1*, 67–71. https://doi.org/10.1016/j.copsyc.2015.01.001

Rheinberg, F., Vollmeyer, R., & Engeser, S. (2003). Die Erfassung des Flow-Erlebens [The assessment of flow experience]. In J. Stiensmeier-Pelster & F. Rheinberg (Eds.), *Diagnostik von Motivation und Selbstkonzept* (pp. 261–279). Hogrefe.

Riva, G., Baños, R. M., Botella, C., Mantovani, F., & Gaggioli, A. (2019). Transforming experience: The potential of augmented reality and virtual reality for enhancing personal and clinical change. *Frontiers in Psychiatry*, *10*, 164. https://doi.org/10.3389/fpsyt.2016.00164

Rosenbaum, S., Vancampfort, D., Steel, Z., Newby, J., Ward, P. B., & Stubbs, B. (2015). Physical activity interventions for people with mental illness: A systematic review and meta-analysis. *Journal of Clinical Psychiatry*, *75*(9), 964–974. https://doi.org/10.4088/jcp.13r08765

Rowland, L., & Curry, O. S. (2019). A range of kindness activities boost happiness. *Journal of Social Psychology*, *159*(3), 340–343. https://doi.org/10.1080/00224545.2018.1469461

Ryan, R. M., & Deci, E. L. (2000). Self-determination theory and the facilitation of intrinsic motivation, social development, and well-being. *American Psychologist*, *55*(1), 68–78. https://doi.org/10.1037//0003-066x.55.1.68

Ryan, R. M., & Deci, E. L. (2001). On happiness and human potentials: A review of research on hedonic and eudaimonic well-being. *Annual Review of Psychology*, *52*(1), 141–166. https://doi.org/10.1146/annurev.psych.52.1.141

Sapolsky, R. M. (1998). *Why zebras don't get ulcers* (2nd ed.). Freeman.

Seligman, M. E. P. (1998). *Learned optimism*. Pocket Books.

Seligman, M. E. P. (2002). *Authentic happiness: Using the new positive psychology to realize your potential for lasting fulfillment.* Free Press.

Seligman, M. E. P. (2008). Positive health. *Applied Psychology*, *57*(1), 3–18. https://doi.org/10.1111/j.1464-0597.2008.00351.x

Seligman, M. E. P. (2011). *Flourish: A visionary new understanding of happiness and well-being*. Free Press.

Seligman, M. E. P., & Csikszentmihalyi, M. (2000). Positive psychology: An introduction. *American Psychologist*, *55*(1), 5–14. https://doi.org/10.1037//0003-066x.55.1.5

Seligman, M. E. P., Ernst, R. M., Gillham, J., Reivich, K., & Linkins, M. (2009). Positive education: Positive psychology and classroom interventions. *Oxford Review of Education*, *35*(3), 293–311. https://doi.org/10.1080/03054980902934563

Seligman, M. E. P., & Schulman, P. (1986). Explanatory style as a predictor of productivity and quitting among life insurance sales agents. *Journal of Personality and Social Psychology*, *50*(4), 832–838. https://doi.org/10.1037//0022-3514.50.4.832

Seligman, M. E. P., Steen, T. A., Park, N., & Peterson, C. (2005). Positive psychology progress: Empirical validation of interventions. *American Psychologist*, *60*(5), 410–421. https://doi.org/10.1037/0003-066x.60.5.410

Sheldon, K. M., & Lyubomirsky, S. (2006). How to increase and sustain positive emotion: The effects of expressing gratitude and visualizing best possible selves. *Journal of Positive Psychology*, *1*(2), 73–82. https://doi.org/10.1080/17439760500510676

Sin, N. L., & Lyubomirsky, S. (2009). Enhancing well-being and alleviating depressive symptoms with positive psychology interventions: A practice-friendly meta-analysis. *Journal of Clinical Psychology*, *65*(5), 467–487. https://doi.org/10.1002/jclp.20593

Stavrou, N. A., Psychountaki, M., Georgiadis, E., Karteroliotis, K., & Zervas, Y. (2015). Flow theory–goal orientation theory: Positive experience is related to athlete's goal orientation. *Frontiers in Psychology*, *6*, 1499. https://doi.org/10.3389/fpsyg.2015.01499

Stein, F. (1986). *The Stress Management Questionnaire (SMQ)*. University of Wisconsin-Milwaukee.

Stein, F., & Cutler, S. (1998). *Psychosocial occupational therapy: A holistic approach*. Singular Publishing.

Stein, F., & Nikolic, S. (1989). Teaching stress management techniques to a schizophrenic patient. *American Journal of Occupational Therapy*, *43*(3), 162–169. https://doi.org/10.5014/ajot.43.3.162

Stein, F., & Smith, J. (1989). Short-term stress management program with acutely depressed inpatients. *Canadian Journal of Occupational Therapy*, *56*(4), 185–192. https://doi.org/10.1177/000841748905600407

Tedeschi, R. G., & Calhoun, L. G. (2004). Posttraumatic growth: Conceptual foundations and empirical evidence. *Psychological Inquiry*, *15*(1), 1–18. https://doi.org/10.1207/s15327965pli1501_01

Tedeschi, R. G., Park, C. L., & Calhoun, L. G. (1998). *Posttraumatic growth: Positive changes in the aftermath of crisis*. Lawrence Erlbaum Associates.

Tennen, H., & Affleck, G. (2005). Benefit-finding and benefit-reminding. In C. R. Snyder & S. J. Lopez (Eds.), *Handbook of positive psychology* (pp. 584–597). Oxford University Press.

Thoits, P. A., & Hewitt, L. N. (2001). Volunteer work and well-being. *Journal of Health and Social Behavior*, *42*(2), 115–131. https://doi.org/10.2307/3090173

Toepfer, S. M., Cichy, K., & Peters, P. (2012). Letters of gratitude: Further evidence for author benefits. *Journal of Happiness Studies*, *13*(1), 187–201. https://doi.org/10.1007/s10902-011-9257-7

Tylka, T. L., & Homan, K. J. (2015). Exercise motives and positive body image in physically active college women and men: Exploring an expanded acceptance model of intuitive eating. *Body Image*, *15*, 90–97. https://doi.org/10.1016/j.bodyim.2015.07.003

Uchida, Y., Norasakkunkit, V., & Kitayama, S. (2004). Cultural constructions of happiness: Theory and empirical evidence. *Journal of Happiness Studies*, *5*(3), 223–239. https://doi.org/10.1007/978-94-007-5702-8_14

Umberson, D., & Montez, J. K. (2010). Social relationships and health: A flashpoint for health policy. *Journal of Health and Social Behavior*, *51*(1_suppl), S54–S66. https://doi.org/10.1177/0022146510383501

van der Kolk, B. (2014). *The body keeps the score: Brain, mind, and body in the healing of trauma*. Viking.

Walker, C. J. (2010). Experiencing flow: Is doing it together better than doing it alone? *Journal of Positive Psychology*, *5*(1), 3–11. https://doi.org/10.1080/17439760903271116

Watkins, P. C., Woodward, K., Stone, T., & Kolts, R. L. (2003). Gratitude and happiness: Development of a measure of gratitude, and relationships with subjective well-being. *Clinical Psychology Review*, *23*(2), 249–266. https://doi.org/10.2224/sbp.2003.31.5.431

Watlington, C. G., & Murphy, C. M. (2006). The roles of religion and spirituality among African American survivors of domestic violence. *Journal of Clinical Psychology*, *62*(7), 837–857. https://doi.org/10.1002/jclp.20268

Watson, D., & Clark, L. A. (1988). Development and validation of brief measures of positive and negative affect: The PANAS scales. *Journal of Personality and Social Psychology*, *54*(6), 1063–1070. https://doi.org/10.1037//0022-3514.54.6.1063

Westerhof, G. J., & Keyes, C. L. M. (2010). Mental illness and mental health: The two continua model across the lifespan. *Journal of Adult Development*, *17*(2), 110–119. https://doi.org/10.1007/s10804-009-9082-y

White, C. A., Uttl, B., & Holder, M. D. (2019). Meta-analyses of positive psychology interventions: The effects are much smaller than previously reported. *PLoS One*, *14*(5), e0216588. https://doi.org/10.1371/journal.pone.0216588

White, M. A., & Waters, L. E. (2015). A case study of 'The Good School:' Examples of the use of Peterson's strengths-based approach with students. *Journal of Positive Psychology*, *10*(1), 69–76. https://doi.org/10.1080/17439760.2014.920408

Zigmond, A. S., & Snaith, R. P. (1983). The Hospital Anxiety and Depression Scale. *Acta Psychiatrica Scandinavica*, *67*(6), 361–370. https://doi.org/10.1111/j.1600-0447.1983.tb09716.x

Chapter 8

Learning New Strategies in Coping with Stress

LEARNING OBJECTIVES

By the end of this chapter, the learner will be able to

1. Describe multiple strategies and approaches to managing stress:
   a. Relaxation therapies
   b. Mindfulness meditation
   c. The relaxation response
   d. Progressive muscle relaxation
   e. Breathing
   f. Guided imagery
   g. Tai chi
   h. Yoga
   i. Prescriptive aerobic exercise
   j. Music and music therapy
   k. Horticulture therapy
   l. Arts therapy
   m. Other (sensory rooms, biofeedback, word/number/video games, sexual activity, animal-assisted therapy and spirituality)
2. Identify research studies evaluating the effectiveness of these approaches.

DOI: 10.4324/9781003671084-8

INTRODUCTION

Occupational therapy practitioners bring a distinct perspective to supporting individuals in managing stress. Rather than viewing stress solely as a collection of physiological or psychological symptoms to be treated, occupational therapy practitioners are trained to recognize it as a factor that can disrupt engagement in the roles, routines and activities that matter to the people we serve. This lens ensures that our interventions address not only stress itself but also its impact on participation in daily living.

In contrast to approaches that focus primarily on symptomatology, occupational therapy emphasizes the functional implications of stress. This perspective shapes the way we develop interventions – prioritizing strategies that are relevant, sustainable and motivating for the individual. We understand that the effectiveness of any stress management strategy depends not only on its clinical merit and evidence base but also on whether the person is genuinely motivated to integrate it into daily life. This means we must take care to identify stress-reducing activities that align with a person's values, interests and capacities – what the Model of Human Occupation describes as volition (Taylor et al., 2023).

A strategy that is externally imposed, overly complex or disconnected from a person's sense of self is unlikely to be sustained and therefore unlikely to be either used or useful. For this reason, occupational therapy practitioners collaborate with clients to explore, test and adapt strategies that fit their identities and circumstances. For one individual, this may involve brief mindfulness practices incorporated into a morning routine; for another, it may mean re-engaging in valued activities such as walking outdoors or preparing meals. For others, those activities may sound unmotivating or impractical, making them unlikely to be a good fit.

By centering interventions on what is both meaningful to and achievable by the people we serve, occupational therapy provides a client-centered approach to stress management that gives distinct value compared to what is offered by others on the care team.

How can we prevent stress from negatively impacting our health by engaging in meaningful and purposeful occupation? As the research has shown, chronic stress can precipitate symptoms in individuals throughout the life span who have specific vulnerabilities such as back pain, migraine headaches and gastrointestinal disorders. In the descriptions below we discuss healthy approaches to stress management that can be incorporated into one's lifestyle or daily habits. The various therapeutic approaches to stress management can augment one's quality of life by improving the individual's health through self-regulation. Meditation, tai-chi, yoga, relaxation exercises and similar therapeutic methods are taught frequently in adult education courses offered by local colleges in the community or demonstrated on YouTube. The exercises and therapeutic methods described below have research evidence that supports their efficacy. Of course, not all of the methods described will fit every individual. These methods are listed to present choices for the individual and occupational therapist to select from, based on one's lifestyle, state of health and resources available in the community. The methods should also be adapted to the individual so as to allow for physical constraints such as being in a wheelchair or having joint limitations or cognitive problems such as early dementia. Good ergonomics means adapting a therapeutic method to the individual's physical and cognitive capacity and emotional state. An important key to the success of introducing and teaching a new therapeutic activity is the individual's motivation to learn the activity and to persist with it. It also should be noted that in our everyday lives many of us use activities or occupations to regulate our stress. For example, taking a deep breath, doing a crossword puzzle or a sudoku, watching a funny movie, reading and immersing yourself in a book that you enjoy, playing Scrabble with a partner, having a chat in a coffee shop with a friend, taking a day trip, walking in a nature area, listening to music in a concert, singing or other experiences that are enjoyable. These experiences make life more livable and reduce our stress.

Besides these everyday activities, in this chapter we introduce more structured activities that have been shown through empirical research to be effective in reducing distress. These techniques, if they are to be successful, have to be learned, practiced on a daily basis and built into the lifestyle of the individual. Thus, the important factor in the effectiveness of the stress management activity is the individual's commitment to engage in the occupation. If the activity is successful in reducing stress or preventing distress, the activity should be enjoyable and have the characteristics of FLOW (Csikszentmihalyi, 1990).

FLOW and Stress Management

One of the most important concepts in stress management is derived from the work of Mihaly Csikszentmihalyi (1990) on FLOW. He conceptualized FLOW activities as being enjoyable. It's often described as being "in the zone." "What makes these activities conducive to flow is that they were designed to make optimal experiences easier to achieve" (p. 72). Examples are engaging in activities that require skills such as playing a musical instrument, competing in a sport, dancing, tai chi, yoga, painting and drawing, writing poetry, cooking, meditating and playing chess. There are many more activities that we engage in that are enjoyable, have our full focus and make time go faster. In self-regulating stress, a fundamental approach is to identify those activities that put us in FLOW. These activities are unique to the individual. The popular expression, "like what you do and do what you like" epitomizes the concept of engaging in an activity that puts us in FLOW. Csikszentmihalyi (1990) stated that it is most positive when we engage in activities that we have a good chance of completing, we give our full concentration to, we have clear goals with feedback, we are distracted from our daily worries, we lose the sense of time and the activity creates a sense of enjoyment (p. 49).

Csikszentmihalyi (1990) introduced the phrase "the autotelic self" to signify an individual who can transform potential threats and adverse experiences into challenges. For example, the individual who has "flunked out of school" can rebound into another career and then perhaps return to school and academically thrive. Or the person who is a survivor from a family death can become more focused to be successful in life. The autotelic self is defined by the author as "A person who is never bored, seldom anxious, involved with what goes on, and in flow most of the time ..." (p. 209). The autotelic self sets clear goals such as learning to play the piano after retirement. Selecting a goal means that the individual is realistic in knowing what skills are necessary in learning a new activity. By setting up realistic goals, the individual has to design a schedule for learning the new activity that fits into a dedicated time, for example, meeting with a piano teacher every Thursday evening at 7 PM. Determination and discipline in organizing and adhering to a time schedule is a key to successful accomplishments. Csikszentmihalyi (1990) also recommended that individuals immerse themselves in the activity by mobilizing their efforts and concentration. In a way it is a commitment to learn a new activity by using all the skills a person possesses and not being discouraged by setbacks. When we are successful in learning a new activity like playing the piano we appreciate our success and it reinforces our enjoyment of engaging in the activity. "Flow drives individuals to creativity and achievement" (Csikszentmihalyi, 1990, p. 213). The concepts of FLOW presage its success as a stress reducer.

Below we discuss specific activities that have research evidence of being effective in a stress management program.

RELAXATION THERAPIES

> Research suggests that multiple forms of relaxation training (e.g., progressive muscle relaxation, meditation, breathing exercises, visualization, and autogenics) can help individuals reduce stress, enhance relaxation states, and improve overall well-being.
>
> (Toussaint et al., 2021, p. 5924040)

After an extensive review of the literature on stress management techniques with children and adolescents who had been diagnosed with a psychiatric disorder, Zisopoulou and Varvogli (2023) found that relaxation was the predominant approach for anxiety and stress reduction. In the following section several distinct approaches to relaxation will be addressed.

Mindfulness Meditation – Definition and Purposes

Meditation rooted in ancient Buddhist traditions has been defined in many ways. Essentially, meditation is training yourself to be in a calm mental state with positive emotions. In this state the individual is in the here and now, focusing on inner mental states that distract from worry and anxiety. Mindfulness meditation is one of the most popular meditation techniques. Typically, it involves focusing your awareness on your breath, your thoughts, the physical sensations in your body and the feelings you are experiencing, without judging them. Mindfulness meditation classes include breathing exercises, yoga and guided imagery to help you become aware of body sensations, thoughts and feelings.

How Meditation Arose in the Western World

There are many definitions of meditation in the literature, with, however, common themes. Western definitions emphasize that meditation is a self-regulating strategy with a particular emphasis on training the mind to focus on the present. Historically there are multiple types of meditation that emphasize mental development, such as bhavana (mental cultivation) in Buddhism and lien-hsin (refining the mind) in Taoism (Walsh & Shapiro, 2006).

> Contrary to the belief that Mindfulness only has Buddhist and Hindu origins, it is also rooted in Jewish, Islamic and Christian religions. Furthermore, western philosophers have described a mindful path to become more

> aware of thoughts, feelings, and bodily sensations. Mindfulness can be considered as a universal human ability embodied to foster clear thinking and open-heartedness. As such, this form of being requires no particular religious or cultural belief system.
>
> (Trousselard et al., 2014, p. 474)

The Insight Meditation Society in Massachusetts was founded in 1975 by Sharon Salzberg, a teacher of meditation, Jack Kornfield, trained as a Buddhist monk, and Joseph Goldstein, author of *Mindfulness: A Practical Guide to Awakening* (2013). These three highly respected meditation teachers introduced mindfulness meditation based on Eastern spiritual practices to Western psychology.

> The main purpose of mindfulness meditation is to achieve a state of relaxation to counteract stressful thoughts and anxiety by focusing your mind on the present moment. Mindfulness meditation can be incorporated into your everyday life by using the principles while sitting quietly, listening to classical music, or accomplishing daily routine tasks like cleaning house or working in the garden. Through mindfulness meditation the body goes into a parasympathetic response where heart rate and systolic blood pressure slows down.
>
> (Pascoe et al., 2017, p. 156)

The American Institute of Stress (http://www.stress.org) provides information on practicing meditation.

Over the years meditation has been adapted and secularized for modern contexts. It is often practiced as part of mindfulness-based stress reduction (MBSR). A heightened, non-judgmental awareness of one's immediate experience is at the heart of MBSR meditation (Huang & Shi, 2016).

Evidence of Effectiveness of Mindfulness Meditation

There have been an enormous number of studies in the literature examining the effectiveness of mindfulness meditation. The research has focused on mindfulness-based stress reduction (MBSR) and mindfulness-based cognitive therapy (MBCT) that combines elements of MBSR and cognitive behavioral therapy (CBT). From 1966 to 2021, 16,581 publications on mindfulness were identified – an exponential growth of publications since 2006 (Baminiwatta & Solangaarachchi, 2021).

One early study was conducted by Kabat-Zinn (1982). It introduced the practice of mindfulness meditation in clinics for people with chronic pain. He deemed it an effective program in self-regulation (Kabat-Zinn, 1982).

In a comprehensive review, Khoury et al. (2013) examined the effects of 209 trials of mindfulness-based interventions among 12,145 patients with a variety of disorders. The authors concluded that meditation-based therapy was more effective in reducing anxiety, depression and stress in people with medical or psychiatric diagnoses compared to psychoeducation, psychotherapy, relaxation training, imagery approaches or controls. The effects were greatest for psychological outcomes (Khoury et al., 2013).

Yang et al. (2018) studied 100 psychiatric nurses (68 females, 32 males) from three hospitals in Hunan province of China. They were randomly assigned to intervention and control groups. The intervention group received MBSR therapy. The authors found that MBSR improved mental health and reduced anxiety, depression and work stress.

Kuyken et al. (2015) designed a single-blind, randomized controlled trial with 424 adult patients having three or more previous major depressive episodes and on maintenance antidepression medication from 94 primary care general practices in urban and rural settings in the UK. MBCT is intended to enable people to learn to become more aware of their bodily sensations, thoughts and feelings associated with depressive relapse or recurrence and to relate constructively to these experiences. Participants learned mindfulness practices and cognitive-behavioral skills both in session and through homework assignments. The authors found that MBCT designed to enable patients to learn skills was effective in the prevention and avoidance of the recurrence of depression.

A recent meta-analysis of stress studies on medical students (da Silva et al., 2023) found that the students receiving mindfulness training saw reduced symptoms of distress and improved well-being, although the authors cautioned about the high variability in the studies (da Silva et al., 2023).

Hofmann and Gómez (2017) drew similar conclusions about mindfulness-based interventions, that they were superior in effects to relaxation therapy, health education and psychotherapy. Their outcomes were also comparable to those of cognitive-behavioral therapy, with which its principles were compatible. Confirming the above results, Ghahari et al. (2020) in a systematic review and meta-analysis declared that MBCT was effective in reducing anxiety.

In short, mindfulness meditation has been shown in numerous studies to be effective in reducing stress, anxiety and depression, improving focus and attention, enhancing emotional regulation and promoting overall resilience and well-being (see also Goldberg et al., 2018; van der Velden, et al., 2023).

Mindfulness classes and interventions are widely available in yoga centers, athletic clubs, hospitals and clinics and are also available online or through smartphone apps.

The Relaxation Response

One of the most common relaxation therapies is the Relaxation Response (Benson, 1975). Herbert Benson, a cardiologist, developed the relaxation response through his interest in religious prayer and the ancient technique of transcendental meditation (TM). The relaxation response is a natural, innate protective mechanism where the individual sits quietly, is focused on the here and now and turns off the anxieties and worries that produce stress. Sitting quietly in a relaxed position decreases heart rate, lowers metabolism and decreases the rate of breathing. In this way, the body is brought back into a healthier balance. He based his technique on the principles of TM, an ancient spiritual practice from India that was made popular in the 1950s by Maharishi Mahesh (Mason, 1994).

The relaxation response as conceived by Benson is based on four basic recommendations:

1. Sit quietly in a comfortable position.
2. Close your eyes and focus on your internal state of being.
3. Try to deeply relax all the muscles of your body.
4. Breathe in through your nose and exhale through your mouth.

Benson suggested, as you relax in this position, to become aware of your breathing. Maintain a passive attitude. If you are distracted, speak the word "ONE" and remain passive (Benson, 1975, pp. 158–163).

Compared to six other relaxation techniques, Benson found that the physiologic changes occurring during the Relaxation Response were similar:

1. Transcendental meditation (Ooi et al., 2017).
2. Yoga (see below).
3. Autogenic Training (AT): AT consists of six relaxation steps: a sense of heaviness in the limbs, sensing warmth, slow breathing, abdominal warmth, reduced heart rate and a cool forehead (Lim & Kim, 2014).

4. Progressive Relaxation (see below).
5. Hypnosis with suggested deep relaxation (Fisch et al., 2017).

Sentic Cycles: Sentics is a field of study exploring the biological basis of emotional communication. Developed by neuroscientist Manfred Clynes (1973), it investigates how emotions are expressed and recognized through various modalities, including touch, voice and even music, suggesting the existence of underlying, universal patterns or "essentic forms" for each emotion.

Benson suggested that the above stress management meditative techniques approximate the same parasympathetic changes elicited by the Relaxation Response. As a scientist, Benson used physiological measurements to assess the effects of the relaxation response. These measurements consisted of oxygen consumption, respiratory rate, heart rate, alpha waves, blood pressure and muscle tension. He also linked the relaxation response to the early Christian ascetics and Jewish mystics who practiced "contemplation" and "recollection" in order to close off the mind from external thoughts and to produce a passive attitude and mental solitude. Harorani et al. (2020) and Zappella et al. (2021) are recent studies that investigated the relaxation response.

Progressive Muscle Relaxation

Progressive muscle relaxation (PMR) as a stress management technique was first developed by Dr. Edmund Jacobson (Jacobson, 1924). This paper introduced the relaxation technique of progressively tensing and relaxing muscle groups to induce a state of deep relaxation. Progressive relaxation was originally used to treat symptoms of anxiety, but more recently it has been found to be effective for treating tension headaches, migraines, temporomandibular joint disorder, neck pain, insomnia, bipolar disorder, anxiety, backaches and high blood pressure (Muhammad Khir et al., 2024).

PMR is a simple technique to learn. It is a two-step process to increase awareness of deep relaxation in muscles. First, create tension through an isometric contraction (little or no movement at the joints). Second, relax the tension and sense what a relaxed muscle feels like (Mirgain & Singles, 2016).

PMR is based on the concept that muscle tension and psychological stress are interconnected. When individuals are stressed or anxious, they often experience physical tension, especially in the muscles. By learning to consciously relax the muscles, individuals can reduce psychological stress. There have been changes over the years to the original recommendations by Jacobsen.

PMR can be done lying down or sitting. One should avoid overly tensing the muscle. Avoid aggravating any pre-existing injury (Mirgain & Singles, 2016). PMR is not recommended if a person has a history of serious injuries, muscle spasms or back problems (Mirgain & Singles, 2016).

If these principles are followed, progressive relaxation provides a structured method to promote physical and psychological calm, making it an effective means for stress management.

Breathing

Breathing exercises are among the most accessible strategies for stress management. Breathing is an activity that every single one of us does every day. As a stress management tool, it takes an automatic and fundamental process we do and turns it into a therapeutic approach through intentional, purposeful action.

By consciously slowing and deepening breathing, people managing stress can activate the parasympathetic nervous system (PSNS), which helps moderate the SNS arousal associated with stress (Bentley, 2023; Magnon et al., 2021). Because breathing is simultaneously automatic and under voluntary control, it is unique among the strategies described in this chapter for its ability to influence physiological arousal and emotional regulation (Ma et al., 2017).

Occupational Therapy Application

While breathing exercises may not be right for every client, they can serve as a valuable component of the occupational therapy toolkit when supporting clients working to better manage their stress. Occupational therapy practitioners can use breathing-related interventions as a strategy to support clients in nearly any practice setting with clients across the lifespan.

Commonly used breathing techniques include box breathing (Jerath et al., 2023; Raj, 2021), 4–7–8 breathing (Aktaş, 2023) and diaphragmatic breathing (Hamasaki, 2020; Kramer et al., 2023; Tsakona et al., 2025).

1. Box breathing: Inhale for a set count (e.g., four), hold the breath for the same count, exhale for the same count, and hold again before repeating. This creates a steady "box" rhythm that helps regulate physiological arousal and promote calm (Jerath et al., 2023; Raj, 2021).

2. 4–7–8 breathing: Inhale quietly through the nose for a count of four, hold the breath for a count of seven, and exhale through the mouth for a count of eight. This technique emphasizes prolonged exhalation, which supports parasympathetic activation and is often used for anxiety or sleep preparation (Aktaş, 2023).
3. Diaphragmatic breathing: Also known as "paced breathing," this technique focuses on deep, slow inhalation that expands the diaphragm, followed by a controlled exhalation. This method reduces respiratory rate, lowers cortisol and can be integrated into daily routines as a portable stress management tool (Hamasaki, 2020; Kramer et al., 2023; Tsakona et al., 2025).
4. Among other advantages, these techniques are useful for their versatility. These can be performed in sitting, lying or standing positions and can be paired with environmental supports such as smartphone apps, timers or guided recordings. They can be taught to individuals or used as a part of a group intervention.

Occupational therapy practitioners understand the importance of aligning intervention strategies with the day-to-day realities and treatment preferences of their clients. Because breathing is so universally accessible, it can be easily embedded into everyday occupations, such as before an exam, while preparing for sleep or during transitions between caregiving tasks. Because it requires no equipment, can be adapted for diverse physical and cognitive abilities and is portable across contexts, it represents a cost-effective and versatile tool that occupational therapy practitioners can help clients integrate into their daily lives.

Equally important, occupational therapy practitioners recognize that the success of any intervention depends on client volition. Breathing strategies must be meaningful and acceptable to the individual. If a client does not perceive the practice as useful or appealing, it is unlikely to be sustained.

Guided Imagery

Guided imagery or visualization is a relaxation technique that many times is combined with mindful meditation. It involves using positive and calming mental imagery, such as visualizing one's blood nourishing parts of the body, a nature scene or building a dream house in a wooded area. In practice, the therapist guides the individual client through a series of steps to create a relaxing scene in their mind. In using guided imagery (usually 20 minutes), the therapist suggests to the individual to use all of one's senses (visual, auditory and even olfactory) in recreating a peaceful scene such as a beach, mountains or wooded area.

Krau (2020) asserted that guided imagery can enhance well-being, reduce stress and bolster the immune system. Morikawa et al. (2023), in a systematic review of progressive muscular relaxation and guided imagery in managing stress and anxiety in adults with cancer, found that these interventions can be used by occupational therapy practitioners to improve quality of life. They recommended that the individuals learning guided imagery should be provided with instructional compact discs for practice at home and integrate guided imagery as well as progressive relaxation into their daily routines. A recent randomized control found that guided imagery has the potential to reduce stress (Zemla et al., 2023). Finally, Gupta and Chakraverty (2022) found that tele-guided imagery was effective in reducing perceived stress among caregivers of persons with a chronic neurological diagnosis.

Occupational Therapy Application

In general, relaxation therapies including meditation, progressive relaxation and guided imagery can be incorporated into a holistic program in occupational therapy for self-regulation strategies in psychoeducation groups. These interventions can be used to support various activities of daily living and social participation.

Tai Chi

Tai chi is a practice that involves a series of slow, gentle movements and physical postures, a meditative state of mind and controlled breathing. Tai chi originated as an ancient martial art in China. Over the years, it has become more focused on rehabilitation and health promotion.

Huston and MacFarlane (2016) undertook a review of the 500 trials and 120 systematic reviews over the preceding 45 years. They found the following strengths of evidence for its benefits (see Table 8.1).

Tai chi was studied specifically for reducing stress levels in older adults by Siva Subramanian et al. (2024). The group receiving two weeks of tai chi had significantly lower levels of perceived stress at post-intervention measurement. The control group showed no reduction. Zou et al. (2018) reviewed RCTs using tai chi or yoga to affect changes in heart rate variability, a marker for autonomic nervous system operation and thus, indirectly, stress and mental health. In 17 studies they noted evidence of beneficial effects on perceived stress and heart rate variability. They attributed the results to the sympathetic/vagal balance influence of mind-body exercises (Zou et al., 2018).

Table 8.1 Strength of Evidence for Benefits from Tai Chi

Evidence Level	Diagnoses	Benefit
Excellent	OA, PD, COPD, Elderly Healthy people	Fall prevention, cognition Balance, aerobic capacity
Good	Dep, CVA, Card, Dem Healthy people	Various Increased LE strength
Fair	CA, Fibro, HT, OP Healthy people	QoL Well-being, sleep
None	Diabetes, RA, CHF	

From results of a systematic review by Huston and MacFarlane (2016)

Note. OA, osteoarthritis; PD, Parkinson's disease; COP D, chronic obstructive pulmonary disorder; Dep, depression; CVA, cerebrovascular accident; Card, cardiac condition; Dem, dementia; CA, cancer; Fibro, fibromyalgia; HT, hypertension; OP, osteoporosis; QoL, quality of life; RA, rheumatoid arthritis; CHF, congestive heart failure

Additional research has shown tai chi's effectiveness for young adults with subthreshold depression through stress-reward complex mechanisms (Wu et al., 2023), and its benefits for blood pressure, stress, fatigue and sleep quality among women with episodic migraine (Wang et al., 2022). Beyond physical and mental health benefits, tai chi offers spiritual dimensions through its roots in Taoist philosophy and meditative movement practices that promote a holistic view of well-being encompassing body, mind and spiritual aspects (Mendo et al., 2022).

Occupational Therapy Application

Occupational therapy practitioners can integrate tai chi into stress management interventions by adapting the practice to individual client needs and capacities. The slow, gentle movements make tai chi accessible for clients with various physical limitations, including those using wheelchairs or experiencing joint restrictions. Practitioners can modify movements to accommodate cognitive challenges such as early dementia by simplifying sequences and providing clear, step-by-step instruction.

The practice aligns well with occupational therapy's emphasis on meaningful activity and client-centered care. Tai chi can be incorporated into daily routines as a morning stress-reduction practice, integrated into workplace wellness programs or used as a calming activity before sleep. Group tai chi sessions can address social participation goals while providing stress management benefits. The meditative movement aspects support both physical and mental health objectives, making it particularly valuable for clients seeking holistic stress management approaches.

Yoga

Yoga is an ancient and complex practice, rooted in Indian philosophy. It began as a spiritual practice but has become popular as a way of promoting physical and mental well-being. Although classical yoga also includes other elements, yoga as practiced in the U.S. typically emphasizes physical postures (asanas), breathing techniques (pranayama) and meditation (dyana). There are many different yoga styles, ranging from gentle practices to physically demanding ones. Differences in the types of yoga used in research studies may affect study results. This makes it challenging to evaluate research on the health effects of yoga. Yoga and two practices of Chinese origin – tai chi and qigong – are sometimes called "meditative movement" practices. All three practices include both meditative elements and physical ones. Studies have suggested possible benefits of yoga for several aspects of wellness, including stress management, mental/emotional health, promoting healthy eating/activity habits, sleep and balance. Wang and Szabo (2020) found from a review of 12 studies on yoga that most types reduced stress in healthy people. Stress levels in Chinese nurses and self-regulation among medical students were improved by yoga, according to two studies reviewed by Cocchiara et al. (2019).

Further research has demonstrated that yoga may help improve general wellness by relieving stress (Pascoe et al., 2017), improve sleep quality (Wang et al., 2020), help with low back pain (Zhu et al., 2020) and assist with anxiety and depression (Saeed et al., 2019). Additional benefits may include supporting good health habits, improving mental/emotional health, sleep and balance, helping with weight management, supporting smoking cessation efforts, helping manage anxiety or depressive symptoms and relieving menopause symptoms.

The comprehensive nature of yoga's benefits stems from its integration of physical movement, breathwork and mindfulness practices. Meta-analyses have shown that yoga interventions consistently reduce physiological markers of stress while improving psychological well-being, making it an evidence-based approach for stress management across diverse populations. Additionally, yoga integrates an individual's physical, mental and spiritual components, supporting not only stress reduction but also spiritual well-being through practices that recognize health as encompassing body, mind and soul (Mendo et al., 2022).

As yet there is insufficient evidence to claim that yoga helps with headaches or arthritis. It is also noteworthy that people with lower incomes and of minority group status have not been proportionally represented to date in the samples of studies.

Yoga is considered to be a safe physical activity for healthy people when done correctly under supervision. There is a modest risk of strains and sprains, particularly of the lower leg and knee (Cramer et al., 2018).

Occupational Therapy Application

Occupational therapy practitioners can effectively integrate yoga into stress management interventions by adapting practices to align with client goals, interests and physical capabilities. The versatility of yoga allows for modifications that accommodate various limitations, from chair-based poses for individuals with mobility restrictions to simplified breathing exercises for those with cognitive challenges.

Practitioners can work with clients to develop personalized yoga routines that fit naturally into daily schedules, such as morning energizing sequences, workplace stress-relief breathing exercises or evening relaxation practices. The emphasis on breath awareness in yoga makes it particularly valuable for clients learning self-regulation techniques. Group yoga sessions can address social participation goals while building stress management skills in a supportive environment.

Yoga's focus on mind-body connection aligns well with occupational therapy's holistic approach to health and wellness. Practitioners can help clients explore different yoga styles to find approaches that resonate with their preferences and lifestyle, ensuring sustained engagement with the practice. The integration of physical movement, breathing and mindfulness in yoga supports multiple therapeutic goals simultaneously, making it an efficient and comprehensive stress management intervention.

Prescriptive Aerobic Exercise

Aerobic exercise is any physical activity that increases your heart rate and breathing. It boosts the circulation of oxygen throughout the body. The term "aerobic" means "with oxygen," emphasizing that the exercise is sustained long enough to require those muscle units that need oxygen to produce energy to be recruited for the activity.

Common examples of aerobic activities include walking, running, cycling (either on a stationary bike or outdoor bicycle), swimming and dancing. There are many other aerobic activities that we do every day, like climbing stairs, mowing the lawn and working around the garden. Prescriptive aerobic exercise refers to exercise programs that are adapted to the abilities, age and limitations of an individual. For example, an 80-year-old individual with Parkinson's disease might benefit from moderate walking in nature for 30 minutes every day. When designing an individualized aerobic exercise program, the factors to be considered are the purpose of the program (such as reducing stress), the type of exercise program (such as walking outside), the frequency (such as five times a week), the duration (30 minutes engaged in the activity) and the intensity (moderate to fast paced).

Aerobic exercise has been researched thoroughly and has been shown to be effective in reducing stress. Research has demonstrated that it is effective because it reduces the level of cortisol (Zschucke et al., 2015); increases sleep quality (Reid et al., 2010); promotes parasympathetic activity (Wan et al., 2023); increases endorphins (Pahlavani, 2024); increases blood flow to the brain (Stern et al., 2019); increases mental health by reducing stress, anxiety and depression (Noetel et al., 2024; Philippot, 2022); and increases cognitive function in individuals with Alzheimer's disease (Ben Ayed et al., 2024; Zhang et al., 2022). So many studies demonstrate the effectiveness of physical activity, such as aerobic exercise, in reducing stress that Singh et al. (2023) recommended that it be a mainstay in managing anxiety, depression and psychological distress.

CHARACTERISTICS OF AEROBIC EXERCISE

1. Moderate Intensity: Typically performed at an intensity that increases heart rate but allows you to sustain the activity for an extended period while maintaining a steady rate of respiration.
2. Sustained Duration: Usually lasts at least ten minutes and often 20–60 minutes or more.
3. Involves Large Muscle Groups: Engages major muscles in the trunk, legs and arms in repetitive, rhythmic movements.

DIRECT HEALTH BENEFITS OF AEROBIC EXERCISE

1. Improves cardiovascular health by strengthening the heart and lungs.
2. Increases endurance and energy levels.
3. Helps with weight management by burning calories and resetting basal metabolism.
4. Enhances mental health by reducing stress, anxiety and depression.
5. Lowers blood pressure and cholesterol levels.
6. Improves blood sugar control and reduces the risk of Type 2 diabetes.
7. Strengthens the immune system.

Aerobic exercise is suitable for all fitness levels and can be adapted to personal preferences and physical abilities. It is a cornerstone of a well-rounded fitness routine.

Aerobic exercise reduces stress through a combination of physiological and psychological mechanisms. A detailed explanation can be found in Table 8.2.

Table 8.2 Effects of Aerobic Exercise on the Body and Mind

1. Release of endorphins ("Feel-Good Hormones")	During aerobic exercise, the body releases endorphins that act as natural painkillers. They can create a feeling of euphoria referred to as the "runner's high."
2. Reduction in stress hormones	Exercise decreases the levels of stress hormones such as cortisol and adrenaline, released during the "fight or flight" response
3. Improved regulation of the hypothalamic-pituitary-adrenal (HPA) axis	The HPA axis has a central part in the body's stress response. Aerobic exercise enhances its regulation, providing a better response to stressors and a faster recovery of homeostasis.
4. Increased brain-derived neurotrophic factor (BDNF)	Aerobic exercise stimulates BDNF, a protein that supports the growth and repair of brain cells, enhancing neuroplasticity, improving resilience to stress.

5. Activates the parasympathetic nervous system (PNS)	Exercise promotes activation of the PNS, responsible for the "rest and digest" state, which quiets the sympathetic nervous system that is activated by stress.
6. Improved circulation	Aerobic exercise increases blood flow and oxygen delivery to the brain and other tissues.
7. Increased sleep quality	Aerobic exercise improves the sleep-wake cycle. Quality sleep is essential for healthy stress management.
8. Cognitive benefits	Aerobic activity can distract attention from stressors, providing mental relief. Improved cognitive function helps people manage stress better.
9. Cannabinoid system stimulation	Exercise activates the endocannabinoid system, which plays a role in mood regulation.
10. Inflammation reduction	Chronic stress is associated with systemic inflammation. Aerobic exercise reduces inflammation, contributing to improved stress management.

Exercise and Depression

In a systematic review and meta-analysis of prior studies, Heissel et al. (2023) found that exercise was effective as an intervention for depression. The effect was primarily seen when the exercise was conducted in groups or supervised and done at moderate intensity. The biophysiological and psychological mechanisms by which exercise has an anti-depressing effect were investigated by Kandola et al. (2019). They focused on the factors of neuroplasticity, inflammation, oxidative stress, the endocrine system, self-esteem, social support and self-efficacy in their review. Subsequently, Nowacka-Chmielewska et al. (2022) identified outcomes from exercise as including neurotrophism and synaptic plasticity and a reduction of inflammation.

Exercise and Anxiety

In a meta-analysis of studies, Stubbs et al. (2017) found that for people diagnosed with anxiety or a stress-related disorder, exercise improved their symptoms. They noted the additional benefits of exercise on cardiovascular health and well-being as further evidence of its suitability for individuals with this diagnosis.

Aerobic Exercise and Work-Related Stress

Restrepo and Lemos (2021) concluded after a systematic review of studies that aerobic exercise may be effective in reducing work-related stress. They noted that most successful interventions were mindfulness-based, and some used bibliotherapy with a possible beneficial effect (Restrepo & Lemos, 2021).

As to whether aerobic exercise is more effective in stress reduction compared to other interventions, Van der Zwan et al. (2015) found that physical activity, mindfulness meditation and heart rate biofeedback were equally successful in reducing stress, as measured by well-being, sleep quality and symptoms of anxiety and depression.

In summary, aerobic exercise provides a multi-faceted approach to stress reduction by directly influencing the body's hormonal balance, nervous system activity, brain health and overall physiological well-being.

Music and Music Therapy

Music is a tool that many intuitively turn to as part of a coping toolbox. From an occupational therapy perspective, creating, playing or listening to music can serve as both a meaningful occupation in itself and as a tool for supporting stress management. At the same time, the research specific to occupational therapy's use of music as a treatment modality is limited. Much of the evidence for music as a professional, clinical intervention originates in the field of music therapy, a separate and distinct healthcare profession. For example, de Witte et al. (2022) completed a systematic review and meta-analysis of studies on music therapy and stress reduction. They found among the 47 studies reviewed that music therapy had a medium to large positive effect size for reducing stress. Better controlled, randomized studies tended to show medium effect sizes (de Witte et al., 2022).

Occupational therapy practitioners must remain attentive to possible scope-of-practice boundaries and overlaps between occupational therapy, music therapy, and other client-facing professions that utilize music as a tool for stress management. Occupational therapy practitioners must ensure that their use of music complements rather than substitutes for the specialized services of licensed music therapists.

Occupational Therapy Application

Occupational therapy practitioners can incorporate music into interventions when it is a match with client goals and routines. For example, supporting a client in developing personalized playlists to reduce stress before sleep, during commutes or when stressful situations occur can foster a meaningful coping strategy.

Music can also be incorporated into both individual and group sessions. Galloway and Rodriguez (2024) highlighted the underuse of and lack of training on music as an intervention for occupational therapy practitioners, pointing toward an opportunity for further study and increased integration into practice.

Horticulture Therapy

Increasing attention has been directed toward non-pharmacological stress management interventions that promote resilience and emotional regulation (Niazi & Niazi, 2011; Umbrello et al., 2019). Horticulture, the practice of cultivating and caring for plants, has been utilized as a method for managing stress and alleviating its symptoms (Kamioka et al., 2014). In horticultural therapy, structured gardening activities are employed to enhance psychological well-being and reduce levels of stress (Lu et al., 2023).

Several studies support the effectiveness of horticultural therapy, citing reductions in cortisol levels and SNS activity, along with improvements in cardiovascular health (Lee et al., 2013; Park et al., 2009; Taran et al., 2023). Researchers have hypothesized that gardening aligns with humans' innate tendency to connect with nature, a concept explored in biophilia theory (Wilson, 1986). There is also substantial evidence for the positive psychological effects of horticultural therapy (Van Den Berg & Custers, 2011). Tu (2022), in a meta-analysis, found a medium effect size toward positive mental health from horticulture activities in some studies.

According to the attention restoration theory, spending time in natural environments after exposure to urban settings can restore cognitive functioning through the mechanism of effortless attention (Kaplan, 1995). Horticulture therapy may also enhance mindfulness and improve reality testing, as it requires sustained focus on strong sensory stimuli such as soil texture, plant colors and changes in growth (Kabat-Zinn, 2003). Group- or community-based horticultural activities may foster social interaction and improve quality of life, thereby further alleviating stress (Kamioka et al., 2014; Soga et al., 2017).

Typical horticulture therapy activities include raking, planting, fertilizing, staking plants, harvesting, sowing seeds, propagation, potting, pruning, washing and arranging flowers. These tasks have shown greater benefits for stress management when performed in low cognitively demanding configurations (Kim & Park, 2023). Additional suggestions for horticultural therapeutic activities are widely documented in the literature (Simson & Straus, 1997; Söderback et al., 2004).

Horticulture therapy is increasingly being adopted as a clinical and community-based approach to stress management in hospitals, mental health centers, clinics and rehabilitation facilities (Detweiler et al., 2012). Horticulture is also being integrated into workplace wellness programs and through school gardening in educational settings as a viable intervention for stress reduction (Ohly et al., 2016).

Arts Therapy

There has been a growing scholarly interest in arts-based interventions as complementary modalities for addressing stress (Stuckey & Nobel, 2010; Tjasink et al., 2023). The therapeutic use of the arts is grounded in expressive and humanistic frameworks, which hypothesize that creativity fosters psychological resilience, emotional regulation and meaning-making (Csikszentmihalyi, 1990; Iguina & Kashan, 2025). Engagement in the arts activates the processes of symbolic representation and embodies cognition, enabling individuals to externalize internal states, reframe stressful experiences and cultivate a sense of mastery (Jones, 2007). Furthermore, neurobiological evidence indicates that creative expression can down-regulate HPA axis activity, thereby reducing the physiological reactions of stress (Kaimal et al., 2016).

Visual arts interventions, including painting, drawing and sculpture, have been shown to significantly reduce cortisol levels and improve affective states, suggesting a direct psychophysiological pathway for stress alleviation (Kaimal et al., 2016). Beyond biochemical outcomes, the creative arts foster mindfulness and flow states, both of which are strongly correlated with stress reduction and enhanced well-being (Csikszentmihalyi, 1990).

Dance and movement therapy integrate somatic awareness with expressive movement, providing a dual pathway of stress reduction through physical activity and symbolic expression. Randomized controlled trials indicate significant reductions in stress-related symptoms and improved psychological resilience following dance-based interventions (Bräuninger, 2012).

Drama therapy and creative writing further extend the scope of arts-based stress management by facilitating narrative reconstruction and cognitive reappraisal. Through storytelling and role-play, individuals are able to process traumatic or stressful experiences in a contained and symbolic manner, thereby reducing psychological distress and enhancing adaptive coping capacities (Jones, 2007).

The efficacy of the arts in stress management can be attributed to several interrelated mechanisms. First, physiological modulation may occur through the reduction of stress biomarkers such as cortisol and heart rate. Second, affective regulation enables the expression, recognition and transformation of emotions. Third, cognitive restructuring allows for the reframing of stressful experiences through metaphor and narrative. Additionally, arts-based interventions foster social connectedness, enhancing interpersonal support and collective resilience. Finally, engagement in the arts may promote mindfulness and flow, encouraging states of presence, absorption and non-judgmental awareness (Abbing et al., 2019; Huet, 2015; Martin et al., 2018; Visnola et al., 2010).

Other Therapeutic Stress Management Approaches

Sensory Rooms

Established initially by Champagne and Stromberg (2004), sensory rooms are spaces with lights, music, weighted items, textures and activities that are designed to help children or adults manage frustration, anxiety and stress. Features can include textured floor squares, fidget toys, noise-canceling headphones and beanbag chairs. Sensory rooms, where an optimal amount of sensory stimulation is provided, can help individuals strengthen coping skills (Doroud et al., 2024; Importance of sensory rooms in mental health crisis intervention for children, n.d.). Furthermore, West et al. (2017) found that Australian adolescents with a history of aggression or anxiety in psychiatric care, or those who were female, benefited the most from access to a sensory room, according to a measure of distress. Finally, among university students in Australia, those who accessed an art-enriched, nature-enhanced sensory room self-reported a decrease in negative emotions, an increase in positive feelings and a reduction in perceived stress levels (Cavanagh et al., 2021).

There is some evidence, therefore, of the effectiveness of sensory rooms for stress management and the exploration of coping skills among children, adolescents and young adults. They could be another tool used by occupational therapists in guiding their clients to better self-regulation during the challenges of life.

Biofeedback

Using biofeedback to achieve health goals began to become widespread in the 1980s in the U.S. Although it has been partly superseded by other techniques of relaxation, it continues to play a role in some settings. Brinkmann et al. (2020) compared a heart rate variability biofeedback approach to mindfulness-based intervention in a workplace setting. The biofeedback was as effective as the mindfulness in improving the outcome measures (stress perception, coping, well-being and symptoms of depression) taken after six weeks of intervention. Where available, biofeedback could be incorporated into the stress management program for an occupational therapy client if it suited the client and was meaningful.

Word, Number and Video Games

The following word, number and video games were selected from a list generated through Chat-GPT artificial intelligence in September, 2025. Popular word games such as Scrabble, Boggle and Wordle; number games such as sudoku, KenKen and 2048; and video games, such as The Legend of Zelda, The Elder Scrolls, Animal Crossing, Super Mario, Tetris and Minecraft, have in common that they not only seem to reduce stress by providing an engaging world of challenges, but many also involve the user in social communication and rule-following that can build resilience for responding to future stressors. In addition, video games requiring whole-body exercise, such as Dance Dance Revolution or those on the Wii platform (bowling, tennis and golf – added to the list by human intelligence), have the additional stress reduction benefits of aerobic exercise.

Word and number games have been experienced by many as providing an immersive distraction from negative thoughts in response to stressors. They may even be effective in inducing a flow-like state in players. Video games have a similar or greater potential for reducing stress (Pallavicini et al., 2021), as they may require total concentration by players in order to follow the rules of the game and achieve success. While a competition or self-competition may drive up the stress reaction, in certain winnable modes they may reduce stress by inducing a flow state.

Pallavicini and Pepe (2020) studied the emotional and self-reported stress response in players of low- and high-movement virtual reality (VR) video games. Overall exposure to the VR world increased positive emotions, reduced negative feelings and led to a lower reported sense of stress in players. Furthermore, a game requiring a higher level of movement (Audioshield) had greater beneficial effects than one calling for less movement (Fruit Ninja VR; Pallavicini & Pepe, 2020).

Sex and Stress Management

A considerable number of studies have been conducted on human sexual activity and its effect on a variety of physiological and psychological constructs. It has been established that orgasm contributes to an increase in dopamine, endorphins, serotonin and oxytocin (pleasure and bonding hormones; Pfaus, 2025), which results post-coitus in a lowering of blood pressure and thus of the stress reaction. Furthermore, sexual activity increases prolactin (sleep inducing; Brody, 2010), and better ongoing sleep tends to reduce stress. Sexual activity also tends to reduce cortisol and adrenaline levels, which correlates with reducing the stress reaction (Brody, 2006). One study found that after heterosexual intercourse, people would later experience a smaller blood pressure increase after encountering a stressor (Brody, 2006). Several studies have found that the effects are strongest for heterosexual intercourse (Brody, 2010), although it is difficult to separate out social disapprobation as a factor in these differences. Indeed, the sensitivity to sexual issues and desires for privacy make high-quality scientific studies on sexual activity and stress challenging.

It has been established that high levels of chronic stress can negatively affect sexual desire and function (Bodenmann et al., 2010). Conversely, the enhancement of emotional connectivity and psychological support fostered by mutually satisfying sexual activity theoretically would buffer the negative effects of stress. Finally, not to be forgotten is that coerced sexual activity or that within a maladjusted relationship would likely cause greater stress. Thus, therapy practitioners should be conservative in claiming that increased sexual activity will result in better stress management. More direct empirical research needs to be done.

Animal-Assisted Therapy

Animal-assisted therapy (or pet therapy) is the use of an animal to enhance human interaction through touch, visual, auditory and emotional pathways. It ranges from a dog or rabbit being brought to an assisted living facility, to therapeutic horseback riding, to swimming with dolphins. The particular benefits are said to be that the animal provides an unconditional positive relation, that the animal facilitates non-verbal communication and that the animal can provide a new perspective for an individual who is mobility-impaired (such as from the back of a horse).

Overall, animal-assisted therapy shows promise as an intervention for promoting well-being, including stress reduction, among varied populations. Pandey et al. (2024) reviewed five studies suggesting benefits for stress reduction. They recommended further research and the establishment of standardized outcome measures to strengthen the body of evidence for animal-assisted therapy.

Specifically, in a children's hospital setting, Feng et al. (2021) found in a review and meta-analysis that animal-assisted therapy reduced pain and improved blood pressure readings in children who were hospitalized. Overall, though, the eight studies reviewed did not provide evidence that this amount of animal interaction reduced anxiety or depression, or "stress" in general among the participants. Richardson et al. (2022) interviewed parents of autistic children and adolescents about the effects of receiving therapy time with a dog. Parents explicitly cited stress and anxiety reduction as one of the apparent effects of the dog's presence. Parents also noted how the dog fostered social communication in their child or teen (Richardson et al., 2022). Better social communication would itself then contribute to positive resources, instilling greater resilience in the individual. Finally, in a small RCT on military veterans with PTSD, Johnson et al. (2018) found that PTSD measures were statistically significantly reduced after six weeks of therapeutic horseback riding. Coping self-efficacy scores, though, were not.

Due to the widespread availability of pets, it is feasible for an occupational therapy practitioner to consider suggesting time with a pet as part of a stress management strategy for many clients.

Spirituality

Individuals incurring an acute disease or those living with a long-term illness or condition may face adjustment concerns surrounding why these events have happened and the ultimate meaning of their lives. For many, spirituality, including both established religions and independent thought and beliefs, can be a potent source of stress relief. Spiritual values may provide a means in the face of serious stressors for people to decouple their stress reactions. Puchalski et al. (2018) found that an important role was played by spiritual issues among people with cancer. They cited studies that demonstrated a positive effect from a client's spirituality on health outcomes, including anxiety, depression and coping. They called on physicians to assess for "spiritual distress" and to work with spiritual care professionals to ensure these needs are addressed (Puchalski et al., 2018). The recommendation could be applied to all health care professionals.

SUMMARY

In this chapter, specific strategies and activities for stress management were described, such as mindfulness meditation, guided imagery, progressive muscle relaxation, breathing, aerobic exercises, tai chi, yoga, music, arts, horticulture therapy, animal-assisted therapy, word/number/video games and many others that have been shown to be effective in reducing distress and improving related outcome measures. Less widely used approaches as yet do not have strong empirical evidence as to their effectiveness, although there are some positive early indications. With so many activities to select from, the occupational therapy practitioner can offer a wide spectrum of activities to clients seeking to manage their stress. *Flow* is an important element of how to use these activities therapeutically in an effective, meaningful and sustainable way.

DISCUSSION QUESTIONS

1. Which activities do you use for stress reduction? Which of them could you use with clients in an OT practice?
2. Which activity categories have the strongest empirical evidence of their effectiveness for stress reduction?
3. Why is it important in OT practice to collaborate with the client in creating a recommended stress reduction strategy?
4. What are the basic mechanisms, physiological and psychological, by which activities create lower stress levels?

REFERENCES

Abbing, A., de Sonneville, L., Baars, E., Bourne, D., & Swaab, H. (2019). Anxiety reduction through art therapy in women: Exploring stress regulation and executive functioning as underlying neurocognitive mechanisms. *PLOS One, 14*(12), e0225200. https://doi.org/10.1371/journal.pone.0225200

Aktaş, Y. Y. (2023). The effect of deep breathing exercise and the 4–7–8 breathing technique on anxiety and quality of life in patients undergoing bariatric surgery: A randomized controlled trial. *Perspectives in Psychiatric Care, 59*(1), 94–102. https://doi.org/10.1111/ppc.13176

American Institute of Stress. https://www.stress.org, accessed 9 October, 2025.

Baminiwatta, A., & Solangaarachchi, I. (2021). Trends and developments in mindfulness research over 55 years: A bibliometric analysis of publications indexed in Web of Science. *Mindfulness*, *12*(9), 2099–2116. https://doi.org/10.1007/s12671-021-01681-x

Ben Ayed, I., Ammar, A., Aouichaoui, C., Mezghani, N., Salem, A., Naija, S., Ben Amor, S., Trabelsi, K., Jahrami, H., Trabelsi, Y., & El Massioui, F. (2024). Does acute aerobic exercise enhance selective attention, working memory, and problem-solving abilities in Alzheimer's patients? A sex-based comparative study. *Frontiers in Sports and Active Living, 6*, 1383119. https://doi.org/10.3389/fspor.2024.1383119

Benson, H. (1975). *The relaxation response*. William Morrow & Co.

Bentley, T. G. K., D'Andrea-Penna, G., Rakic, M., Arce, N., LaFaille, M., Berman, R., Cooley, K., & Sprimont, P. (2023). Breathing practices for stress and anxiety reduction: Conceptual framework of implementation guidelines based on a systematic review of the published literature. *Brain Sciences*, *13*(12), 1612. https://doi.org/10.3390/brainsci13121612

Bodenmann, G., Atkins, D. C., Schär, M., & Poffet, V. (2010). The association between daily stress and sexual activity. *Journal of Family Psychology, 24*(3), 271–279. https://doi.org/10.1037/a0019365

Bräuninger, I. (2012). Dance movement therapy group intervention in stress treatment: A randomized controlled trial (RCT). *Arts in Psychotherapy, 39*(5), 443–450. https://doi.org/10.1016/j.aip.2012.07.002

Brinkmann, A. E., Press, S. A., Helmert, E., Hautzinger, M., Khazan, I., & Vagedes, J. (2020). Comparing effectiveness of HRV-biofeedback and mindfulness for workplace stress reduction: A randomized controlled trial. *Applied Psychophysiological Biofeedback, 45*(4), 307–322. https://doi.org/10.1007/s10484-020-09477-w

Brody, S. (2006). Blood pressure reactivity to stress is better for people who recently had penile-vaginal intercourse than for people who had other or no sexual activity. *Biological Psychology, 71*(2), 214–222. https://doi.org/10.1016/j.biopsycho.2005.03.005

Brody S. (2010). The relative health benefits of different sexual activities. *Journal of Sexual Medicine, 7*, 1336–1361. https://doi.org/10.1111/j.1743-6109.2009.01677.x

Cavanagh, B., Haracz, K., Lawry, M., Wales, K., & James, C. (2021). Changes in emotions and perceived stress following time spent in an artistically designed multisensory environment. *Medical Humanities*, *47*(4), e13. https://doi.org/10.1136/medhum-2020-011876

Champagne, T., & Stromberg, N. (2004). Sensory approaches in inpatient psychiatric settings: Innovative alternatives to seclusion & restraint. *Journal of Psychosocial Nursing and Mental Health Services*, *42*(9), 34–44. https://doi.org/10.3928/02793695-20040901-06

Clynes, M. (1973). Sentics: Biocybernetics of emotion communication. *Annals of the New York Academy of Sciences, 220*(3), 55–131. https://doi.org/10.1111/j.1749-6632.1973.tb40248.x

Cocchiara, R. A., Peruzzo, M., Mannocci, A., Ottolenghi, L., Villari, P., Polimeni, A., Guerra, F., & La Torre, G. (2019). The use of yoga to manage stress and burnout in healthcare workers: A systematic review. *Journal of Clinical Medicine, 8*(3), 284. https://doi.org/10.3390/jcm8030284

Cramer, H., Ostermann, T., & Dobos, G. (2018). Injuries and other adverse events associated with yoga practice: A systematic review of epidemiological studies. *Journal of Science and Medicine in Sport, 21*(2), 147–154. https://doi.org/10.1016/j.jsams.2017.08.026

Csikszentmihalyi, M. (1990). *Flow: The psychology of optimal experience*. Harper and Row.

da Silva, C. C. G., Bolognani, C. V., Amorim, F. F., & Imoto, A. M. (2023). Effectiveness of training programs based on mindfulness in reducing psychological distress and promoting well-being in medical students: A systematic review and meta-analysis. *Systematic Reviews, 12*(1), 79. https://doi.org/10.1186/s13643-023-02244-y

de Witte, M., Pinho, A. D. S., Stams, G. J., Moonen, X., Bos, A. E. R., & van Hooren, S. (2022). Music therapy for stress reduction: A systematic review and meta-analysis. *Health Psychology Review, 16*(1), 134–159. https://doi.org/10.1080/17437199.2020.1846580

Detweiler, M. B., Sharma, T., Detweiler, J. G., Murphy, P. F., Lane, S., Carman, J., Chudhary, A. S., Halling, M. H., & Kim, K. Y. (2012). What is the evidence to support the use of therapeutic gardens for the elderly? *Psychiatry Investigation, 9*(2), 100–110. https://doi.org/10.4306/pi.2012.9.2.100

Doroud, N., Cappy, M., Grant, K., Scopelliti, M., McKinstry, C., & McMahon, D. (2024). Sensory rooms within mental health settings: A systematic scoping review. *Occupational Therapy in Mental Health, 41*(1), 38–58. https://doi.org/10.1080/0164212X.2024.2308290

Feng, Y., Lin, Y., Zhang, N., Jiang, X., & Zhang, L. (2021). Effects of animal-assisted therapy on hospitalized children and teenagers: A systematic review and meta-analysis. *Journal of Pediatric Nursing, 60*, 11–23. https://doi.org/10.1016/j.pedn.2021.01.020

Fisch, S., Brinkhaus, B., & Teut, M. (2017). Hypnosis in patients with perceived stress: A systematic review. *BMC Complementary and Alternative Medicine, 17*(1), 323. https://doi.org/10.1186/s12906-017-1806-0

Galloway, A. B., & Rodriguez, A. K. (2024). Intentional uses of music in occupational therapy practice: The effectiveness of a workshop. *Journal of Occupational Therapy Education, 8*(4). https://doi.org/10.26681/jote.2024.080418

Ghahari, S., Mohammadi-Hasel, K., Malakouti, S. K., & Roshanpajouh, M. (2020). Mindfulness-based cognitive therapy for generalised anxiety disorder: A systematic review and meta-analysis. *East Asian Archives of Psychiatry, 30*(2), 52–56. https://doi.org/10.12809/eaap1885

Goldberg, S. B., Tucker, R. P., Greene, P. A., Davidson, R. J., Wampold, B. E., Kearney, D. J., & Simpson, T. L. (2018). Mindfulness-based interventions for psychiatric disorders: A systematic review and meta-analysis. *Clinical Psychology Review, 59*, 52–60. https://doi.org/10.1016/j.cpr.2017.10.011

Goldstein, J. (2013). *Mindfulness: A practical guide to awakening.* Sounds True.

Gupta, M., & Chakraverty, S. (2022). Effect of tele-guided imagery on stress among caregivers of chronic neurological patients: A randomized controlled trial. *Journal of Neurosciences in Rural Practice, 13*(2), 333–335. https://doi.org/10.1055/s-0042-1744119

Hamasaki, H. (2020). Effects of diaphragmatic breathing on health: A narrative review. *Medicines, 7*(10), 65. https://doi.org/10.3390/medicines7100065

Harorani, M., Davodabady, F., Farahani, Z., Hezave, A. K., & Rafiei, F. (2020). The effect of Benson's relaxation response on sleep quality and anorexia in cancer patients undergoing chemotherapy: A randomized controlled trial. *Complementary Therapies in Medicine, 50*, 102344. https://doi.org/10.1016/j.ctim.2020.102344

Heissel, A., Heinen, D., Brokmeier, L. L., Skarabis, N., Kangas, M., Vancampfort, D., Stubbs, B., Firth, J., Ward, P. B., Rosenbaum, S., Hallgren, M., & Schuch, F. (2023). Exercise as medicine for depressive symptoms? A systematic review and meta-analysis with meta-regression. *British Journal of Sports Medicine, 57*(16), 1049–1057. https://doi.org/10.1136/bjsports-2022-106282

Hofmann, S. G., & Gómez, A. F. (2017). Mindfulness-based interventions for anxiety and depression. *Psychiatric Clinics of North America*, *40*(4), 739–749. https://doi.org/10.1016/j.psc.2017.08.008

Huang, J., & Shi, L. (2016). The effectiveness of mindfulness-based stress reduction (MBSR) for survivors of breast cancer: Study protocol for a randomized controlled trial. *Trials, 17*, 209. https://doi.org/10.1186/s13063-016-1335-z

Huet, V. (2015). Literature review of art therapy-based interventions for work-related stress. *International Journal of Art Therapy, 20*(2), 66–76. https://doi.org/10.1080/17454832.2015.1023323

Huston, P., & McFarlane, B. (2016). Health benefits of tai chi: What is the evidence? *Canadian Family Physician/Medecin de Famille Canadien, 62*(11), 881–890. [no doi].

Iguina, M. M., & Kashan, S. (2025). Art therapy. In *StatPearls*. StatPearls Publishing.

Importance of sensory rooms in mental health crisis intervention for children. (n.d.). Retrieved from https://monarchnc.org/the-importance-of-sensory-rooms-in-mental-health-crisis-intervention-for-children/#:~:text=A%20sensory%20room%20is%20a,cuddle%20ball%20to%20reduce%20anxiety

Jacobson, E. (1924). The technic of progressive relaxation. *Journal of Nervous and Mental Disease, 60*(6), 568–578. [no doi].

Jacobson, E. (1929). *Progressive relaxation*. University of Chicago Press.

Jerath, R., Crawford, M.W., Barnes, V.A., & Harden, K. (2023). Brief structured respiration practices enhance mood and reduce physiological stress: A review of box breathing and related techniques. *Frontiers in Psychology, 14*, 9873947. https://doi.org/10.3389/fpsyg.2023.9873947

Johnson, R. A., Albright, D. L., Marzolf, J. R., Bibbo, J. L., Yaglom, H. D., Crowder, S. M., Carlisle, G. K., Willard, A., Russell, C. L., Grindler, K., Osterlind, S., Wassman, M., & Harms, N. (2018). Effects of therapeutic horseback riding on post-traumatic stress disorder in military veterans. *Military Medical Research*, *5*(1), 3. https://doi.org/10.1186/s40779-018-0149-6

Jones, P. (2007). *Drama as therapy: Theory, practice and research* (Vol. 1). Routledge.

Kabat-Zinn, J. (1982). An outpatient program in behavioral medicine for chronic pain patients based on the practice of mindfulness meditation: Theoretical considerations and preliminary results. *General Hospital Psychiatry*, *4*(1), 33–47. https://doi.org/10.1016/0163-8343(82)90026-3

Kabat-Zinn, J. (2003). Mindfulness-based interventions in context: Past, present, and future. *Clinical Psychology: Science and Practice, 10*(2), 144–156. https://doi.org/10.1093/clipsy.bpg016

Kaimal, G., Ray, K., & Muniz, J. (2016). Reduction of cortisol levels and participants' responses following art making. *Art Therapy, 33*(2), 74–80. https://doi.org/10.1080/07421656.2016.1166832

Kamioka, H., Tsutani, K., Yamada, M., Park, H., Okuizumi, H., Honda, T., Okada, S., Park, S.-J., Kitayuguchi, J., Abe, T., Handa, S., & Mutoh, Y. (2014). Effectiveness of horticultural therapy: A systematic review of randomized controlled trials. *Complementary Therapies in Medicine*, *22*(5), 930–943. https://doi.org/10.1016/j.ctim.2014.08.009

Kandola, A., Ashdown-Franks, G., Hendrikse, J., Sabiston, C. M., & Stubbs, B. (2019). Physical activity and depression: Towards understanding the antidepressant mechanisms of physical activity. *Neuroscience Biobehavioral Review, 107*, 525–539. https://doi.org/10.1016/j.neubiorev.2019.09.040

Kaplan, S. (1995). The restorative benefits of nature: Toward an integrative framework. *Journal of Environmental Psychology, 15*(3), 169–182. https://doi.org/10.1016/0272-4944(95)90001-2

Khoury, B., Lecomte, T., Fortin, G., Masse, M., Therien, P., Bouchard, V., Chapleau, M. A., Paquin, K., & Hofmann, S. G. (2013). Mindfulness-based therapy: A comprehensive meta-analysis. *Clinical Psychology Review, 33*(6), 763–771. https://doi.org/10.1016/j.cpr.2013.05.005

Kim, Y.-J., & Park, S.-A. (2023). Effects of cognitive demand levels for various horticultural activities on psychophysiological responses in adults. *Horticultural Science, 58*(11), 1450–1458. https://doi.org/10.21273/HORTSCI17272-23

Kramer, J., Litschel, R., Schöbi, N., Tschacher, W., & Hilt, N. (2023). Effects of slow-paced diaphragmatic breathing on negative affect and relaxation in children: A microrandomized trial. *Journal of Pediatric Psychology, 48*(7), 683–694. https://doi.org/10.1093/jpepsy/jsad037

Krau, S. D. (2020). The multiple uses of guided imagery. *Nursing Clinics of North America, 55*(4), 467–474. https://doi.org/10.1016/j.cnur.2020.06.013

Kuyken, W., Hayes, R., Barrett, B., Byng, R., Dalgleish, T., Kessler, D., Lewis, G., Watkins, E., Brejcha, C., Cardy, J., Causley, A., Cowderoy, S., Evans, A., Gradinger, F., Kaur, S., Lanham, P., Morant, N., Richards, J., Shah, P., Sutton, H., … Byford, S. (2015). Effectiveness and cost-effectiveness of mindfulness-based cognitive therapy compared with maintenance antidepressant treatment in the prevention of depressive relapse or recurrence (PREVENT): A randomised controlled trial. *Lancet, 386*(9988), 63–73. https://doi.org/10.1016/S0140-6736(14)62222-4

Lee, M.-s., Park, B.-j., Lee, J., Park, K.-t., Ku, J.-h., Lee, J.-w., Oh, K.-o., & Miyazaki, Y. (2013). Physiological relaxation induced by horticultural activity: Transplanting work using flowering plants. *Journal of Physiological Anthropology, 32*(1), 15. https://doi.org/10.1186/1880-6805-32-15

Lim, S. J., & Kim, C. (2014). Effects of autogenic training on stress response and heart rate variability in nursing students. *Asian Nursing Research*, *8*(4), 286–292. https://doi.org/10.1016/j.anr.2014.06.003

Lu, S., Liu, J., Xu, M., & Xu, F. (2023). Horticultural therapy for stress reduction: A systematic review and meta-analysis. *Frontiers in Psychology, 14*, 1086121. https://doi.org/10.3389/fpsyg.2023.1086121

Ma, X., Yue, Z. Q., Gong, Z. Q., Zhang, H., Duan, N. Y., Shi, Y. T., Wei, G. X., & Li, Y. F. (2017). The effect of diaphragmatic breathing on attention, negative affect and stress in healthy adults. *Frontiers in Psychology, 8*, 874. https://doi.org/10.3389/fpsyg.2017.00874

Magnon, V., Dutheil, F., & Vallet, G. T. (2021). Benefits from one session of deep and slow breathing on vagal tone and anxiety in young and older adults. *Scientific Reports, 11*, 19267. https://doi.org/10.1038/s41598-021-98736-9

Martin, L., Oepen, R., Bauer, K., Nottensteiner, A., Mergheim, K., Gruber, H., & Koch, S. C. J. B. S. (2018). Creative arts interventions for stress management and prevention: A systematic review. *Behavioral Sciences, 8*(2), 28. https://doi.org/10.3390/bs8020028

Mason, P. (1994). *The Marashi: The biography of the man who gave Transcendental Meditation to the world*. Element.

Mendo, B., Gonçalves, M., Lopes, L., Matos, L. C., & Machado, J. (2022). Can yoga, qigong, and tai chi breathing work support the psycho-immune homeostasis during and after the

COVID-19 pandemic? A narrative review. *Healthcare, 10*(10), 1934. https://doi.org/10.3390/healthcare10101934

Mirgain, S. A., & Singles, J. (2016). *Progressive muscle relaxation*. https://www.va.gov/WHOLE-HEALTHLIBRARY/tools/progressive-muscle-relaxation.asp

Morikawa, S., Newman, R., & Amanat, Y. (2023). Relaxation and guided imagery for adults living with and beyond breast cancer (2018–2022). *American Journal of Occupational Therapy, 77*(Supplement 1), 7710393300. https://doi.org/10.5014/ajot.2023.77S10030

Muhammad Khir, S., Wan Mohd Yunus, W. M. A., Mahmud, N., Wang, R., Panatik, S. A., Mohd Sukor, M. S., & Nordin, N. A. (2024). Efficacy of progressive muscle relaxation in adults for stress, anxiety, and depression: A systematic review. *Psychology Research and Behavior Management, 17*, 345–365. https://doi.org/10.2147/PRBM.S437277

Niazi, A. K., & Niazi, S. K. (2011). Mindfulness-based stress reduction: A non-pharmacological approach for chronic illnesses. *North American Journal of Medical Sciences, 3*(1), 20. https://doi.org/10.4297/najms.2011.320

Noetel, M., Sanders, T., Gallardo-Gómez, D., Taylor, P., Del Pozo Cruz, B., van den Hoek, D., Smith, J. J., Mahoney, J., Spathis, J., Moresi, M., Pagano, R., Pagano, L., Vasconcellos, R., Arnott, H., Varley, B., Parker, P., Biddle, S., & Lonsdale, C. (2024). Effect of exercise for depression: Systematic review and network meta-analysis of randomised controlled trials. *BMJ (Clinical Research ed.), 384*, e075847. https://doi.org/10.1136/bmj-2023-075847

Nowacka-Chmielewska, M., Grabowska, K., Grabowski, M., Meybohm, P., Burek, M., & Małecki, A. (2022). Running from stress: Neurobiological mechanisms of exercise-induced stress resilience. *International Journal of Molecular Sciences, 23*(21), 13348. https://doi.org/10.3390/ijms232113348

Ohly, H., Gentry, S., Wigglesworth, R., Bethel, A., Lovell, R., & Garside, R. (2016). A systematic review of the health and well-being impacts of school gardening: Synthesis of quantitative and qualitative evidence. *BMC Public Health, 16*(1), 286. https://doi.org/10.1186/s12889-016-2941-0

Ooi, S. L., Giovino, M., & Pak, S. C. (2017). Transcendental meditation for lowering blood pressure: An overview of systematic reviews and meta-analyses. *Complementary Therapies in Medicine, 34*, 26–34. https://doi.org/10.1016/j.ctim.2017.07.008

Pahlavani, H. A. (2024). Possible role of exercise therapy on depression: Effector neurotransmitters as key players. *Behavioural Brain Research, 459*, 114791. https://doi.org/10.1016/j.bbr.2023.114791

Pallavicini, F., & Pepe, A. (2020). Virtual reality games and the role of body involvement in enhancing positive emotions and decreasing anxiety: Within-subjects pilot study. *JMIR Serious Games, 8*(2), e15635. https://doi.org/10.2196/15635

Pallavicini, F., Pepe, A., & Mantovani, F. (2021). Commercial off-the-shelf video games for reducing stress and anxiety: Systematic review. *JMIR Mental Health, 8*(8), e28150. https://doi.org/10.2196/28150

Pandey, R. P., Himanshu, G., Mukherjee, R., & Chang, C. M. (2024). The role of animal-assisted therapy in enhancing patients' well-being: Systematic study of the qualitative and quantitative evidence. *JMIRx Med, 5*, e51787. https://doi.org/10.2196/51787

Park, S.-A., Shoemaker, C. A., & Haub, M. D. (2009). Physical and psychological health conditions of older adults classified as gardeners or nongardeners. *Horticultural Science, 44*(1), 206–210. https://doi.org/10.21273/HORTSCI.44.1.206

Pascoe, M. C., Thompson, D. R., Jenkins, Z. M., & Ski, C. F. (2017). Mindfulness mediates the physiological markers of stress: Systematic review and meta-analysis. *Journal of Psychiatric Research, 95*, 156–178. https://doi.org/10.1016/j.jpsychires.2017.08.004

Pascoe, M. C., Thompson, D. R., & Ski, C. F. (2017). Yoga, mindfulness-based stress reduction and stress-related physiological measures: A meta-analysis. *Psychoneuroendocrinology, 86*, 152–168. https://doi.org/10.1016/j.psyneuen.2017.08.008

Pfaus, J. G. (2025). Orgasms, sexual pleasure, and opioid reward mechanisms. *Sexual Medicine Reviews, 13*(3), 381–393. https://doi.org/10.1093/sxmrev/qeaf023

Philippot, A., Dubois, V., Lambrechts, K., Grogna, D., Robert, A., Jonckheer, U., Chakib, W., Beine, A., Bleyenheuft, Y., & De Volder, A. G. (2022). Impact of physical exercise on depression and anxiety in adolescent inpatients: A randomized controlled trial. *Journal of Affective Disorders, 301*, 145–153. https://doi.org/10.1016/j.jad.2022.01.011

Puchalski, C. M., King, S. D. W., & Ferrell, B. R. (2018). Spiritual considerations. *Hematology/Oncology Clinics of North America, 32*(3), 505–517. https://doi.org/10.1016/j.hoc.2018.01.011

Raj, N. (2021). Effect of box breathing technique on lung function test in healthy individuals. *Journal of Pharmaceutical Research International, 33*(46B), 191–197. https://doi.org/10.9734/jpri/2021/v33i46B32917

Reid, K. J., Baron, K. G., Lu, B., Naylor, E., Wolfe, L., & Zee, P. C. (2010). Aerobic exercise improves self-reported sleep and quality of life in older adults with insomnia. *Sleep Medicine, 11*(9), 934–940. https://doi.org/10.1016/j.sleep.2010.04.0143

Restrepo, J., & Lemos, M. (2021). Addressing psychosocial work-related stress interventions: A systematic review. *Work, 70*(1), 53–62. https://doi.org/10.3233/WOR-213577

Richardson, K., Mackenzie, L., Lovarini, M., & Dickson, C. (2022). Occupational therapy incorporating dogs for autistic children and young people: Parent perspectives. *British Journal of Occupational Therapy, 85*(11), 859–868. https://doi.org/10.1177/03080226221086217

Saeed, S. A., Cunningham, K., & Bloch, R. M. (2019). Depression and anxiety disorders: Benefits of exercise, yoga, and meditation. *American Family Physician, 99*(10), 620–627. [no doi; PMID: 31083878].

Sapolsky, R. (1998). *Why zebras don't get ulcers: An updated guide to stress, stress-related disease and coping*. W. H. Freeman & Co.

Sharma, M., & Haider, T. (2015). Tai chi as an alternative and complimentary therapy for anxiety: A systematic review. *Journal of Evidence-based Complementary & Alternative Medicine, 20*(2), 143–153. https://doi.org/10.1177/2156587214561327

Simson, S., & Straus, M. (1997). *Horticulture as therapy: Principles and practice*. CRC Press.

Singh, B., Olds, T., Curtis, R., Dumuid, D., Virgara, R., Watson, A., Szeto, K., O'Connor, E., Ferguson, T., Eglitis, E., Miatke, A., Simpson, C. E., & Maher, C. (2023). Effectiveness of physical activity interventions for improving depression, anxiety and distress: An overview of systematic reviews. *British Journal of Sports Medicine, 57*(18), 1203–1209. https://doi.org/10.1136/bjsports-2022-106195

Siva Subramanian, N., Hareshbhai, M. Z., Santhi, S., Bhaskaran, R., Jamuna Rani, P., & Mahalakshmi, B. (2024). Evaluating the impact of tai chi therapy on stress reduction among older adults. *Bioinformation, 20*(12), 1877–1880. https://doi.org/10.6026/9732063002001877

Soga, M., Gaston, K. J., & Yamaura, Y. (2017). Gardening is beneficial for health: A meta-analysis. *Preventive Medicine Reports, 5*, 92–99. https://doi.org/10.1016/j.pmedr.2016.11.007

Stern, Y., MacKay-Brandt, A., Lee, S., McKinley, P., McIntyre, K., Razlighi, Q., Agarunov, E., Bartels, M., & Sloan, R. P. (2019). Effect of aerobic exercise on cognition in younger adults: A randomized clinical trial. *Neurology, 92*(9), e905–e916. https://doi.org/10.1212/WNL.0000000000007003

Stubbs, B., Vancampfort, D., Rosenbaum, S., Firth, J., Cosco, T., Veronese, N., Salum, G. A., & Schuch, F. B. (2017). An examination of the anxiolytic effects of exercise for people with anxiety and stress-related disorders: A meta-analysis. *Psychiatry Research, 249*, 102–108. https://doi.org/10.1016/j.psychres.2016.12.020

Stuckey, H. L., & Nobel, J. (2010). The connection between art, healing, and public health: A review of current literature. *American Journal of Public Health, 100*(2), 254–263. https://doi.org/10.2105/AJPH.2008.156497

Söderback, I., Söderström, M., & Schälander, E. (2004). Horticultural therapy: The 'healing garden' and gardening in rehabilitation measures at Danderyd Hospital Rehabilitation Clinic, Sweden. *Pediatric Rehabilitation, 7*(4), 245–260. https://doi.org/10.1080/13638490410001711416

Taran, N., Batsmanova, L., Kosyk, O., & Zyma, I. (2023). Effect of gardening on the human psychological and physiological state. *Bulletin of Taras Shevchenko National University of Kyiv, Psychology, 2*(18), 78–83. https://doi.org/10.17721/BPSY.2023.2(18).11

Taylor, R. R., Bowyer, P., & Fisher, G. (2023). *Kielhofner's model of human occupation: Theory and application (6th ed.)*. Wolters Kluwer.

Thoma, M. V., Ryf, S., Mohiyeddini, C., Ehlert, U., & Nater, U. M. (2012). Emotion regulation through listening to music in everyday situations. *Cognition & Emotion, 26*(3), 550–560. https://doi.org/10.1080/02699931.2011.595390

Tjasink, M., Keiller, E., Stephens, M., Carr, C. E., & Priebe, S. (2023). Art therapy-based interventions to address burnout and psychosocial distress in healthcare workers: A systematic review. *BMC Health Services Research, 23*(1), 1059. https://doi.org/10.1186/s12913-023-09958-8

Toussaint, L., Nguyen, Q. A., Roettger, C., Dixon, K., Offenbächer, M., Kohls, N., Hirsch, J., & Sirois, F. (2021). Effectiveness of progressive muscle relaxation, deep breathing, and guided imagery in promoting psychological and physiological states of relaxation. *Evidence-based Complementary and Alternative Medicine, 2021*, 5924040. https://doi.org/10.1155/2021/5924040

Trousselard, M., Steiler, D., Claverie, D., & Canini, F. (2014). L'histoire de la Mindfulness à l'épreuve des données actuelles de la littérature: questions en suspens [The history of Mindfulness put to the test of current scientific data: Unresolved questions]. *L'Encephale*, *40*(6), 474–480. https://doi.org/10.1016/j.encep.2014.08.006

Tsakona, P., Mourouzis, I., Tesseromatis, C., & Pantos, C. (2025). Diaphragmatic breathing as a therapeutic intervention: A systematic review. *Children, 12*(1), 59. https://doi.org/10.3390/children12010059

Tu, H. M. (2022). Effect of horticultural therapy on mental health: A meta-analysis of randomized controlled trials. *Journal of Psychiatric Mental Health Nursing, 29*(4), 603–615. https://doi.org/10.1111/jpm.12818

Umbrello, M., Sorrenti, T., Mistraletti, G., Formenti, P., Chiumello, D., & Terzoni, S. (2019). Music therapy reduces stress and anxiety in critically ill patients: A systematic review of randomized clinical trials. *Minerva Anestesiologica, 85*(8), 886–898. https://doi.org/10.23736/s0375-9393.19.13526-2

Van Den Berg, A. E., & Custers, M. H. (2011). Gardening promotes neuroendocrine and affective restoration from stress. *Journal of Health Psychology, 16*(1), 3–11. https://doi.org/10.1177/1359105310365577

van der Velden, A. M., Scholl, J., Elmholdt, E. M., Fjorback, L. O., Harmer, C. J., Lazar, S. W., O'Toole, M. S., Smallwood, J., Roepstorff, A., & Kuyken, W. (2023). Mindfulness training changes brain dynamics during depressive rumination: A randomized controlled trial. *Biological Psychiatry, 93*(3), 233–242. https://doi.org/10.1016/j.biopsych.2022.06.038

van der Zwan, J. E., de Vente, W., Huizink, A. C., Bögels, S. M., & de Bruin, E. I. (2015). Physical activity, mindfulness meditation, or heart rate variability biofeedback for stress reduction: A randomized controlled trial. *Applied Psychophysiology and Biofeedback, 40*(4), 257–268. https://doi.org/10.1007/s10484-015-9293-x

Visnola, D., Sprudza, D., Arija, M. B., & Pike, A. (2010). Effects of art therapy on stress and anxiety of employees. *Proceedings of the Latvian Academy of Sciences, Section B. Natural, Exact, and Applied Sciences, 64*(1–2), 85–91. https://doi.org/10.2478/v10046-010-0020-y

Walsh, R., & Shapiro, S. L. (2006). The meeting of meditative disciplines and western psychology: A mutually enriching dialogue. *American Psychologist, 61*(3), 227–239. https://doi.org/10.1037/0003-066X.61.3.227

Wan, H. Y., Bunsawat, K., & Amann, M. (2023). Autonomic cardiovascular control during exercise. *American Journal of Physiology: Heart and Circulatory Physiology, 325*(4), H675–H686. https://doi.org/10.1152/ajpheart.00303.2023

Wang, F., & Szabo, A. (2020). Effects of yoga on stress among healthy adults: A systematic review. *Alternative Therapies in Health and Medicine, 26*(4), AT6214. [no doi]

Wang, S., Tian, L., Ma, T., Wong, Y. T., Yan, L. J., Gao, Y., Zhang, D., Hui, S. S., & Xie, Y. J. (2022). Effectiveness of tai chi on blood pressure, stress, fatigue, and sleep quality among Chinese women with episodic migraine: A randomised controlled trial. *Evidence-based Complementary and Alternative Medicine, 2022*, 2089139. https://doi.org/10.1155/2022/2089139

Wang, W. L., Chen, K. H., Pan, Y. C., Yang, S. N., & Chan, Y. Y. (2020). The effect of yoga on sleep quality and insomnia in women with sleep problems: A systematic review and meta-analysis. *BMC Psychiatry, 20*(1), 195. https://doi.org/10.1186/s12888-020-02566-4

Webster, C. S., Luo, A. Y., Krägeloh, C., Moir, F., & Henning, M. (2015). A systematic review of the health benefits of tai chi for students in higher education. *Preventive Medicine Reports, 3*, 103–112. https://doi.org/10.1016/j.pmedr.2015.12.006

West, M., Melvin, G., McNamara, F., & Gordon, M. (2017). An evaluation of the use and efficacy of a sensory room within an adolescent psychiatric inpatient unit. *Australian Occupational Therapy Journal, 64*(3), 253–263. https://doi.org/10.1111/1440-1630.12358

Wilson, E. O. (1986). *Biophilia*. Harvard University Press.

Wood, J., Henderson, W., & Foster, E. R. (2022). Occupational therapy practice guidelines for people with Parkinson's disease. *American Journal of Occupational Therapy, 76*(3), 7603397010. https://doi.org/10.5014/ajot.2022.763001

Wu, J., Song, J., He, Y., Li, Z., Deng, H., Huang, Z., Xie, X., Wong, N. M. L., Tao, J., Lee, T. M. C., & Chan, C. C. H. (2023). Effect of tai chi on young adults with subthreshold depression via a stress-reward complex: A randomized controlled trial. *Sports Medicine- Open, 9*(1), 90. https://doi.org/10.1186/s40798-023-00637-w

Yang, J., Tang, S., & Zhou, W. (2018). Effect of mindfulness-based stress reduction therapy on work stress and mental health of psychiatric nurses. *Psychiatria Danubina, 30*(2), 189–196. https://doi.org/10.24869/psyd.2018.189

Zappella, M., Biamonte, F., Balzamino, B. O., Manieri, R., Cortes, M., Santucci, D., Di Stasio, E., Rizzuto, M., & Micera, A. (2021). Relaxation response in stressed volunteers: Psychometric tests and neurotrophin changes in biological fluids. *Frontiers in Psychiatry, 12*, 655453. https://doi.org/10.3389/fpsyt.2021.655453

Zemla, K., Sedek, G., Wróbel, K., Postepski, F., & Wojcik, G. M. (2023). Investigating the impact of guided imagery on stress, brain functions, and attention: A randomized trial. *Sensors, 23*(13), 6210. https://doi.org/10.3390/s23136210

Zhang, S., Zhen, K., Su, Q., Chen, Y., Lv, Y., & Yu, L. (2022). The effect of aerobic exercise on cognitive function in people with Alzheimer's disease: A systematic review and meta-analysis of randomized controlled trials. *International Journal of Environmental Research and Public Health, 19*(23), 15700. https://doi.org/10.3390/ijerph192315700

Zhu, F., Zhang, M., Wang, D., Hong, Q., Zeng, C., & Chen, W. (2020). Yoga compared to non-exercise or physical therapy exercise on pain, disability, and quality of life for patients with chronic low back pain: A systematic review and meta-analysis of randomized controlled trials. *PLOS One, 15*(9), e0238544. https://doi.org/10.1371/journal.pone.0238544

Zisopoulou, T., & Varvogli, L. (2023). Stress management methods in children and adolescents: Past, present, and future. *Hormone Research in Paediatrics, 96*(1), 97–107. https://doi.org/10.1159/000526946

Zou, L., Sasaki, J. E., Wei, G. X., Huang, T., Yeung, A. S., Neto, O. B., Chen, K. W., & Hui, S. S. (2018). Effects of mind-body exercises (tai chi/yoga) on heart rate variability parameters and perceived stress: A systematic review with meta-analysis of randomized controlled trials. *Journal of Clinical Medicine, 7*(11), 404. https://doi.org/10.3390/jcm7110404

Zschucke, E., Renneberg, B., Dimeo, F., Wüstenberg, T., & Ströhle, A. (2015). The stress-buffering effect of acute exercise: Evidence for HPA axis negative feedback. *Psychoneuroendocrinology, 51*, 414–425. https://doi.org/10.1016/j.psyneuen.2014.10.019

Chapter 9

Beyond Everyday Stress: Stress-Related Disorders through an Occupational Therapy Lens

LEARNING OBJECTIVES

By the end of this chapter, the reader will be able to

1. Distinguish between everyday stress responses and stress that meet criteria for clinical disorders.
2. Identify common stress-related disorders (e.g., PTSD, acute stress disorder, adjustment disorders) and their key features.
3. Examine the impact of stress-related disorders on occupational participation, routines and roles.

INTRODUCTION

Stress is an unavoidable feature of life as a human being. From managing schoolwork, to pressure to succeed at work, to managing personal relationships, most activities of day-to-day life carry with them at least the possibility of contributing to stress. Stress is something we all must learn to manage to get through life, and in most cases, with proper support and coping strategies, we can do just that.

What happens, though, when we cannot? What does it look like when stress can no longer be managed? What does it look like when stress begins to have an impact on one's ability to participate in the activities they need to, want to, and must do as a part of life? When this happens, it represents the crossing of a line – on one side is everyday stress that we all must experience as a part of the human condition, and on the other is pathological stress.

DOI: 10.4324/9781003671084-9

PATHOLOGICAL STRESS

Compared to everyday stress pathological stress differs in its intensity and impact on health. Everyday stress is a normal part of life, often triggered by daily events or challenges and usually does not cause significant health problems. Pathological stress, however, is chronic and can lead to negative health outcomes by affecting the body through autonomic and neuroendocrine responses. This type of stress can directly impact health or do so indirectly by leading to changes in the way that someone experiencing pathological stress manages their health (O'Connor et al., 2021).

Before getting further into the distinctions between everyday stress and pathological stress as concepts, it is useful to consider what this distinction may look like in a real person. The following case study invites you to consider the differences between everyday stressors and pathological stress by learning about Sarah and her relationship with stress.

BOX 9.1 CASE STUDY: SARAH'S STRUGGLE WITH STRESS

Sarah, a 32-year-old project manager working for an IT company, balances a demanding career with her roles as a spouse and mother of two young children. Like many working parents, she juggles tight project deadlines, school drop-offs, meal preparation, kids' activities and household responsibilities. Although the pace is often intense, Sarah generally manages these everyday stressors with the help of her supportive spouse, close friends, and coping practices such as yoga and reading. These strategies help her stay productive at work and engaged in family routines, even when things are demanding at work.

Over time, however, Sarah's workload begins to escalate. Project deadlines grow more frequent and demanding, leaving her little opportunity to recover between high-pressure periods. To "stay ahead," she starts checking work emails on weekends, during family events, and at just about any moment she has time to do so. Sleep becomes harder, and she experiences constant fatigue, irritability, and heightened anxiety. She skips meals, loses weight, and begins withdrawing from friends and extended family. At home, her spouse notices her distractedness, and her children comment on her frequent mood changes and irritability

This shift marks a progression from everyday stress – which is generally temporary and manageable – to pathological stress, characterized by chronic intensity, persistent physical and emotional symptoms and significant interference with daily functioning. Sarah's occupational performance is increasingly affected: her work efficiency declines due to fatigue and poor concentration, participation in family and social life decreases and self-care routines are neglected.

Sarah's case illustrates several distinguishing features of pathological stress discussed earlier in this chapter:

- Intensity and duration – Stress is prolonged and unrelenting, with no recovery periods.
- Physical and emotional symptoms – Insomnia, irritability, anxiety and neglect of health.
- Social and relationship impact – Withdrawal from social supports and strain on close relationships.
- Denial and overcommitment – Minimizing the seriousness of her condition while overinvesting in work at the expense of other life roles.

By reframing Sarah's situation through an occupational therapy lens, it becomes clear how prolonged, unmanaged stress can compromise multiple areas of occupational performance and participation. This case underscores the importance of early identification, timely intervention and strategies that address both the individual and environmental contributors to stress.

DISORDERS RELATED TO STRESS AND TRAUMA

To better understand the distinguishing features of pathological stress, it is critical to understand the variety of stress-related disorders that have been identified and categorized (Maercker & Eberle, 2022). Such disorders have been cataloged in diverse sources, including the *Diagnostic and Statistical Manual of Mental Health Disorders*, Fifth Edition, which is widely used in the USA (American Psychiatric Association, 2013). For the purpose of this text, however, we will utilize language from the World Health Organization's International Classification of Diseases, 11th revision (ICD-11; World Health Organization, 2019).

As a part of the revision from the 10th edition of the ICD to the ICD-11, a new grouping of mental health disorders that are specifically related to stress was formed. Perhaps not surprisingly, this grouping is titled "disorders specifically associated with stress." The ICD-11 collectively describes these disorders as follows:

> Disorders specifically associated with stress are directly related to exposure to a stressful or traumatic event, or a series of such events or adverse experiences. For each of the disorders in this grouping, an identifiable stressor is a necessary, though not sufficient, causal factor. Although not all individuals exposed to an identified stressor will develop a disorder, the disorders in this grouping would not have occurred without experiencing the stressor. Stressful events for some disorders in this grouping are within the normal range of life experiences (e.g., divorce, socio-economic problems, bereavement). Other disorders require the experience of a stressor of an extremely threatening or horrific nature (i.e., potentially traumatic events). With all disorders in this grouping, it is the nature, pattern, and duration of the symptoms that arise in response to the stressful events- together with associated functional impairment- that distinguishes the disorders.
>
> (World Health Organization, 2019)

This definition is worth reading in its entirety. It makes clear several key features of stress-related disorders. Among the key features described are

1. These disorders must be directly related to a specifically identified stressful or traumatic event(s).
2. Exposure to a stressful or traumatic event will not necessarily develop a pathological disorder as described by the ICD-11.
3. While some of the most extreme stressors and traumas that we can imagine such as war, famine or violence are certainly events that may lead to stress-related disorders, "everyday stressors" such as divorce or bereavement can also lead to a diagnosis.

Furthermore, these diagnoses are defined in part by the degree to which they impair function. As occupational therapy practitioners, our interest in these disorders is rooted in their impact on the everyday functioning of the people we serve.

As occupational therapy practitioners, we are of course not responsible for *diagnosing* these disorders. In the USA, this task is left to professionals such as physicians, psychologists and clinical social workers. As occupational therapy practitioners, we are rightly more concerned with function than specific diagnostic criteria.

As such, this section will focus on basic definitions of these disorders along with the impact they can have on occupational performance and participation. In addition to using terminology from the ICD-11, this section will use language from the Occupational Therapy Practice Framework – Fourth Edition (OTPF-4; *Occupational Therapy Practice Framework: Domain and Process* – Fourth Edition, 2020). As you read, please take time to consider how these conditions might impact those living with chronic conditions such as the aftereffects of stroke, chronic pain, diabetes or other conditions or diseases.

POST-TRAUMATIC STRESS DISORDER

Definition and Key Features

Post-traumatic stress disorder (PTSD) is defined as the experience of a traumatic event or series of events that are perceived to be threatening, frightening or horrific. The event can be personally experienced or witnessed firsthand and usually involves actual or threatened violence, death, serious injury or sexual violence (World Health Organization, 2019).

While PTSD (and all psychiatric disorders) will present differently among different individuals, there are a number of key features to be aware of.

1. **Re-experiencing the Traumatic Event**. Individuals with PTSD often report "re-experiencing" the traumatic event, causing them to experience the stress of the event repeatedly. This may include flashbacks, nightmares and other ways in which the affected person feels or acts as if the traumatic event(s) is/are occurring again.
2. **Avoidance**. Individuals with PTSD often make active efforts to avoid thoughts, feelings, activities, situations or people reminiscent of the traumatic event(s).
3. **Perception of Threat**. Many individuals report heightened perceptions of threat, which can be evidenced by increased startle response, hypervigilance or a general state of fear related to cues that the person associates with the traumatic event (e.g., reacting to fireworks as gunfire, "jumping" at loud noises, fear/avoidance of men). This increased "fight or flight" response is often noticed by others.

Impacts on Performance and Participation

PTSD can have an impact on nearly all areas of occupation, and it would be impossible to develop an exhaustive and definitive list of the condition's potential impact on performance and participation. It is a certainty that PTSD has the potential to, in some way, impact one's ability to participate in any conceivable area of occupation. However, select examples of areas of occupation that may be impacted by PTSD are listed below:

1. **Rest and sleep**. Due to symptoms such as nightmares and recurrent negative thoughts, individuals may find it difficult to engage in sleep (Germain, 2013).
2. **Education and work**. Symptoms of PTSD may interfere with concentration, memory and one's ability to handle stress and pressure, which can significantly impact one's ability to engage in pursuits related to work or school (Edgelow et al., 2020).
3. **Social participation**. For example, a person may avoid people and social situations or may present as irritable, withdrawn or hostile (Harker, 2018).

BOX 9.2 CASE STUDY: OCCUPATIONAL THERAPY AND PTSD

Alex, a 29-year-old former emergency medical technician (EMT), was known for his calm approach in high-pressure situations. He volunteered regularly at a food bank, enjoyed hiking, and participated in a book club with friends. Six months ago, Alex experienced a traumatic call involving an unsuccessful attempt to resuscitate a child, leading to a diagnosis of post-traumatic stress disorder (PTSD).

Following the event, Alex began experiencing flashbacks, hyperarousal, and severe anxiety. He avoided crowded places, withdrew from social activities that once mattered to him, and stopped participating in his hobbies. Sleep disturbances led to chronic fatigue, further limiting his ability to engage in work, leisure, and community roles. His primary care provider referred him to an occupational therapist specializing in behavioral health as part of an interdisciplinary care plan that also included more traditional talk therapy.

The occupational therapy assessment identified that before the trauma, Alex's life included multiple valued roles and routines, supported by strong social connections and meaningful activity. After the trauma, his occupational participation narrowed considerably. Avoidance behaviors, reduced social contact, and loss of leisure routines were compounded by difficulty concentrating and heightened anxiety.

Therapeutic goals included reducing PTSD symptoms to enable participation in daily activities, reintroducing previously enjoyed occupations using graded exposure, and exploring new occupations aligned with Alex's abilities and interests. Interventions included education about PTSD and its effects; sensory-based and environmental strategies to increase tolerance to distressing stimuli; cognitive–behavioral strategies applied in the context of daily activities; graded exposure to meaningful activities such as hiking and book discussions; and lifestyle redesign to create a balanced weekly routine that incorporated rest, leisure, self-care, and new pursuits like painting and yoga.

After six months of occupational therapy, in combination with psychological support, Alex reported a significant decrease in PTSD symptoms. He resumed hiking in quiet areas, joined an online book club, and developed effective coping strategies for anxiety. Although he chose not to return to EMT work, his engagement in occupational therapy supported his transition to new vocational goals, including enrolling in courses to teach medical terminology. This case demonstrates how occupational therapy can use meaningful activity, gradual re-engagement and life redesign to restore participation and support role transitions following trauma.

COMPLEX POST-TRAUMATIC STRESS DISORDER

Definition and Key Features

Complex post-traumatic stress disorder (CPTSD) is closely related to PTSD. Like PTSD, CPTSD may develop during exposure to traumatic events. According to the ICD-11, CPTSD develops from repeated exposure to particularly horrifying or threatening events such as torture, genocide or slavery.

In addition to the additional nuance regarding the degree of trauma in the precipitating event, CPTSD has a unique set of symptoms compared to PTSD.

CPTSD features "(1) problems in affect regulation; (2) beliefs about oneself as diminished, defeated or worthless, accompanied by feelings of shame, guilt or failure related to the traumatic event; and (3) difficulties in sustaining relationships and in feeling close to others" (World Health Organization, 2019).

Impacts on Performance and Participation

Given the required features described above, the potential impact of CPTSD on performance and participation in valued occupations may be immense. Among others, the following areas of occupation may be affected:

1. **Activities of daily living**. Tasks such as grooming and oral hygiene may be neglected due to depressive symptoms that are often associated with CPTSD (Tagger-Green et al., 2022).
2. **Health management**. Everyday tasks such as medication management may become **overwhelming** and difficult to complete without significant additional effort (Taggart Wasson et al., 2018).

See also Chapter 7 on PTSD and post-traumatic growth (PTG).

PROLONGED GRIEF DISORDER

Definition and Key Features

Prolonged grief disorder may develop following the death of a loved one. While grief is a normal and expected behavior following a loss of a parent, child, or other family member, prolonged grief disorder may be at play when this grief is unusual in both its length and intensity (World Health Organization, 2019). According to the ICD-11, a diagnosis of prolonged grief disorder requires at least six months of intense grieving and must "clearly [exceed] expected social, cultural, or religious norms for the individual's culture and context" (World Health Organization, 2019).

Impacts on Performance and Participation

Individuals experiencing prolonged grief disorder may experience significant occupational disruption or imbalance. Areas of occupation that may be affected include but are not limited to:

1. **Social participation**. Individuals with this condition may have difficulty forming secure and meaningful attachments with others (Al-Gamal et al., 2019).

2. **Activities of daily living**. Many individuals experiencing profound grief disorder may experience severe depressive symptoms and may lose the motivation to engage in activities such as bathing and grooming (Sekowski & Prigerson, 2022).

ADJUSTMENT DISORDER

Definition and Key Features

Like PTSD and CPTSD, adjustment disorder may develop after a negative life event such as the loss of a job or ending of a relationship. Unlike those disorders, adjustment disorder can be triggered by "everyday" undesirable life events and diagnosis does not require a severe trauma such as war, slavery or sexual violence (World Health Organization, 2019).

Key symptoms of adjustment disorder include a

> preoccupation with the stressor or its consequences, including excessive worry, recurrent and distressing thoughts about the stressor, or constant rumination about its implications, as well as by failure to adapt to the stressor that causes significant impairment in personal, family, social, educational, occupational, or other important areas of functioning.
>
> (World Health Organization, 2019)

To meet the criteria for adjustment disorder, these symptoms typically must last six months or less.

Impacts on Performance and Participation

As with the other conditions discussed in this chapter, adjustment disorder can have a negative impact on occupational functioning. Areas of occupation that may be impacted include:

1. **Social participation**. Individuals experiencing adjustment disorder may become withdrawn or distrustful of others (Casey, 2008).
2. **Work and education**. Preoccupation with the precipitating event of adjustment disorder may make engagement in work and educational ventures difficult or impossible.

OTHER STRESS-RELATED DISORDERS

Because this book is focused primarily on the impact of stress on adults living with chronic conditions, our focus will remain primarily on the adult population. However, the ICD-11 also categorizes two pediatric disorders as related to stress: disinhibited social engagement disorder and reactive attachment disorder. For more information on these disorders, please see the ICD-11 (World Health Organization, 2019).

DIAGNOSES AND THEIR ROLE IN OCCUPATIONAL THERAPY PRACTICE

Over the last several pages, you have read about numerous stress-related disorders, their diagnostic criteria and their potential impacts on occupational performance. To be an effective, evidence-based practitioner, it is critical to understand these basic aspects of psychiatric illness so that you can make fully informed decisions when evaluating, treating and supporting clients with these diagnoses.

It must be stressed, however, that as occupational therapy practitioners, we should not reduce the people we serve to a particular diagnosis or category of illness. Everyone comes with their own vastly different experiences of life, preferences and needs. These differences can dramatically impact the way that a given disease or diagnosis presents in a particular person.

Former President of the American Occupational Therapy Association Virginia "Ginny" Stoffel articulated this key concept well when she stated that "occupational therapy practitioners ask, 'what matters to you?' not 'what's the matter with you?'" (Stoffel, 2015). This perspective is critical to keep in mind as you read about the various diagnoses and conditions that the people you serve as an occupational therapy practitioner have, whether you read about them in textbooks as a student or in chart reviews as an occupational therapy practitioner.

SUMMARY

It is important to understand that the content in this chapter has focused specifically on stress-related disorders or pathological stress, in contrast to everyday stress. In the context of supporting those whom we work with as occupational therapy practitioners, it is necessary to recognize that both every day and pathological stress can have an impact on people's ability to participate in and engage with their preferred occupations. As you continue to read this text, please consider the potential impact of elevated levels of stress on those living with chronic conditions, whether that stress meets the criteria for diagnosis of a specific condition or not.

DISCUSSION QUESTIONS

1. How would you describe the difference between everyday stress and pathological stress?
2. Consider one of the stress-related disorders described in this chapter. How can you imagine that the experience of this disorder might affect one's ability to engage in meaningful occupation?
3. How do you imagine that the presence of one of these stress-related disorders might impact occupational therapy practice in non-mental health settings? For example, how could these conditions impact someone's progress in an inpatient rehabilitation or school setting in which OT treatment does not specifically focus on the condition?

REFERENCES

Al-Gamal, E., Saeed, S. B., Victor, A., & Long, T. (2019). Prolonged grief disorder and its relationship with perceived social support and depression among university students. *Journal of Psychosocial Nursing and Mental Health Services*, *57*(2), 44–51. https://doi.org/10.3928/02793695-20181023-03

American Psychiatric Association (2013). *Diagnostic and statistical manual of mental disorders* (5th ed.). https://doi.org/10.1176/appi.books.9780890425596

Casey, P. (2008). Diagnosing adjustment disorder with depressive features. *Expert Review of Neurotherapeutics*, *8*(8), 1203–1208. https://doi.org/10.1586/14737175.8.8.1203

Edgelow, M., Harrison, L., Miceli, M., & Cramm, H. (2020). Occupational therapy return to work interventions for persons with trauma and stress-related mental health conditions: A scoping review. *Work*, *65*(4), 821–836. https://doi.org/10.3233/WOR-203134

Germain, A. (2013). Sleep disturbances as the hallmark of PTSD: Where are we now? *American Journal of Psychiatry*, *170*(4), 372–382. https://doi.org/10.1176/appi.ajp.2012.12040432

Harker, A. (2018). Chapter 16- Social dysfunction: The effects of early trauma and adversity on socialization and brain development. In R. Gibb & B. Kolb (Eds.), *The neurobiology of brain and behavioral development* (pp. 439–467). Academic Press. https://doi.org/10.1016/B978-0-12-804036-2.00016-9

Maercker, A., & Eberle, D. J. (2022). Disorders specifically associated with stress in ICD-11. *Clinical Psychology in Europe*, *4*(Spec Issue), e9711. https://doi.org/10.32872/cpe.9711

Occupational Therapy Practice Framework: Domain and Process-4th Edition. (2020). *American Journal of Occupational Therapy*, *74*(Supplement_2), 7412410010p1–7412410010p87. https://doi.org/10.5014/ajot.2020.74S2001

O'Connor, D. B., Thayer, J. F., & Vedhara, K. (2021). Stress and health: A review of psychobiological processes. *Annual Review of Psychology, 72*, 663–688. https://doi.org/10.1146/annurev-psych-062520-122331

Sekowski, M., & Prigerson, H. G. (2022). Associations between symptoms of prolonged grief disorder and depression and suicidal ideation. *British Journal of Clinical Psychology*, *61*(4), 1211–1218. https://doi.org/10.1111/bjc.12381

Stoffel, V. (2015). Engagement, exploration, and empowerment. *American Journal of Occupational Therapy*, *69*(6), 6906140010p1–6906140010p8. https://doi.org/10.5014/ajot.2015.696002

Taggart Wasson, L., Shaffer, J. A., Edmondson, D., Bring, R., Brondolo, E., Falzon, L., Konrad, B., & Kronish, I. M. (2018). Posttraumatic stress disorder and nonadherence to medications prescribed for chronic medical conditions: A meta-analysis. *Journal of Psychiatric Research*, *102*, 102–109. https://doi.org/10.1016/j.jpsychires.2018.02.013

Tagger-Green, N., Nemcovsky, C., Fridenberg, N., Green, O., Chaushu, L., & Kolerman, R. (2022). Oral and dental considerations of combat-induced post -traumatic stress disorder (PTSD)-A cross-sectional study. *Journal of Clinical Medicine*, *11*(11), 3249. https://doi.org/10.3390/jcm11113249

World Health Organization. (2019). *International classification of diseases for mortality and morbidity statistics* (11th Revision). https://icd.who.int/browse11/l-m/en

Chapter 10

Caring for the Caregiver: Self-Care, Burnout Prevention and Resilience in OT Education and Practice

LEARNING OBJECTIVES

By the end of this chapter, the reader will be able to

1. Identify potential sources of stress experienced by occupational therapy students and practitioners, including stress in the classroom, the demands of fieldwork and the challenges of professional practice.
2. Understand the symptoms of burnout and its potential impact on personal well-being, professional performance and the quality of patient care.
3. Explore and implement various stress management strategies, including self-care practices, mindfulness techniques and seeking professional support, to enhance personal resilience and professional effectiveness.

INTRODUCTION

Imagine a time when you had to take care of someone who was sick or in pain. Perhaps this person was a family member or a friend. Reflect on the emotional and physical demands of that experience. How did you feel trying to provide care and support? For most of us, providing care is something that requires considerable energy.

Now consider, have you ever had to take care of someone when you were also sick? If you are a parent, the answer is very likely yes! You may have also had this experience in other contexts as well. How much more challenging was it to care

DOI: 10.4324/9781003671084-10

for others when you yourself needed care, rest or support? If you are like most people, the answer is probably "a lot!" If you were a parent in your example, the answer may be even stronger.

This reflection brings to light the reality that providing care to others as an occupational therapy practitioner is made even more difficult by unmanaged stress, mental health challenges or burnout. These factors can significantly impact your ability to provide effective and compassionate care to those you serve.

As we approach the end of this text, we hope you have learned a great deal about how you can help those you serve manage their stress. In this chapter, we invite you to consider the ways in which stress can influence not only the people you serve but also your own performance in your job and your overall well-being. The insights and strategies discussed in this chapter are designed to help you be aware of and manage your stress, prioritize your own self-care, and enhance your ability to care for the people you serve.

By acknowledging and addressing the challenges you may face as an occupational therapy practitioner, you can better prepare yourself to meet the demands of both your personal and professional life, ensuring that you can provide the highest quality of care to those who rely on you.

STRESS IN OCCUPATIONAL THERAPY

Occupational therapy students and practitioners often face significant stress due to the demanding nature of their educational and professional environments. Stress is a critical factor that can influence both success and well-being in both academic and clinical settings (Andonian, 2013; Greenstein, 1983; Mitchell & Kampfe, 1990, 1993; Pfeifer et al., 2008; Yuen, 1990). Graduate students, such as those pursuing careers in occupational therapy, are especially susceptible to mental health challenges such as depression and anxiety, with rates higher than people in the general population (Evans et al., 2018; Hoying et al., 2020).

Participation in graduate and professional programs has been linked to worsened sleep, poor diet and exercise, worsened mental health and heightened levels of stress (Smith & Brooks, 2015). For students, this stress may occur in either the classroom or on fieldwork, which often carries with it elevated levels of stress (Compton et al., 2008; Thomure, 2023).

Factors such as the pressure to succeed academically and the pursuit of career plans following graduation may significantly contribute to stress in higher education (Beiter et al., 2015). The competitive nature of admissions into occupational therapy programs means that many students have consistently achieved high levels of success throughout their academic careers. The transition from academic learning to clinical practice requires a shift to different skills and often comes with an expectation of growth through struggle that is not necessarily present in classroom learning, often leading to increased stress levels that previously utilized coping methods cannot manage (Karp, 2020).

Occupational therapy practitioners may also face substantial stressors in their roles as healthcare providers following completion of their degree and licensure. The demands of client care, productivity requirements that are often excessive and the emotional toll of working with individuals and families with chronic and debilitating conditions can have a significant impact on one's own mental health. It is safe to say that most practitioners are in this field because they care about others – that care can sometimes come with an emotional cost.

The implications of that emotional cost and the stress it can cause can be significant. Elevated stress levels can adversely affect both the training process (Almhdawi et al., 2018; Barton et al., 2012; Beiter et al., 2015; Hoying et al., 2020; Jones et al., 2018; Pascoe et al., 2020; Smith & Brooks, 2015) and the delivery of care by both students and practitioners (Ardıç et al., 2022; Çelmeçe & Menekay, 2020; Jones et al., 2018; Sabo, 2011). Therefore, understanding and managing stress is critical not just for maintenance of one's own well-being but for providing good care to others. It isn't selfish to be concerned about your own self-care – we cannot help others if we cannot help ourselves.

While existing research has identified various factors contributing to stress and strategies for coping specific to the field of occupational therapy, much of this research is outdated (Mitchell & Kampfe, 1990, 1993). More recent studies have explored stress management in higher education broadly (Chao, 2012; Kumar & Bhukar, 2013), but research with specific focus on occupational therapy students and practitioners remains limited. Recent findings suggest opportunities for enhanced collaboration between academic programs and clinical sites to support success (Karp, 2020). Leaders in the occupational therapy profession have highlighted the need for increased attention to stress management in occupational therapy education and practice (Zeman & Harvison, 2017).

In this chapter, the experience of both occupational therapy students and practitioners with regard to stress will be explored – both how they experience it and how they might attempt to manage it. By understanding both the unique challenges of working in this field and strategies that can help manage those challenges, it is our hope that you will be better prepared to manage your own stress and, as a result, be better able to serve the people you work with.

BURNOUT: A PERVASIVE ISSUE IN HEALTHCARE

Burnout is a condition emerging as a prolonged response to chronic stressors on the job. Burnout can be characterized by three main components: (1) emotional exhaustion, (2) cynicism and (3) a reduced sense of personal accomplishment (Maslach & Leiter, 2016). Due to its pervasiveness and potential impacts on both job satisfaction and quality of care, it is a critical issue for both occupational therapy students and practitioners to understand.

Burnout is not just an issue for occupational therapy practitioners, but healthcare providers more broadly. A national study of over 7,000 physicians found that over 50% reported at least some level of burnout (Shanafelt et al., 2015). Similarly, a survey of nurses revealed that over 30% of nurses in various settings reported some degree of burnout (Cimiotti et al., 2012). The prevalence of burnout among occupational therapists is also significant, with studies indicating that approximately 40% of occupational therapy practitioners report having experienced burnout (Gupta et al., 2012). Burnout can also affect patient care. Burnout is associated with decreased job performance, poor job satisfaction, and lower reported patient satisfaction (Dyrbye et al., 2017).

It is crucial that healthcare providers, including occupational therapy practitioners, recognize the signs of burnout and take proactive steps to address it (Soper, 2022). Strategies such as seeking professional support, engaging in self-care and maintaining a healthy and sustainable work-life balance can be valuable tools in the fight against burnout. Employers of occupational therapy practitioners, such as hospitals, schools and clinics, can also play a vital role in preventing burnout by fostering supportive work environments and promoting self-care for employees. Ultimately, one cannot "self-care" their way out of unrealistic job demands or unhealthy work environments.

By understanding the nature and consequences of burnout, occupational therapy students and practitioners can better navigate the challenges of their chosen profession and maintain their mental and physical health while providing high-quality care. Awareness and proactive management of burnout can help ensure the longevity, efficacy and well-being of those dedicated to caring for others.

THE STRESS OF OCCUPATIONAL THERAPY EDUCATION

Occupational therapy students, along with other students in health education programs, face unique challenges that can contribute to increased stress throughout their education. This stress can impact both their overall well-being and academic performance, making it essential to understand and address the factors contributing to it. The following section will explore the stress experienced by occupational therapy students in both didactic (classroom) settings and the unique stressors of fieldwork. It will highlight both key potential stressors and, most importantly, potential strategies to manage them.

STRESS IN THE CLASSROOM

Graduate students, such as those studying to become occupational therapists, are particularly susceptible to stress, depression and anxiety relative to the general population (Evans et al., 2018; Hoying et al., 2020). Participation in graduate and professional programs has also been linked to disruption in sleep, poor diet, impacted health routines, worsened mental health and elevated levels of reported stress (Smith & Brooks, 2015). The pressure to perform academically, maintain grades and learn new, complex concepts can lead to the creation of a high-stress environment, whether or not that is the intention of faculty involved in developing that learning environment.

KEY STRESSORS IN THE CLASSROOM

Three categories of stressors operate in the environment of professional studies.

1. **Academic performance.** The competitive nature of occupational therapy programs means that students often feel immense pressure to excel academically and have felt such pressure before beginning their programs as they worked to achieve the grades necessary to gain acceptance. Further, they have often not had to experience anything other than success, as evidenced by the types of grades and achievements that are required to gain admittance to occupational therapy school in the first place. These high expectations and the rigorous coursework associated with occupational therapy training can lead to significant stress (Beiter et al., 2015).

2. **Time management.** Balancing demanding and complex coursework, the need to learn critical occupational therapy skills from splinting to interpersonal communication and personal responsibilities can be overwhelming. Many students struggle to manage their time and competing demands effectively, which may lead to increased stress (Conneeley, 2005).
3. **Financial concerns.** The increasingly high cost of higher education and related expenses can add to the stress experienced by occupational therapy students. Financial strain and preoccupation with day-to-day finances can impact students' ability to succeed both in the classroom and on fieldwork (Moore et al., 2021).

STRESS ON FIELDWORK

Fieldwork is a critical component of occupational therapy education, required for all entry-level programs by the Accreditation Council for Occupational Therapy Education (ACOTE; "2018 Accreditation Council for Occupational Therapy Education Standards and Interpretive Guide," 2018) in the United States. However, this transition from the classroom to the clinical environment brings its own set of stressors that may contribute to later burnout (Bell et al., 2014; Robins et al., 2018). A significant majority of occupational therapy students report having experienced fieldwork-related stress during at least one Level II fieldwork placements (Thomure, 2023).

KEY STRESSORS IN FIELDWORK

There are three key sources of stressors in fieldwork placements.

1. **Transition to clinical practice**. Moving from a controlled academic environment to a dynamic clinical setting requires students to adapt to new routines, work under close supervision and meet professional standards (Grenier, 2015; Gurková & Zeleníková, 2018; Pfeifer et al., 2008).
2. **High workload and fast pace**. The demanding nature of clinical work, coupled with high expectations for performance, can be overwhelming for students. Students must manage a full-time, client-facing schedule and complete documentation and other administrative tasks critical to day-to-day occupational therapy practice (Grenier, 2015; Thomure, 2023). This can represent a significant shift from classroom learning, which often offers more flexibility and autonomy.
3. **Personal factors**. Mental health issues and a lack of confidence in one's abilities are significant contributors to stress during fieldwork. Many students

face challenges in managing work-life balance, further exacerbating their stress levels (Thomure, 2023).

COPING STRATEGIES

Effective stress management is crucial for occupational therapy students to thrive in both academic and clinical environments. Research has identified various formal and informal strategies that students use to cope with stress.

Formal Strategies

1. **Engagement with Fieldwork Educators and Academic Fieldwork Coordinators**. Although underutilized, consulting with fieldwork educators and academic fieldwork coordinators can provide significant support. These key fieldwork stakeholders can offer guidance, resources and reassurance to help students navigate their fieldwork experiences (Thomure, 2023).
2. **Professional mental health services**. Seeking help from mental health professionals, such as counselors or therapists, can be beneficial. These services can help students develop new coping mechanisms and manage their stress more effectively (Thomure, 2023).
3. **Consultation with other faculty**. Consultation with other faculty members in the student's academic program, especially faculty members who have practiced in similar clinical environments, may be of support to some students.
4. **Use of disability-related accommodations**. Some students may find it helpful to work with their academic program and university disability resource centers to create a letter of accommodation to support success on fieldwork.

Informal Strategies

1. **Self-care practices**. Engaging in activities that promote physical and mental well-being, such as regular exercise, sufficient sleep, and healthy eating, can help reduce stress levels. Students often rely on socialization with family and friends and engaging in hobbies to manage stress (Thomure, 2023).
2. **Peer support.** Connecting with peers who are going through similar experiences can provide emotional support and practical advice. Peer interaction can help students feel less isolated and more understood (Thomure, 2023).

3. **Mindfulness and relaxation techniques**. Practicing mindfulness, meditation and other relaxation techniques may help some students manage their stress (Dweck, 2006; Moscaritolo, 2009; Palase et al., 2019).

STRESS FACED BY PROFESSIONAL OCCUPATIONAL THERAPY PRACTITIONERS

Occupational therapy practitioners, like occupational therapy students and many other healthcare providers, may also face significant stress in their professional roles (Barton et al., 2012; Beiter et al., 2015; Bridgeman et al., 2018; Hoying et al., 2020; Jones et al., 2018; Smith & Brooks, 2015). The demands of client care, productivity requirements that are often excessive and the emotional toll of working with individuals with chronic conditions can significantly impact mental health and lead to burnout. These stressors are compounded by the need to stay current with professional standards, evidence-based practice and continuing education requirements, all while managing personal and professional responsibilities.

High productivity standards often require practitioners to see a high volume of clients within limited time frames, contributing to high-pressure, demanding work environments (Adib Ibrahim et al., 2019). Moreover, the nature of occupational therapy work, which involves supporting clients, families and caregivers with diverse and often complex needs, can be emotionally challenging. Occupational therapy practitioners frequently work with individuals dealing with severe physical, cognitive and emotional issues, which can be draining and lead to compassion fatigue and burnout (Bridgeman et al., 2018).

KEY STRESSORS FOR OCCUPATIONAL THERAPY PRACTITIONERS

The following five categories have been identified as important sources of stress for practitioners. See Box 10.1 for a case study describing how these may play out in an inpatient rehabilitation setting.

1. **Client care demands**. Managing a diverse caseload and addressing the complex needs of clients requires significant emotional, cognitive and physical energy. The responsibility to provide high-quality care consistently can be overwhelming and may lead to unmanageable stress. This challenge can be exacerbated in times of crisis, such as the COVID-19 pandemic (Sung et al., 2021).

2. **Productivity requirements**. Many occupational therapy practitioners face high productivity standards that necessitate seeing a specific number of clients or billable hours. This constant pressure to meet targets can lead to increased stress and potential burnout (Adib Ibrahim et al., 2019; Bridgeman et al., 2018).
3. **Emotional toll**. Working with individuals with chronic conditions or severe injuries or disabilities can be emotionally taxing. Practitioners may experience secondary traumatic stress or compassion fatigue, impacting their mental health and stress levels (Bridgeman et al., 2018; Sung et al., 2021).
4. **Professional development**. The need to stay current with evolving practices, new research, and continuing education requirements adds another layer of stress. Balancing professional growth with day-to-day responsibilities can be challenging.
5. **Work-life balance**. The demands of the profession may extend beyond typical working hours, as practitioners often stay late to complete documentation or work shifts on evenings and weekends. This may affect practitioners' ability to maintain a healthy work-life balance. Personal time may be sacrificed to meet professional obligations, which can contribute to increased stress (Bridgeman et al., 2018).

BOX 10.1 CASE STUDY: ANNA, AN OCCUPATIONAL THERAPIST IN INPATIENT REHABILITATION

Anna, a 32-year-old occupational therapist, has been working in an inpatient rehabilitation setting for the past six years. Known for her empathy and care for her clients, Anna has increasingly been feeling overwhelmed by her caseload. With a daily schedule consistently packed with back-to-back patient sessions, administrative duties and interdisciplinary and team meetings, Anna finds little time for breaks, personal reflection or even biological needs like eating lunch and using the restroom.

In the past year, Anna has noticed a significant increase in her stress levels. She often feels irritable, has trouble sleeping and experiences persistent fatigue, which she initially dismissed as an everyday reality of a demanding job. However, these symptoms have begun to affect both her satisfaction with her work and the quality of that work. Anna noticed her patience wearing thin in sessions, particularly with patients requiring significant physical assistance and external motivation. Her focus during sessions has declined, and she feels it may be impacting her clients' progress. Recently, she accidentally overlooked a patient's allergy to latex, a mistake caught just in time by a colleague.

Colleagues, supervisors and friends have suggested she may be experiencing burnout, a possibility that Anna has dismissed until a client gently pointed out her apparent distraction during a therapy session. Realizing the impact her stress was having not only on her well-being but also on her clients, Anna decided it was time to seek help and implement serious changes.

STRATEGIES FOR MANAGING STRESS

Occupational therapy practitioners must be mindful of their own stress and have strategies to manage it in order to provide the best possible care to their clients. The following strategies can help practitioners manage stress effectively.

Organizational Strategies

1. **Professional support**: Seeking support from colleagues, supervisors, or professional organizations can provide a valuable outlet for stress. Peer support groups and mentorship programs can offer practical advice and emotional support (Gilstrap & Bernier, 2017; Maslach & Leiter, 2016). Advocating for healthier work environments and realistic expectations around productivity may also lead to a greater sense of self-efficacy and improved working conditions for all.
2. **Time management**: Implementing effective time management techniques, such as prioritizing tasks appropriately, delegating responsibilities and setting realistic goals, can help reduce stress levels. Scheduling (and taking) regular breaks and avoiding overcommitment are also important strategies (Alziyadat & Obidat, 2022).
3. **Continuing education**: Engaging in professional development activities that are of personal interest and relevance can enhance job satisfaction and reduce stress. Staying informed about the latest practices and techniques can also increase confidence and competence.

Personal Strategies

1. **Self-care**. Prioritizing self-care activities, such as regular exercise, healthy eating and sufficient sleep, can be essential for managing stress. Practitioners may also benefit from engagement in hobbies and other activities that they enjoy and find relaxing, such as reading, journaling or spending time with

family and friends (Kuhn & Flanagan, 2017; Gilstrap & Bernier, 2017; Posluns & Gall, 2020).

2. **Mindfulness and relaxation**. Practicing mindfulness techniques, such as meditation, deep breathing exercises and yoga, can help reduce stress and improve overall well-being. These practices can help practitioners stay grounded and present, which may reduce stress (Moscaritolo, 2009).
3. **Professional help**. Mental health professionals, such as counselors or therapists, can be valuable tools in the fight against stress. Professional help can also offer a safe space to discuss challenges and develop coping mechanisms (Wu et al., 2017).

Workplace Support

1. **Supportive work environment**. Employers of occupational therapy practitioners, such as hospitals, clinics and home health agencies, can play a significant role in reducing stress by fostering a supportive work environment. This includes providing access to mental health resources, offering flexible work schedules and promoting a culture of open communication (Gilstrap & Bernier, 2017; Moscaritolo, 2009; Shanafelt et al., 2015). Organizations cannot expect their employees to be healthy, happy and maximally productive if they are not provided with a supportive work environment.
2. **Professional development opportunities**. Employers should encourage and support ongoing professional development, including offering paid time off for continuing education and providing access to relevant training programs (Farahmand et al., 2022; Rankin & Armstrong, 2017).
3. **Recognition and rewards**. Recognizing and rewarding the hard work and dedication of occupational therapy practitioners can boost morale and reduce stress. This can include formal recognition programs, bonuses and other incentives (Dyrbye et al., 2017; Gilstrap & Bernier, 2017).

See Box 10.2 for a description of how a stress management strategy was implemented for the therapist in the case study of Box 10.1.

BOX 10.2 ANNA MANAGING STRESS

CASE STUDY: ANNA'S JOURNEY TO MANAGING STRESS

Anna, who we met early in this chapter, may benefit from the implementation of stress reduction strategies.

IMPLEMENTATION OF SELF-CARE STRATEGIES

Recognizing the impact of unmanaged stress on her professional and personal life, Anna decided to take proactive steps to manage her stress. She implemented several self-care and stress management strategies:

1. Re-engaging in meaningful occupation: Anna returned to gardening, a leisure activity she valued but set aside due to work demands. This helped provide restorative time away from the responsibilities of her job and aligned with her belief that engagement in occupation can be a source of well-being.
2. Mindfulness and emotional regulation: Anna began each workday by engaging in brief mindfulness meditation and utilized deep breathing techniques that she had once taught to clients before beginning challenging sessions. This helped her improve focus and emotional regulation.
3. Peer support and professional connection: Anna joined a workplace peer support group where she learned from colleagues facing similar pressures and challenges. This provided validation to her struggles and taught her practical solutions.
4. Time and energy management: She applied time management techniques from her OT toolkit, prioritizing essential responsibilities, setting realistic goals, and scheduling short breaks whenever able.
5. Professional advocacy: Recognizing that burnout cannot be solved simply by "self-caring" your way out of it, she met with supervisors to discuss opportunities for workload distribution and flexible scheduling. This helped address systemic contributors to stress rather than simply trying to cope her way through them.

POSITIVE OUTCOMES

After several months of consistently applying these strategies, Anna noticed significant improvements, including better sleep and energy, increased patience and empathy during sessions, and more effective engagement with clients. Her re-engagement in gardening provided a tangible sense of balance outside of work, and her advocacy efforts resulted in modest but meaningful workplace adjustments. Most importantly, her renewed focus helped her clients do their best work under her care.

Anna's journey underscores two key points. First, that occupational therapy practitioners can benefit from applying the same person-centered, occupation-based approaches to their own self-care that they use with clients. Second, that sustainable stress management requires implementation of both personal strategies and organizational support and recognition of the challenges of this work. Without those, burnout is a significant risk.

SUMMARY

Managing stress is critical for occupational therapy students and practitioners to maintain their well-being and continue providing high-quality care. Stressors arising from the pressures of didactic coursework, fieldwork, productivity expectations and compassion fatigue increase the risk of burnout, especially under unusually challenging conditions, such as the COVID-19 pandemic. Resources and practices that support resilience and self-care, including rest, exercise, mindfulness, boundary-setting, time management, peer connection, mentoring and advocacy for reasonable workloads, were presented. By understanding the unique stressors of the profession and implementing effective strategies for stress management, practitioners can have more satisfying and fulfilled careers, ultimately contributing to better outcomes for the people they serve.

DISCUSSION QUESTIONS

1. Consider a time when you experienced significant stress or burnout in your academic or professional life. What were the main sources of that stress? How did it affect your well-being and the quality of your work? What strategies did you use to manage it, and what could you have done differently to better support your mental health?
2. Reflect on your current self-care practices. How do you prioritize self-care? Are there specific activities or strategies that you find particularly useful to manage stress? Identify areas where you could

improve or incorporate new strategies to better manage stress and prevent burnout.

3. Reflect on the support systems available in your educational or professional environment. Have you utilized these systems? Why or why not? How effective are these systems in helping you manage stress and avoid burnout? Are there any additional resources you are aware of that you haven't used?

REFERENCES

2018 Accreditation Council for Occupational Therapy Education (ACOTE®) Standards and Interpretive Guide (effective July 31, 2020). (2018). *American Journal of Occupational Therapy*, *72*(Supplement_2), 7212410005p1–7212410005p83. https://doi.org/10.5014/ajot.2018.72S217

Adib Ibrahim, M., Abdul Aziz, A., Suhaili, N.-A., Zahid Daud, A., Naing, L., & Abdul Rahman, H. (2019). A study into psychosocial work stressors and health care productivity. *International Journal of Occupational and Environmental Medicine*, *10*(4), 185–193. https://doi.org/10.15171/ijoem.2019.1610

Almhdawi, K. A., Kanaan, S. F., Khader, Y., Al-Hourani, Z., Almomani, F., & Nazzal, M. (2018). Study-related mental health symptoms and their correlates among allied health professions students. *Work*, *61*(3), 391–401. https://doi.org/10.3233/WOR-182815

Alziyadat, Z., & Obidat, A. (2022). The relationship between time management, job satisfaction, and job burnout among Jordanian medical staff during COVID-19. *Problems and Perspectives in Management*, *20*(4), 396–406. https://doi.org/10.21511/ppm.20(4).2022.30

Andonian, L. (2013). Emotional intelligence, self-efficacy, and occupational therapy students' fieldwork performance. *Occupational Therapy in Health Care*, *27*(3), 201–215. https://doi.org/10.3109/07380577.2012.763199

Ardıç, M., Ünal, Ö., & Türktemiz, H. (2022). The effect of stress levels of nurses on performance during the COVID-19 pandemic: The mediating role of motivation. *Journal of Research in Nursing*, *27*(4), 330–340. https://doi.org/10.1177/17449871211070982

Barton, J., Griffin, M., & Pretty, J. (2012). Exercise-, nature- and socially interactive-based initiatives improve mood and self-esteem in the clinical population. *Perspectives in Public Health*, *132*(2), 89–96. https://doi.org/10.1177/1757913910393862

Beiter, R., Nash, R., McCrady, M., Rhoades, D., Linscomb, M., Clarahan, M., & Sammut, S. (2015). The prevalence and correlates of depression, anxiety, and stress in a sample of college students. *Journal of Affective Disorders*, *173*, 90–96. https://doi.org/10.1016/j.jad.2014.10.054

Bell, J., Cox, D., & Marcangelo, C. (2014). Master's level occupational therapy students on placement: An exploration of perceptions and expectations. *British Journal of Occupational Therapy*, *77*(4), 181–188. https://doi.org/10.4276/030802214X13968769798755

Bridgeman, P. J., Bridgeman, M. B., & Barone, J. (2018). Burnout syndrome among healthcare professionals. *American Journal of Health-System Pharmacy*, *75*(3), 147–152. https://doi.org/10.2146/ajhp170460

Çelmeçe, N., & Menekay, M. (2020). The effect of stress, anxiety and burnout levels of healthcare professionals caring for COVID-19 patients on their quality of life. *Frontiers in Psychology*, *11*, 597624. https://doi.org/10.3389/fpsyg.2020.597624

Chao, R. C.-L. (2012). Managing perceived stress among college students: The roles of social support and dysfunctional coping. *Journal of College Counseling*, *15*(1), 5–21. https://doi.org/10.1002/j.2161-1882.2012.00002.x

Cimiotti, J. P., Aiken, L. H., Sloane, D. M., & Wu, E. S. (2012). Nurse staffing, burnout, and health care–associated infection. *American Journal of Infection Control*, *40*(6), 486–490. https://doi.org/10.1016/j.ajic.2012.02.029

Compton, M. T., Carrera, J., & Frank, E. (2008). Stress and depressive symptoms/dysphoria among US medical students: Results from a large, nationally representative survey. *Journal of Nervous and Mental Disease*, *196*(12), 891–897. https://doi.org/10.1097/NMD.0b013e3181924d03

Conneeley, A. L. (2005). Study at master's level: A qualitative study exploring the experience of students. *British Journal of Occupational Therapy*, *68*(3), 104–109. https://doi.org/10.1177/030802260506800302

Dweck, C. S. (2006). *Mindset: The new psychology of success* (1st ed). Random House.

Dyrbye, L. N., West, C. P., Satele, D., Boone, S., Tan, L., Sloan, J., & Shanafelt, T. D. (2017). Burnout among U.S. medical students, residents, and early career physicians relative to the general U.S. *Population: Academic Medicine*, *89*(3), 443–451. https://doi.org/10.1097/ACM.0000000000000134

Evans, T. M., Bira, L., Gastelum, J. B., Weiss, L. T., & Vanderford, N. L. (2018). Evidence for a mental health crisis in graduate education. *Nature Biotechnology*, *36*(3), 282–284. https://doi.org/10.1038/nbt.4089

Farahmand, S., Rad, E., & Keshmiri, F. (2022). Exploring the effective elements on the personal and professional development among health-care providers: A qualitative study. *Journal of Education and Health Promotion*, *11*(1), 256. https://doi.org/10.4103/jehp.jehp_1405_21

Gilstrap, C. M., & Bernier, D. (2017). Dealing with the demands: Strategies healthcare communication professionals use to cope with workplace stress. *Qualitative Research Reports in Communication*, *18*(1), 73–81. https://doi.org/10.1080/17459435.2017.1330277

Greenstein, L. R. (1983). Student anxiety toward Level II Fieldwork. *American Journal of Occupational Therapy*, *37*(2), 89–95. https://doi.org/10.5014/ajot.37.2.89

Grenier, M.-L. (2015). Facilitators and barriers to learning in occupational therapy fieldwork education: Student perspectives. *American Journal of Occupational Therapy*, *69*(Supplement_2), 6912185070p1. https://doi.org/10.5014/ajot.2015.015180

Gupta, S., Paterson, M. L., Lysaght, R. M., & von Zweck, C. M. (2012). Experiences of burnout and coping strategies utilized by occupational therapists. *Canadian Journal of Occupational Therapy. Revue Canadienne d'Ergotherapie*, *79*(2), 86–95. https://doi.org/10.2182/cjot.2012.79.2.4

Gurková, E., & Zeleníková, R. (2018). Nursing students' perceived stress, coping strategies, health and supervisory approaches in clinical practice: A Slovak and Czech perspective. *Nurse Education Today*, *65*, 4–10. https://doi.org/10.1016/j.nedt.2018.02.023

Hoying, J., Melnyk, B. M., Hutson, E., & Tan, A. (2020). Prevalence and correlates of depression, anxiety, stress, healthy beliefs, and lifestyle behaviors in first-year graduate health sciences students. *Worldviews on Evidence-based Nursing*, *17*(1), 49–59. https://doi.org/10.1111/wvn.12415

Jones, P. J., Park, S. Y., & Lefevor, G. T. (2018). Contemporary college student anxiety: The role of academic distress, financial stress, and support. *Journal of College Counseling*, *21*(3), 252–264. https://doi.org/10.1002/jocc.12107

Karp, P. (2020). Occupational therapy student readiness for transition to the fieldwork environment: A pilot case study. *Open Journal of Occupational Therapy*, *8*(4), 1–14. https://doi.org/10.15453/2168-6408.1719

Kuhn, C. M., & Flanagan, E. M. (2017). Self-care as a professional imperative: Physician burnout, depression, and suicide. *Canadian Journal of Anesthesia/Journal Canadien d'Anesthésie*, *64*(2), 158–168. https://doi.org/10.1007/s12630-016-0781-0

Kumar, S., & Bhukar, J. P. (2013). Stress level and coping strategies of college students. *Journal of Physical Education and Sports Management*, *4*(1), 7. https://doi.org/10.5897/JPESM12.001

Maslach, C., & Leiter, M. P. (2016). Understanding the burnout experience: Recent research and its implications for psychiatry. *World Psychiatry*, *15*(2), 103–111. https://doi.org/10.1002/wps.20311

Mitchell, M. M., & Kampfe, C. M. (1990). Coping strategies used by occupational therapy students during fieldwork: An exploratory study. *American Journal of Occupational Therapy*, *44*(6), 543–550. https://doi.org/10.5014/ajot.44.6.543

Mitchell, M. M., & Kampfe, C. M. (1993). Student coping strategies and perceptions of fieldwork. *American Journal of Occupational Therapy*, *47*(6), 535–540. https://doi.org/10.5014/ajot.47.6.535

Moore, A., Nguyen, A., Rivas, S., Bany-Mohammed, A., Majeika, J., & Martinez, L. (2021). A qualitative examination of the impacts of financial stress on college students' well-being: Insights from a large, private institution. *Sage Open Medicine*, *9*, 205031212110181. https://doi.org/10.1177/20503121211018122

Moscaritolo, L. M. (2009). Interventional strategies to decrease nursing student anxiety in the clinical learning environment. *Journal of Nursing Education*, *48*(1), 17–23. https://doi.org/10.3928/01484834-20090101-08

Palase, N., Lopes, A., Rigney, C., Walsh-Roche, M., & Garbarini, J. (2019). Pilot study: The effects of mindfulness practices among graduate OT students. *American Journal of Occupational Therapy*, *73*(4_Supplement_1), 7311515371p1. https://doi.org/10.5014/ajot.2019.73S1-PO6030

Pascoe, M. C., Hetrick, S. E., & Parker, A. G. (2020). The impact of stress on students in secondary school and higher education. *International Journal of Adolescence and Youth*, *25*(1), 104–112. https://doi.org/10.1080/02673843.2019.1596823

Pfeifer, T. A., Kranz, P. L., & Scoggin, A. E. (2008). Perceived stress in occupational therapy students. *Occupational Therapy International*, *15*(4), 221–231. https://doi.org/10.1002/oti.256

Posluns, K., & Gall, T. L. (2020). Dear mental health practitioners, take care of yourselves: A literature review on self-care. *International Journal for the Advancement of Counselling*, *42*(1), 1–20. https://doi.org/10.1007/s10447-019-09382-w

Rankin, J., & Armstrong, A. (2017). Continuing Professional Development: Integral to the role for everyday practice in healthcare. *Digital Library,* 148152. https://doi.org/10.5176/2315-4330_WNC17.123

Robins, T. G., Roberts, R. M., & Sarris, A. (2018). The role of student burnout in predicting future burnout: Exploring the transition from university to the workplace. *Higher Education Research & Development*, *37*(1), 115–130. https://doi.org/10.1080/07294360.2017.1344827

Sabo, B. (2011). Reflecting on the concept of compassion fatigue. *Online Journal of Issues in Nursing*, *16*(1), 1. https://doi.org/10.3912/OJIN.Vol16No01Man01

Shanafelt, T. D., Hasan, O., Dyrbye, L. N., Sinsky, C., Satele, D., Sloan, J., & West, C. P. (2015). Changes in burnout and satisfaction with work-life balance in physicians and the general US working population between 2011 and 2014. *Mayo Clinic Proceedings*, *90*(12), 1600–1613. https://doi.org/10.1016/j.mayocp.2015.08.023

Smith, E., & Brooks, Z. (2015). *Graduate student mental health 2015*. National Association of Professional Graduate Students. https://nagps.org/wordpress/wp-content/uploads/2015/06/NAGPS_Institute_mental_health_survey_report_2015.pdf

Soper, K. (2022). Reducing burnout and promoting professional development in the palliative care service. *Journal of Hospice & Palliative Nursing*, *24*(3), 181–185. https://journals.lww.com/jhpn/fulltext/2022/06000/reducing_burnout_and_promoting_professional.7.aspx

Sung, C.-W., Chen, C.-H., Fan, C.-Y., Chang, J.-H., Hung, C. C., Fu, C.-M., Wong, L. P., Huang, E. P.-C., & Lee, T. S.-H. (2021). Mental health crisis in healthcare providers in the COVID-19 pandemic: A cross-sectional facility-based survey. *BMJ Open*, *11*(7), e052184. https://doi.org/10.1136/bmjopen-2021-052184

Thomure, R. (2023). Use of formal and informal strategies to manage stress during Level II occupational therapy fieldwork. *Open Journal of Occupational Therapy, 11*(4), 1–9. https://doi.org/10.15453/2168-6408.2158

Wu, I. H. C., Bathje, G. J., Kalibatseva, Z., Sung, D., Leong, F. T. L., & Collins-Eaglin, J. (2017). Stigma, mental health, and counseling service use: A person-centered approach to mental health stigma profiles. *Psychological Services*, *14*(4), 490–501. https://doi.org/10.1037/ser0000165

Yuen, H. K. (1990). Fieldwork students under stress. *American Journal of Occupational Therapy*, *44*(1), 80–81. https://doi.org/10.5014/ajot.44.1.80

Zeman, E., & Harvison, N. (2017). Burnout, stress, and compassion fatigue in occupational therapy practice and education: A call for mindful, self-care protocols. *National Academy of Medicine Perspectives*, *7*(3), 1–4. https://nam.edu/wp-content/uploads/2017/03/Burnout-Stress-and-Compassion-Fatigue-in-Occupational-Therapy-Practice-and-Education-A-Call-for-Mindful-Self-Care-Protocols.pdf

Chapter 11

Group Interventions for Stress Management

"What is most personal is most universal."

Carl Rogers (1961)

LEARNING OBJECTIVES

By the end of this chapter, the reader will be able to

1. Analyze the theoretical foundations and benefits of group therapy in occupational therapy practice.
2. Apply principles from Cole's Seven Steps of Group Leadership to design and facilitate groups focused on stress management.
3. Recognize different approaches to group intervention.

INTRODUCTION

Have you ever been in a situation where you felt alone? When facing stress, it is common to feel isolated. It can feel as though no one else truly understands what you are going through – or that simply feeling the way you feel is, in itself, some kind of personal failure (it is not!). However, as this book has outlined, stress is a *universal human experience!* While no two people navigate life and its many challenges in precisely the same way, we have all encountered someone who has been through something similar or who can relate to our emotions in ways we hadn't previously realized. When we come across those people, it can help us realize that we are not alone and that we haven't failed – we are just human beings.

DOI: 10.4324/9781003671084-11

One of the most powerful aspects of group therapy is its ability to pull the curtain back on this shared reality. Group interventions have the potential to create spaces where individuals can connect, recognize common struggles and learn from and support one another.

Part of what can make group therapy so useful is the fact that it can create that sense of universality – the realization that others share similar thoughts, feelings and challenges (Yalom & Leszcz, 2020). This shared experience can reduce feelings of isolation and help to combat the tempting idea that experiencing excessive stress and not quite knowing how to handle it represents a unique, personal failing. When individuals recognize that others are also navigating stress, encountering and overcoming associated obstacles and utilizing specific strategies to manage it, they are more likely to feel understood, validated and motivated to engage in positive coping strategies, including techniques they might learn about in the group itself.

Beyond whatever support a group participant may receive from the facilitator, group therapy provides an opportunity for peer support. Participants not only receive guidance from the facilitator but also can share experiences, work through problems and learn about different approaches to managing stress. Participants can and should learn from the facilitator, but these peer interactions are often where the "magic" of group therapy happens (Farr et al., 2021; Ranasinghe et al., 2023; Won et al., 2021). Professional credentials and training only go so far – evidence of success by those with similar lived experience can go even further.

By fostering a safe and supportive environment rooted in shared experience and collective problem-solving, group therapy can empower individuals to share their own story, learn from those who have had similar experiences and gain tools to better manage stress. Groups can help shine a light on the fact that one's struggles are not singular, but an experience faced by many.

While professionals from many disciplines can and do facilitate group interventions, occupational therapy practitioners are uniquely equipped to lead groups that emphasize practical skill-building. Rather than focusing solely on discussion or emotional exploration, occupational therapy-led groups engage participants in problem-solving and collaboration grounded in real-world tasks, helping them develop techniques they can apply in their daily lives (Ikiugu et al., 2017; Lambdin-Pattavina & Pyatak, 2022; Swarbrick & Noyes, 2018). For example, a group might work together to plan and cook a simple meal, manage a weekly schedule or practice communication strategies for navigating stress – activities that directly support the skills of managing stress with increased independence.

BACKGROUND AND RATIONALE FOR GROUP INTERVENTIONS

Group therapy is a commonly utilized intervention in many behavioral health settings (Velasquez et al., 2015). In occupational therapy, group interventions provide structured opportunities for individuals to develop and refine coping strategies through active participation, social interaction and engagement in some kind of meaningful activity. The effectiveness of group therapy is supported by various theoretical frameworks, including Social Learning Theory (Bandura, 1982), which helps explain how individuals acquire new behaviors, strategies and coping mechanisms through observation of and interaction with others.

There are a variety of ways that we learn from and through others. These means of learning can be especially relevant in group therapy, where participants are provided with the opportunity to observe others navigate stress, practice coping techniques and adjust behaviors based on feedback from the group.

Some of the mechanisms through which social learning can occur, along with examples relevant to the context of stress management, are listed below.

1. **Observational learning**. Individuals learn effective stress management techniques by seeing peers successfully use coping strategies (Goubert et al., 2011).
2. **Vicarious reinforcement**. When participants see others benefit from adaptive behaviors (e.g., relaxation exercises, cognitive reframing), they may become more interested in how they can potentially apply those strategies in their own lives (Coates & Rooke, 2008).
3. **Guided mastery**. Group leaders, including occupational therapy practitioners, can provide structured opportunities for participants to practice and refine specific skills (such as meditation, deep breathing or other coping skills) in a supportive environment (Bandura, 2019).
4. **Self-efficacy development**. As individuals learn that their peers have overcome challenges that are not unlike their own, they can gain confidence in their own ability to manage similar challenges (Bandura, 1982).

Seeing others successfully manage stress can help to foster the belief that better outcomes are possible, a potentially transformative revelation. Challenges such as managing chronic illness or caregiving can be isolating and can feel "unconquerable." Seeing others overcome challenges can help foster a sense of self-efficacy that allows an individual to overcome challenges that they once thought to be unmanageable.

Beyond the mechanisms of social learning, group therapy provides additional benefits that support stress reduction. One of the most significant is the power of shared experience (Marogna & Caccamo, 2015; Robak et al., 2022). Stress, especially in the context of managing a chronic condition, can be an isolating experience, leading individuals to feel that they are struggling alone (Bertollo et al., 2023; Campagne, 2019). Group therapy can help normalize these experiences, fostering a sense of connection and validation (Hoang et al., 2022). Through structured discussions and meaningful activities, participants learn that stress is universal, that others share similar struggles and that they are not alone in their journey toward finding better ways to cope.

Occupational therapy is not the only discipline that facilitates stress management groups, but occupational therapy practitioners stand apart in their use of meaningful activity as a central intervention strategy (Ikiugu et al., 2017; Swarbrick & Noyes, 2018). Rather than relying solely on discussion or verbal support, occupational therapy-led groups promote active participation in purposeful tasks that help individuals build coping skills, restore routines and manage stress through real-life engagement.

Engagement in activities such as mindfulness exercises, journaling, role-playing, creative expression or physical activity enable group participants to engage in and learn stress management strategies that they can apply in their day-to-day lives. When considering what occupational therapy's "distinct value" is, given that social workers, psychologists, nurses and others can run similar groups, we must place an emphasis on this active participation – the "doing" of such strategies – as a means of ensuring that coping strategies are both practical, sustainable and relevant to the needs of a given person.

Our profession brings distinct frameworks that ensure group interventions are rooted in occupation and aligned with client goals. One such framework is Cole's Seven Steps of Group Leadership, which offers a clear structure for designing and facilitating activity-based groups. This model helps occupational therapy practitioners lead groups that are purposeful, client-centered and grounded in therapeutic intent.

In addition to this framework, occupation-based models such as the Person-Environment-Occupation-Performance (PEOP) model and the Model of Human Occupation (MOHO) provide theoretical grounding that helps practitioners develop groups that are occupation- and activity-based. These models help practitioners analyze how group participation affects occupational performance and participation by considering the interactions among personal factors, environmental conditions and meaningful activity. Together, these tools can help guide the development of groups that are not only broadly therapeutic but also distinctly occupation-focused, helping carve out a distinct space for our profession.

THEORETICAL FOUNDATIONS FOR OCCUPATION-FOCUSED GROUPS

Applying Occupation-based Models to Group Therapy

Occupational therapy is grounded in the belief that engagement in meaningful occupation promotes health and well-being, both as a means and an end in treatment ("Occupational Therapy Practice Framework: Domain and Process-Fourth Edition," 2020). While broader psychological and behavioral theories such as cognitive-behavioral therapy provide insight into how groups might function and strategies to create change, occupation-focused models offer a lens for thinking about why our profession uses groups in the first place and the distinct role that occupational therapy practitioners can play. Models like the Person–Environment–Occupation–Performance (PEOP) Model and the Model of Human Occupation (MOHO) can help us connect group participation to broader goals of occupational engagement and daily functioning. While other occupation-based models can certainly be applied to group practice, this text will explore these two models as examples.

Person–Environment–Occupation-Performance Model

The PEOP model describes occupational performance as the result of interactions between a person, their environment, their occupations and their performance of those occupations (Baum et al., 2015). From this perspective, group interventions can be seen as an opportunity to create environments that support engagement, using shared engagement in occupation as a means of addressing stress or other challenges.

Each person who enters a group brings their own values, abilities and experiences. These personal factors interact with the structure and norms of the group environment and with the tasks and occupations being used as interventions. Whether the focus is on mindfulness, leisure, social participation or daily routines, the occupations selected for group intervention can either support or hinder participation and performance depending on the fit between the person, the environment and the occupation.

For example, a stress management group that utilizes interventions such as guided imagery, reflective journaling and group discussion might offer meaningful and accessible ways for participants to engage in new coping strategies. A participant with limited literacy may benefit from modifications to the journaling task or from alternative modes of expression, while someone with difficulty trusting others might need more time to engage in discussion-based activities. The PEOP model encourages occupational therapy practitioners to consider these interactions and to adapt the environment or the occupation itself to support each person's ability to participate in a way that is both personally meaningful and practically accessible.

Model of Human Occupation

MOHO provides another way to view group intervention through an occupation-focused lens (Taylor et al., 2023). Group intervention can address key concepts from the model, such as volition, habituation and performance capacity. Volition can be supported when the group content is meaningful to participants, encouraging genuine interest and participation. Habituation might be addressed by helping group members establish routines, explore new roles or reflect on existing patterns of behavior. Performance capacity can be strengthened through structured practice, facilitator and peer feedback and skill-building.

For example, a community reintegration group might include activities that help participants build routines for managing time, navigating public transportation or attending appointments. These tasks can be practiced within the group, while the occupational therapy practitioner observes how participants organize themselves, follow through and respond to challenges. At the same time, participants reflect on what these experiences mean to them – what they're learning about their own capabilities and what kind of person they want to become. This process, emphasized in MOHO, supports the development of occupational identity and promotes lasting change.

Cole's Seven Steps of Group Leadership

Distinct from any specific occupation-based model, occupational therapy practitioners commonly use Cole's Seven Steps of Group Leadership as a structured framework for designing and facilitating effective group sessions (Cole, 2025). This model ensures that group therapy remains goal-directed, client-centered and therapeutic, while still allowing space for discussion and peer learning. These steps help create structure, creating a sense of predictability for both group facilitators and participants. They are also a helpful "guardrail" for group facilitators, ensuring that groups are activity-based and with real-world application in mind.

While Cole's Seven Steps are applicable to group treatment in any occupational therapy practice setting, they have the potential to be especially effective in behavioral health contexts, including in stress management. This is true in part because designing a group with the steps in mind can create a group environment that encourages participants to move from exploration to application, ensuring that the strategies discussed in the group do not stay in the group setting. Rather, the focus is on ensuring that participants have the tools needed to apply the tools of stress management in the "real world," outside the safety of the group.

The following is an overview of each step, framed in the context of a stress management group.

1. **Introduction**. Establishing the purpose of group and creating a safe space
   The introduction helps set the tone, expectations and purpose of the group. Facilitators begin by explaining the goals of the session, clarifying the structure and establishing group norms such as respect and confidentiality (e.g., "what happens in group, stays in group").
   For stress management groups, this might include a "warmup" exercise – such as deep breathing, mindfulness or a simple check-in – allowing participants to share how their stress management routine is going. This introduction helps create a safe atmosphere and fosters an opportunity for vulnerability, accountability and support.
2. **Activity**. Engaging in meaningful activity
   The activity component is at the core of what makes an occupational therapy-led group unique compared to those led by other disciplines. It should be carefully selected to align with the group's overall purpose and goals, as well as the needs and abilities of participants (e.g., it should adhere to the "just right challenge"). For stress management groups, activities might include:
   - Guided relaxation exercises (e.g., progressive muscle relaxation, visualization).
   - Journaling prompts to explore stressors and coping mechanisms.
   - Cognitive restructuring exercises based on cognitive-behavioral techniques.
   - Art-based interventions, such as drawing, sculpting or painting.
   - Movement-based activities, such as stretching or mindful walking.

The key to an effective activity is balancing structure and flexibility – it should provide enough guidance to support therapeutic engagement while allowing for individual interpretation and participation.

3. **Sharing**. Encouraging expression and disclosure
   After the activity, participants are encouraged to share their experiences, thoughts or reactions. Sharing allows group members to connect, find commonalities and learn from one another's experiences.
   In stress management groups, facilitators might ask:
   - What was this experience like for you?
   - Did anything about this exercise surprise you?
   - How does this strategy compare to ones you've used before?
   - How could you see yourself using this strategy?

   Some participants may be hesitant to share, especially early in the group process. Facilitators can encourage participation by modeling openness and using alternative sharing formats, such as writing reflections, using technology like virtual whiteboards or using creative methods like drawing or symbolic objects.
4. **Processing**. Exploring and reflecting
   This step goes deeper than simply sharing responses — it examines emotions, group dynamics and interpersonal interactions. It allows participants to reflect on their reactions to the group experience and how those reactions relate to broader patterns in their lives.
   For stress management, facilitators might guide discussion with questions like:
   - What emotions came up for you during the activity?
   - Did anything feel challenging? Why?
   - How does stress affect your ability to engage in activities like this outside the group?

   This phase helps participants gain self-awareness and recognize how their emotional responses impact their coping strategies. It also can strengthen the group's cohesion, as members build trust through deeper reflection and shared experiences.
5. **Generalizing**. Identifying commonalities
   Generalizing helps participants connect their own experiences to those of their peers. The facilitator helps the group identify common themes, patterns and insights from the session.
   For a stress management group, this could include:
   - Recognizing common stressors and coping strategies.
   - Identifying barriers to stress management and how others overcome them.
   - Discovering shared challenges and successes in implementing self-care.

Rather than reflecting only on individual experiences, this step shifts the focus to universal lessons that can be applied outside of the group.

6. **Application**. Translating tools into daily life (answering the question of "so what?")
   Application is one of the most critical steps in group therapy. It ensures that the lessons learned during the session are translated into everyday life. The facilitator helps participants identify specific, actionable ways to use the skills and insights gained from the group.
   For stress management, this might involve:
   - Setting a small, realistic goal (e.g., "I will practice deep breathing for five minutes before bed").
   - Identifying situations where a strategy can be applied (e.g., "I will use progressive muscle relaxation before a big presentation").
   - Encouraging accountability by having members share how they plan to integrate what they've learned into their day-to-day routine

   Facilitators can also normalize setbacks and encourage self-compassion, reminding participants that progress is rarely linear.
7. **Summary**. Reinforcing takeaways and closure
   The final step involves wrapping up the session with a summary of key insights, themes and takeaways. This helps solidify learning, provides closure and reinforces a sense of accomplishment.
   A strong summary in a stress management group might include:
   - Highlighting key themes from the discussion and encouraging participants to reflect on what felt most useful or interesting for them.
   - Expressing appreciation for the group's contributions.
   - Reviewing how concepts from the group can and should be applied "in real life."

   Facilitators should also check in to ensure participants feel supported as they leave the group, particularly if emotionally intense topics were discussed.

APPLICATION FOR STRESS MANAGEMENT

Cole's Seven Steps provide a structured yet flexible approach to group therapy, ensuring that sessions remain goal-oriented, engaging and focused on engagement in meaningful activity. For stress management groups, this structure is particularly beneficial because:

1. It ensures a balance of activity, discussion and reflection, keeping participants engaged while ensuring that facilitators have a framework that encourages occupation-based, activity-focused practice.

2. It creates a safe, predictable framework, which can be calming and reassuring for individuals experiencing high stress.
3. It guides participants toward application outside of the context of the group, helping them translate insights into real-world coping strategies.

By utilizing this model, occupational therapy practitioners can facilitate meaningful, evidence-based group interventions that support stress reduction, self-awareness and long-term well-being. See Box 11.1 for a case study description of such a group used for a client.

BOX 11.1 CASE STUDY OF A STRESS MANAGEMENT GROUP

CASE STUDY: SPOUSAL CAREGIVER STRESS MANAGEMENT GROUP

Elena is a 56-year-old elementary school teacher whose husband was diagnosed with early-onset Parkinson's disease. In addition to maintaining her full-time job, Elena manages her husband's medication schedule, drives him to weekly appointments and takes on most household responsibilities. Over time, she noticed feeling exhausted, frequent headaches and a sense of resentment that left her guilty and isolated.

Her neurologist referred her to an occupational therapy-led stress management group for caregivers. The group met weekly for eight sessions, using **Cole's Seven Steps of Group Leadership** to structure participation.

- **Introduction:** Each session began with a grounding exercise, such as mindful breathing, to model simple strategies for daily use.
- **Activity:** Members practiced task-management tools, including visual schedules and activity prioritization, to manage competing demands. Sessions also included role-plays of difficult conversations with healthcare providers and guided relaxation activities.
- **Sharing/Processing:** Elena admitted struggling with guilt when asking her adult children for support. Hearing other spouses describe similar dilemmas reduced her sense of isolation and allowed her to reframe her request for help as part of healthy family functioning.

- **Generalizing/Application:** Elena committed to two strategies: using a weekly meal-planning chart (developed during a session) and scheduling a standing weekend-walk with a friend.
- **Summary:** By the final session, Elena reported improved sleep, fewer headaches, and greater confidence in balancing her professional and caregiving roles. Her Perceived Stress Scale scores decreased, and she described feeling "like myself again, not just a caregiver."

This case showcases how occupational therapy-led groups can enable caregivers to practice stress management in context. The occupational therapy lens ensured strategies were tied to routines, roles and meaningful occupations – making them practical, sustainable and, most importantly, transferable to daily life.

See Box 11.2 for a sample template for the use of these steps in the context of stress management.

BOX 11.2 GROUP THERAPY TEMPLATE USING COLE'S SEVEN STEPS

Group title:	
Facilitator(s):	
Date:	
Duration:	
Population/target audience:	
Session goal(s):	

1. Introduction

   Objective: Establish the purpose of the session, set expectations and create a welcoming environment.

Key points:	
Guided questions/discussion points:	
Strategies/activities:	
Expected duration:	

2. Activity

   Objective: Engage participants in a structured task relevant to the session's goals.

Key points:	
ww	
Strategies/activities:	
Expected duration:	

3. Sharing

   Objective: Provide participants an opportunity to share their experiences or reflections.

Key points:	
Guided questions/discussion points:	
Strategies/activities:	
Expected duration:	

4. Processing
   Objective: Explore emotional responses and group dynamics related to the activity.

Key points:	
Guided questions/discussion points:	
Strategies/activities:	
Expected duration:	

5. Generalizing
   Objective: Identify key takeaways and themes that emerged from the session.

Key points:	
Guided questions/discussion points:	
Strategies/activities:	
Expected duration:	

6. Application
   Objective: Help participants integrate content from the session into their daily lives.

Key points:	
Guided questions/discussion points:	
Strategies/activities:	
Expected duration:	

7. Summary
Objective: Reinforce key takeaways and provide closure to the session.

Key points:	
Guided questions/discussion points:	
Strategies/activities:	
Expected duration:	

Facilitator notes and reflections

What worked well?	
What challenges emerged?	
Adjustments for future sessions:	

EXAMPLES OF GROUP THERAPY APPROACHES

Within the specifications of a framework like Cole's Steps of Group Leadership (or similar tools), stress management groups can take many forms. While this text cannot describe every possible approach to group therapy, it is worth digging into some of the most common approaches, including psychoeducation groups (see Chapter 12 on Psychoeducation) and activity-based groups.

ACTIVITY-BASED STRESS MANAGEMENT GROUPS

Activity-based groups emphasize "learning by doing," creating a space for participants to engage in activities that promote relaxation, self-expression and development of coping skill. Compared to more traditional "talk therapy" groups, activity-based groups are focused on practicing skills and engaging in real-world tasks, role plays or activities (Bullock & Bannigan, 2011).

Such groups align well with occupational therapy's focus on the use of occupation as both a means and an end in treatment, giving participants practical tools to manage stress (Bullock & Bannigan, 2011). If occupational therapy is to carve out a unique niche in this arena, its expertise in the "doing" of skills like task management represents a strong starting point.

Potential Activities

1. **Creative expression**. Art-based interventions such as painting, journaling or sculpting (Jean-Berluche, 2024; Sohal et al., 2022)
2. **Physical movement**. Stretching, yoga or low-intensity exercise (Padvamathi et al., 2023; Smith & Merwin, 2021)
3. **Mindfulness practices**. Guided meditation, progressive muscle relaxation, body scanning or mindful movement (e.g., walking meditation; Fazia et al., 2023; Menardo et al., 2022)
4. **Sensory modulation**. Engaging in tactile, auditory or other sensory experiences for stress relief (e.g., aromatherapy, use of fidget tools, listening to calming music; Craswell & Ghanouni, 2021).
5. **Engagement in leisure occupations**. Exploring hobbies that promote relaxation, such as gardening, knitting or collaborative tabletop games (Chen et al., 2022)

Benefits

1. Provides an experiential approach to stress management
2. Helps participants discover personalized coping strategies
3. Reinforces the use of meaningful activities as stress-relief tools

Key Takeaways

1. Different group formats, including psychoeducational and activity-based approaches, can support stress management in different ways.
2. Occupational therapy's role in stress management groups often emphasizes active participation and skill-building (the "doing" of stress management) rather than passive discussion alone (Bullock & Bannigan, 2011).

3. Facilitators can tailor groups based on participant needs, interests and functional goals while maintaining a strong occupation-based focus.
4. By incorporating a variety of group approaches, occupational therapy practitioners can create engaging, effective interventions that empower individuals to build resilience, develop coping skills and improve their overall well-being.

LOGISTICAL CONSIDERATIONS FOR GROUP THERAPY

Successful group therapy requires more than clinical expertise on the part of the facilitator. Groups require careful planning of logistical factors to ensure an effective and supportive environment for participants. A facilitator can come prepared with all the best in evidence-based strategies to manage stress, but if there aren't enough chairs for participants to sit comfortably, the group is unlikely to be a success. Simple logistical factors such as physical space, group size, session length and other factors can play a key role in the success of any group intervention.

Group Size and Composition

The size of groups can vary widely across different settings and contexts. Sometimes, a group may be smaller (two participants) or larger (fifteen participants) than is ideal, especially if the group is an "open" group, potentially removing some degree of facilitator control. The optimal number of participants is typically 5–10, to maintain engagement while ensuring opportunities for individual participation (Erickson, 1982; Thorn & Kuhajda, 2006; Yalom & Leszcz, 2020).

Homogeneous groups (e.g., all participants who are dealing with stress resulting from a specific chronic illness) may provide shared understanding and faster trust-building. Heterogeneous groups can offer diverse perspectives and peer learning but may require additional facilitation strategies to help participants understand the nature of their commonalities.

Participant readiness for group intervention is a critical item to assess prior to starting a group. The occupational therapy practitioner must assess individual needs, social skills and ability to participate in group dynamics to ensure that all members are able to benefit from the group intervention. While it is tempting to say that facilitators should maximize openness and welcome all newcomers, incompatible group dynamics or abilities can significantly impact the effectiveness of a group intervention.

Open vs. Closed Groups

An important consideration in group design is whether a group should be "open" or "closed." Open groups allow new members to join at any time, making the group more flexible and accessible. Closed groups have a set membership from the beginning, meaning no new participants are permitted to join after the group starts.

Each of these configurations has its own advantages and drawbacks. Open groups allow for rolling admission and greater accessibility. However, group cohesion and trust may be harder to establish, and facilitators will likely need to frequently reintroduce group norms and rules to ensure that all participants are on "the same page" regarding group expectations.

Closed groups offer the potential for more stability, stronger group cohesion and the opportunity for greater trust among participants. However, they also result in limited flexibility compared to open groups. If participants drop out, or if there is not enough initial interest, group size may be smaller than ideal.

Length and Frequency of Sessions

Most group therapy sessions last between 30 and 90 minutes, allowing a balance of engagement and cognitive load, on top of making it logistically more accessible for people with competing demands. Shorter sessions (30–45 minutes) may be suitable for populations with cognitive or attentional challenges.

Weekly sessions are common in group therapy, but biweekly or intensive formats (e.g., daily) may be appropriate in certain settings such as intensive outpatient therapy.

Physical Space and Environment

Because groups necessarily take up quite a bit more space than individual sessions, the physical environment can be a key factor. Privacy and confidentiality are essential; groups should be held in quiet, private spaces to promote a sense of safety and to allow for open discussion.

Seating arrangement should be considered based on the goals of the group. Many people think of group therapy as being conducted in a large room with chairs arranged in a circle. Such an arrangement may foster connection and encourage verbal participation but may be less well-suited to activity-based groups that could require a tabletop or other flat surface for drawing, writing or other activities.

Other considerations include lighting, noise control and accessibility. Natural light can enhance comfort, while dimmable lights may be helpful for relaxation-based activities. External noise should be minimized, and the space should be wheelchair accessible and adaptable for participants with sensory or mobility needs.

ONLINE/TELEHEALTH GROUPS

In recent years, especially following the onset of the COVID-19 pandemic, the use of online platforms such as Zoom to facilitate therapeutic intervention has increased markedly. The pandemic forced many practitioners who might not otherwise have thought to offer their services remotely to switch to online platforms, at least temporarily. These platforms offer both opportunities and challenges for occupational therapy practitioners who wish to implement group interventions for stress management.

Platform selection should prioritize legally compliant (e.g., HIPAA in the USA) video conferencing platforms designed for use in healthcare settings. Technical accessibility should be ensured for both facilitators and participants *before* sessions begin. This includes stable internet access, clear audio and familiarity with the platform. Trying to troubleshoot these issues in real time can drain valuable time that could otherwise be spent engaging in the group process.

Common challenges and potential solutions for online groups include:

1. Nonverbal communication may be limited. Use chat features, reaction buttons and structured check-ins.
2. Group cohesion can take longer to develop. Consider longer introductions, icebreakers and structured participation prompts.
3. Confidentiality concerns. Encourage participants to join from private locations with headphones.

By heeding these important logistical factors that are nonetheless easy to lose sight of, occupational therapy practitioners can increase the likelihood of group success. Attention to these factors enables structured, effective and engaging group therapy sessions that maximize participant benefit and long-term success.

SUMMARY

Group therapy can be a powerful tool to help people more effectively manage their stress. Group interventions can offer participants the opportunity to share experiences, learn new coping strategies and build connections, fostering a sense of self-efficacy. Through the use of engagement in occupation, structured activities and guided discussions, group interventions can foster self-awareness, social support and the development of meaningful, practical strategies to manage stress. Occupational therapy, with the profession's unique focus on engagement in occupation as both a means and an end in treatment, is particularly well-suited to facilitate these groups in a way that moves beyond discussion and into actionable skill-building.

DISCUSSION QUESTIONS

1. What unique benefits does group therapy offer in stress management that individual interventions may not provide?
2. How can occupational therapy practitioners use group leadership skills to facilitate effective stress management interventions?
3. What logistical factors (e.g., group size, session structure, environment) are most important when designing a stress management group?
4. Imagine you were tasked with developing a stress management group. What might such a group look like? How would you ensure that it is grounded in evidence-based strategies?

REFERENCES

Bandura, A. (1982). Self-efficacy mechanism in human agency. *American Psychologist*, *37*(2), 122–147. https://doi.org/10.1037/0003-066X.37.2.122

Bandura, A. (2019). Applying theory for human betterment. *Perspectives on Psychological Science*, *14*(1), 12–15. https://doi.org/10.1177/1745691618815165

Baum, C. M., Christiansen, C. H., & Bass-Haugen, J. D. (2015). *Person–Environment–Occupation-Performance model*. In C. H. Christiansen, C. M. Baum, & J. D. Bass-Haugen (Eds.), *Occupational therapy: Performance, participation, and well-being* (4th ed., pp. 49–56). SLACK.

Bertollo, A. G., Braga, G. D. C., Tonin, P. T., Luzardo, A. R., Bagatini, M. D., & Ignácio, Z. M. (2023). The impact of stress from social isolation during the COVID-19 pandemic on psychiatric disorders: An analysis from the scientific literature. *Brain Sciences*, *13*(10), 1414. https://doi.org/10.3390/brainsci13101414

Bullock, A., & Bannigan, K. (2011). Effectiveness of activity-based group work in community mental health: A systematic review. *American Journal of Occupational Therapy*, *65*(3), 257–266. https://doi.org/10.5014/ajot.2011.001305

Campagne, D. M. (2019). Stress and perceived social isolation (loneliness). *Archives of Gerontology and Geriatrics*, *82*, 192–199. https://doi.org/10.1016/j.archger.2019.02.007

Chen, F., Zang, Y., Dong, H., Wang, X., Bian, J., & Lin, X. (2022). Effects of a hospital-based leisure activities programme on nurses' stress, self-perceived anxiety and depression: A mixed methods study. *Journal of Nursing Management*, *30*(1), 243–251. https://doi.org/10.1111/jonm.13484

Coates, C., Malouff, J., & Rooke, S. E. (2008). Efficacy of written modeling and vicarious reinforcement in increasing use of problem-solving methods by distressed individuals. *Journal of Psychology*, *142*(4), 413–426. https://doi.org/10.3200/JRPL.142.4.413-426

Cole, M. B. (2025). *Group dynamics in occupational therapy: The theoretical basis and practice application of group intervention* (6th ed.). Routledge.

Craswell, G., Dieleman, C., & Ghanouni, P. (2021). An integrative review of sensory approaches in adult inpatient mental health: Implications for occupational therapy in prison-based mental health services. *Occupational Therapy in Mental Health*, *37*(2), 130–157. https://doi.org/10.1080/0164212X.2020.1853654

Erickson, R. C. (1982). Inpatient small group psychotherapy: A survey. *Clinical Psychology Review*, *2*(2), 137–151. https://doi.org/10.1016/0272-7358(82)90008-3

Farr, M., Brant, H., Patel, R., Linton, M.-J., Ambler, N., Vyas, S., Wedge, H., Watkins, S., & Horwood, J. (2021). Experiences of patient-led chronic pain peer support groups after pain management programs: A qualitative study. *Pain Medicine*, *22*(12), 2884–2895. https://doi.org/10.1093/pm/pnab189

Fazia, T., Bubbico, F., Nova, A., Buizza, C., Cela, H., Iozzi, D., Calgan, B., Maggi, F., Floris, V., Sutti, I., Bruno, S., Ghilardi, A., & Bernardinelli, L. (2023). Improving stress management, anxiety, and mental well-being in medical students through an online mindfulness-based intervention: A randomized study. *Scientific Reports*, *13*(1), 8214. https://doi.org/10.1038/s41598-023-35483-z

Goubert, L., Vlaeyen, J. W. S., Crombez, G., & Craig, K. D. (2011). Learning about pain from others: An observational learning account. *Journal of Pain*, *12*(2), 167–174. https://doi.org/10.1016/j.jpain.2010.10.001

Hoang, P., King, J. A., Moore, S., Moore, K., Reich, K., Sidhu, H., Tan, C. V., Whaley, C., & McMillan, J. (2022). Interventions associated with reduced loneliness and social isolation in older adults: A systematic review and meta-analysis. *JAMA Network Open*, *5*(10), e2236676. https://doi.org/10.1001/jamanetworkopen.2022.36676

Ikiugu, M. N., Nissen, R. M., Bellar, C., Maassen, A., & Van Peursem, K. (2017). Clinical effectiveness of occupational therapy in mental health: A meta-analysis. *American Journal of Occupational Therapy*, *71*(5), 7105100020p1–7105100020p10. https://doi.org/10.5014/ajot.2017.024588

Jean-Berluche, D. (2024). Creative expression and mental health. *Journal of Creativity*, *34*(2), 100083. https://doi.org/10.1016/j.yjoc.2024.100083

Lambdin-Pattavina, C., & Pyatak, E. (2022). Occupational therapy's role in chronic conditions. *American Journal of Occupational Therapy*, *76*(Supplement_3), 7613410220. https://doi.org/10.5014/ajot.2022.76S3003

Marogna, C., & Caccamo, F. (2015). Analysis of the process in brief psychotherapy group: The role of therapeutic factors. *Research in Psychotherapy: Psychopathology, Process and Outcome*, *17*(1), 43–51. https://doi.org/10.4081/ripppo.2014.161

Menardo, E., Di Marco, D., Ramos, S., Brondino, M., Arenas, A., Costa, P., Vaz De Carvalho, C., & Pasini, M. (2022). Nature and mindfulness to cope with work-related stress: A narrative review. *International Journal of Environmental Research and Public Health*, *19*(10), 5948. https://doi.org/10.3390/ijerph19105948

Padvamathi, R., Kumar, A. P., Dhamodhini, K. S, Venugopal, V., Silambanan, S. K. M., & Shah, P. (2023). Role of yoga in stress management and implications in major depression disorder. *Journal of Ayurveda and Integrative Medicine*, *14*(5), 100767. https://doi.org/10.1016/j.jaim.2023.100767

Ranasinghe, B. A., Balasuriya, A., Wijeyaratne, C. N., & Fernando, N. (2023). The impact of peer-led support groups on health-related quality of life, coping skills and depressive symptomatology for women with PCOS. *Psychology, Health & Medicine*, *28*(3), 564–573. https://doi.org/10.1080/13548506.2021.2019805

Robak, R. W., Doshi, P. V., & Tursi, M. M. (2022). Exploring key group counseling processes: Implications for group counselor training. *Journal of Counselor Preparation and Supervision*, *15*(2). https://research.library.kutztown.edu/jcps/vol15/iss2/8

Rogers, C. R. (1961). *On becoming a person: A therapist's view of psychotherapy*. Houghton Mifflin.

Smith, P. J., & Merwin, R. M. (2021). The role of exercise in management of mental health disorders: An integrative review. *Annual Review of Medicine*, *72*(1), 45–62. https://doi.org/10.1146/annurev-med-060619-022943

Sohal, M., Singh, P., Dhillon, B. S., & Gill, H. S. (2022). Efficacy of journaling in the management of mental illness: A systematic review and meta-analysis. *Family Medicine and Community Health*, *10*(1), e001154. https://doi.org/10.1136/fmch-2021-001154

Swarbrick, M., & Noyes, S. (2018). Effectiveness of occupational therapy services in mental health practice. *American Journal of Occupational Therapy*, *72*(5), 7205170010p1–7205170010p4. https://doi.org/10.5014/ajot.2018.725001

Taylor, R. R., Bowyer, P., & Fisher, G. (2023). *Kielhofner's model of human occupation: Theory and application* (6th ed.). Wolters Kluwer.

Thorn, B. E., & Kuhajda, M. C. (2006). Group cognitive therapy for chronic pain. *Journal of Clinical Psychology*, *62*(11), 1355–1366. https://doi.org/10.1002/jclp.20315

Velasquez, M. M., Crouch, C., Stephens, N. S., & DiClemente, C. C. (2015). *Group therapy for substance abuse: A stage-of-change therapy manual* (2nd ed.). Guilford Press.

Won, P., Bello, M. S., Stoycos, S. A., Carrera, B. T., Kurakazu, D. M., Briere, J., Garner, W. L., Gillenwater, J., & Yenikomshian, H. A. (2021). The impact of peer support group programs on psychosocial outcomes for burn survivors and caregivers: A review of the literature. *Journal of Burn Care & Research*, *42*(4), 600–609. https://doi.org/10.1093/jbcr/irab042

Yalom, I. D., & Leszcz, M. (2020). *The theory and practice of group psychotherapy* (6th ed.). Basic Books.

Chapter 12

Designing a Group Psychoeducation Model for Stress Management

LEARNING OBJECTIVES

By the end of reading this chapter, the reader will be able to

1. Define psychoeducation.
2. Design a group psychoeducation program for stress management.
3. Become familiar with the current literature on applying psychoeducation to a diverse number of clinical groups.
4. Evaluate the effectiveness of a psychoeducation program.

OVERVIEW AND DEFINITION OF PSYCHOEDUCATION

As Steed wrote,

> Psychoeducation… is instruction intended to improve the client's emotional regulation and related behavioral skills. In the psychiatric literature, the term 'psychoeducation' usually refers to a component of an illness management program and is limited to instruction in medication and disease processes.
>
> (2014, p. 129)

DOI: 10.4324/9781003671084-12

Psychoeducation groups for stress management in occupational therapy contain a combination of didactic education and practical skill-building. The dual approach is to help participants both understand stress and develop strategies to manage it effectively (Cowls & Hale, 2005; Günaydin, 2022; Mirhosseini et al., 2025). The groups can include interactive discussions and problem-solving exercises (Hale & Cowls, 2009).

In this type of group, the leader plays the role of both facilitator and something resembling a teacher. A strong grasp of the content being discussed (e.g., stress management strategies) is a must – facilitators need to be prepared to educate, answer questions and generally be a resource for participants. Few things have the potential to derail a psychoeducation group more than a facilitator who does not have a grasp of group content.

In general, psychoeducational approaches have been used to increase patient knowledge of, and insight into, their illness and its treatment (Xia et al., 2011). Psychoeducation has been applied therapeutically to many conditions, such as anxiety and depression (Dolan et al., 2021; Donker et al., 2009; Tursi et al., 2013), schizophrenia (Pekkala & Merinder, 2002), multiple sclerosis (Oz & Oz, 2020), breast cancer (Setyowibowo et al., 2022) and facilitating return to work for individuals on sick leave (Pedersen et al., 2015).

OTHER POTENTIAL TOPICS AND ACTIVITIES IN PSYCHOEDUCATION GROUPS

1. Understanding the stress response and its effects on the body (American Psychological Association, 2018; James et al., 2023)
2. Identifying personal stressors and triggers (Riachi et al., 2022)
3. Learning cognitive-behavioral strategies (problem-solving skills, reframing negative thoughts; Fogarty et al., 2019; Thimm & Antonsen, 2014)
4. Practicing time management, goal setting, boundary-setting techniques (Chernata, 2024)

BENEFITS OF PSYCHOEDUCATION GROUPS FOR STRESS MANAGEMENT

Psychoeducation groups can provide participants with knowledge about symptoms of stress, stressors and effective coping mechanisms. They can encourage self-awareness and proactive stress management. Finally, they can create a supportive space for discussion.

A psychoeducational approach can be incorporated into a stress management intervention. In this approach, the occupational therapist uses educational technology, integrating lecture, discussion, role playing, behavioral rehearsal, homework and laboratory experiences.

GROUP DESIGN AND PROTOCOL

A prototype of a psychoeducational model for individuals diagnosed with depression is described below from the first author's clinical experiences (Stein & Cutler, 2002, pp. 431–444). Although the focus of the example is individuals with depression, it can be adapted for other individuals with mental health issues, such as schizophrenia or severe anxiety. Here the focus could be to develop positive health strategies so that the individual can self-regulate stress to prevent it from precipitating a recurrence of symptoms.

In the following specific example, a psychoeducation group approach was used with individuals who had either been hospitalized for depression or had been treated for depression in the community. Participants in the course came from the local chapter of a mental health support group. All participants volunteered to participate in the group after receiving a letter of invitation that described the purposes of the group and the sessions involved. The course description, objectives and outline of the sessions were distributed to the participants on the first day of the course.

The following discussion topics as well as handouts were distributed to the group members over the duration of the course:

a. Stress management as a critical life skill
b. Sleep hygiene
c. Humor
d. Getting up in the morning
e. Breakfast
f. Mindfulness meditation
g. Exercise for alleviating depression
h. Adherence to the stress management program

PSYCHOEDUCATIONAL COURSE ON STRESS MANAGEMENT: TECHNIQUES TO PREVENT RECURRENCE OF DEPRESSION

Course Outline and Description of the Course

This course is intended to help individuals who have experienced clinical depression. The course is divided into lectures, discussions and practical demonstrations. The course will meet for eight consecutive weeks for approximately one and a half hours. The content of the course will be discussions of the causes, symptoms and treatment of depression; the effects of stressors and coping skills; and practical demonstrations of relaxation techniques.

Specific Objectives of the Course

By the end of the course the adult learner will

1. understand the dynamics of depression as a biopsychosocial illness
2. understand the symptoms of stress, the stressors that trigger stress and the coping activities that are effective in managing stress
3. gain insight in how distress can precipitate symptoms of depression in individuals who are vulnerable
4. be able to incorporate a stress management program into his or her everyday life.
5. learn the Benson Relaxation Response
6. learn how to do the Jacobson Progressive Relaxation Technique
7. use visual imagery as a relaxation strategy
6. learn how to use cognitive behavioral strategies to cope with the symptoms of depression, such as with insomnia, eating disturbance, difficulty getting up in the morning, sad mood, low energy, low self-esteem, poor concentration and inability to feel pleasure
7. practice other techniques such as listening to calm music and meditation to prevent and cope with depression.
8. initiate an exercise program incorporated into a daily schedule.

Schedule for Class

Session 1

1. Introduction and objectives of course
2. Discussion of causes of depression and its relationship to stress
3. Benson Relaxation Response – demonstration and practice

Session 2

1. Discussion of the relationship between stress and the onset of symptoms (Diathesis-Stress Model of Colodro-Conde et al., 2018)
2. Progressive relaxation demonstration and practice
3. Getting up in the morning (Handout and Discussion)

Session 3

1. Discussion of the everyday stressors that can trigger symptoms of depression
2. Visual imagery – demonstration and practice
3. Sleep hygiene (Handout and Discussion)

Session 4

1. Discussion of individual coping activities and resources in managing stress
2. Physiological symptoms that are triggered by stress
3. Daily physical exercise as a method to prevent distress and anxiety

Session 5

1. Discussion of pleasant activities in one's life
2. Role playing stressful situations that may trigger stress
3. Understanding the relationship between a healthy diet (Mediterranean diet) and positive health

Session 6

1. Setting up an Individualized Stress Management Program via group discussion
2. Learning how to control feelings by self-talk
3. Activities to increase concentration such as cross-word puzzles, sudoku, video games

Session 7

1. Techniques to interrupt negative thoughts, such as relaxing music, concentrating on an enjoyable arts and crafts activity, taking part in sports and other activities that increase FLOW (Salonen et al., 2022)
2. Paradoxical intention by Frankl (1975) consists of consciously producing anxiety and depression so as to be able to control the feelings – Demonstration and Practice.

Session 8

1. Closure activity – individual evaluation of the experience
2. Reinforcing a positive experience of the group through a potluck picnic or dinner or whatever the group decides

PARTICIPANT HOMEWORK ASSIGNMENTS

1. Complete the Stress Management Questionnaire (SMQ)
2. Practice relaxation techniques every day
3. Set up a daily schedule for including positive health habits (exercise, meditation, healthy diet, socialization) to prevent depression
4. Keep daily diary of symptoms, stressors and coping activities
5. Write a first-person account of a stressful experience and response

HANDOUTS TO PARTICIPANTS ON STRESS MANAGEMENT

These handouts are meant to encourage discussion in the group. They are based on the authors' personal experiences and a search of the research literature. They are guidelines meant to be adapted to the needs of the individual.

a. Handout on Stress Management as a Critical Life Skill

STRESS MANAGEMENT AS A CRITICAL LIFE SKILL

What is stress and what is its relationship to illness?

Stress can be defined as both a cause and an effect. As a cause, stress is a common part of everyday life. Examples include the pressure to perform well on an exam when unprepared, fear of rejection by a friend, job loss or anxiety about the future. These are everyday stressors that trigger physiological responses in the body.

When exposed to a stressor, the autonomic nervous system (specifically the sympathetic response) activates: heart rate increases, blood pressure rises and metabolism speeds up. The body mobilizes as if under threat. If this response is intense or prolonged, it can lead to physical or psychological symptoms such as headaches, back pain, heartburn, blurred vision or anxiety – often depending on the individual's vulnerabilities.

The key to managing stress lies in how an individual responds to stressors. For instance:

1. Talking about a stressful event with a good listener can relieve stress.
2. Physical exercise dissipates built-up tension and releases endorphins.
3. Activities such as listening to music, writing, cleaning, doing puzzles or any relaxing hobby can reduce stress.

Managing stress should be as routine as brushing your teeth or eating regularly. Since stress is an unavoidable part of life, individuals need to be prepared to deal with it effectively.

BUILDING RESILIENCE TO STRESS

One way to deal with stress is to toughen ourselves physically and mentally. This means developing confidence and resources both within ourselves and through our relationships. Physical resilience can be built through exercise and sports, which condition the body to better handle stress and boost the immune system. Emotional resilience can be developed through positive relationships or support groups, which create a network of resources – especially important for individuals vulnerable to mental health issues.

In cases of severe stress, such as living in a war zone, individuals, no matter how resilient, may develop post-traumatic stress disorder (PTSD), which can trigger depression and physical symptoms.

RECENT RESEARCH

According to LeMoult et al. (2023), major mental illnesses like depression are episodic and marked by intense symptoms followed by periods of remission. These episodes are often triggered by distress, either external (e.g., loss of a loved one) or internal (e.g., negative self-thoughts).

Preventing episodes of mental illness involves coping with stress before it becomes overwhelming. This includes adopting healthy daily habits, such as

1. Talking with someone you trust
2. Listening to relaxing music

3. Exercising
4. Reading
5. Engaging in enjoyable activities

We are best able to handle stress when we are physically and mentally healthy. Developing a daily wellness strategy can help build resilience and maintain mental health.

CREATING YOUR STRESS STRATEGY

Stress management can be viewed as a self-hardening exercise – preparation for life's daily challenges. Begin by answering these three questions:

1. What are the symptoms and problems I experience when I'm stressed?
2. Which everyday hassles or triggers cause my stress?
3. What coping methods have helped me in the past?

Each individual will have unique responses. Stress symptoms generally fall into four categories:

1. Cognitive – difficulty concentrating or learning
2. Emotional – feeling anxious or sad
3. Physiological – physical symptoms like back pain
4. Behavioral – changes like insomnia

Common daily stressors include (1) too many tasks, not enough time, (2) conflicts with friends or family and (3) feelings of rejection.

Helpful coping strategies ("copers") can include:

1. Talking to a supportive person
2. Listening to music
3. Walking in nature
4. Doing a hobby
5. Playing with a pet

Keeping a stress diary is also a great tool to identify your stress triggers and what helps you manage them. By understanding and handling your stress, you promote your own mental well-being.

FINAL THOUGHT

Use Humor and Perspective – Learning to laugh at yourself and with others adds balance and perspective. A good laugh a day may be even better than the proverbial apple.

b. Handout on Sleep Hygiene

SELF-REGULATING RESTFUL SLEEP

Set a specific time for going to bed, such as 10:30 PM, and getting up in the morning, such as 6:30 AM. Give yourself a little leeway on the weekends. As a rule, go to bed when you are drowsy. Your body will become conditioned to a specific bedtime.

Do not take afternoon naps. If you feel tired during the day, try meditating for 10–15 minutes or take a short walk. This should make you feel more energetic.

Exercise in the morning with a walk and/or in the early evening, such as before dinner, is desirable. Do not exercise two hours before bedtime. Vigorous exercise will arouse your body.

Maintain a cool temperature in the bedroom. Preferably keep a window open during the times of year when it is possible and the noise isn't disturbing. As a rule, use blankets to keep warm rather than overheating the room.

Use an air purifier or dehumidifier if it is helpful in getting to sleep.

A warm bath before going to bed may make you feel drowsy, especially if the bedroom is cool.

A light snack before going to bed is sometimes helpful. However, chocolate or excessive sweets may keep you awake. A glass of low-fat milk and some crackers may be sufficient.

Do not drink alcohol within two hours of your bedtime. Although alcohol is a depressant and may initially make you feel drowsy, it has a delayed effect that may lead to restlessness during the night. It also may upset your stomach. In addition, if you are on medication, there may be an interactive effect that could be detrimental.

Coffee, caffeinated tea, energy drinks and soda serve as stimulants and could keep you awake. The effect of caffeine takes about six hours to wear off.

Some people become drowsy by reading or listening to music. Other people need a completely quiet and dark room to fall asleep. Try to find out what the best environment is for you.

Visualization of pleasant experiences, past or future, has been helpful for some individuals in falling asleep, especially when feeling tense, stressed or preoccupied with disturbing thoughts. The individual is encouraged to think of a past scene in life that is serene and or pleasurable such as a walk in nature. The individual then tries to recapture the sensory experiences surrounding the event.

Another example of a sleep hygiene protocol was presented by Tucker et al. (2021).

c. Handout on Humor

HUMOR AS A MEANS TO COUNTERACT DEPRESSION: GUIDE FOR DISCUSSION

1. What is humor?
2. What makes us laugh?
3. What is a funny story?
4. Why does humor make us feel good?
5. What are different types of humor?
6. How do you develop a sense of humor?
7. Can we learn how to tell a funny story?
8. Comedy styles
    - The wit, thinks while he is talking
    - Satirist finds humor in the daily news
    - Punster has fun with words
    - Clown exaggerates life
    - Joke teller has a stock of stories
    - Kidder loves to tease
    - Masochist loves to put him- or herself down, à la Rodney Dangerfield
9. Collect funny stories from books, magazines, videos, movies and friends
10. Take a philosophical view of life

d. Handout on Getting up in the Morning

GETTING UP IN THE MORNING

A morning ritual should be established that arouses the body and activates the individual. Many individuals with depression have difficulty getting up in the morning. This includes:

1. Getting up at a set time every day such as 6:30 AM.
2. Putting on a bright light as soon as the alarm goes off. The light arouses the neurological system. Research on Seasonal Affective Disorders (SAD) verifies the importance of light in countering depression (Wirz-Justice, 2018).
3. Listening to a melodic and pleasant piece of music such as Bach's Brandenburg Concerti, Mozart, Vivaldi or other pieces that are stimulating is another way to arouse the neurological system.
4. Taking a stimulating shower for 10–15 minutes. Water and heat increase circulation in the muscles and joints of the body while reducing muscle tension. The individual is now prepared to do morning exercises.
5. Morning exercises should be conservative in nature in that they do not put undue stress on the muscles, joints and cardiovascular system. The main purpose of the exercises is to tone the muscles and joints. Exercise is an excellent activity to counteract depression. The morning stretching exercise of about ten minutes should be seen as preventative to back injuries and as helping to build muscle strength and to maintain range of motion in the joints. The stress management exercise of tensing and releasing the muscles of the face is a good starting activity.

e. Handout on Breakfast and Nutrition

BREAKFAST AND IMPLICATIONS FOR NUTRITION

Research has shown that a Mediterranean diet (Finicelli et al., 2022) containing fruit and vegetables, whole grains and lean meats and devoid of ultra-processed foods (with high levels of fats, sugar and salt) is the healthiest diet for most individuals. It is probably a good idea to take a multivitamin every day. This way you are assured of obtaining essential vitamins for sustaining health and preventing disease. This is a prudent approach. On the other hand, megavitamins, some supplements or massive doses of vitamins can be harmful.

Breakfast may be the most important meal of the day, especially for someone with a tendency toward depression. The suggested breakfast should include a citrus fruit (vitamin C), grains (vitamin B), nuts (protein), dairy (plain yogurt) and coffee or tea (stimulant).

f. Handout: Recommendations to Clients Using Mindfulness Meditation

APPLICATION FOR MINDFULNESS MEDITATION

Mindfulness meditation is a practice that involves focusing your mind on the present moment while calmly acknowledging and accepting your feelings, thoughts and bodily sensations. The main purpose of mindfulness meditation is to achieve a state of relaxation to counteract stressful thoughts and anxiety by focusing your mind on the present moment. Through mindfulness meditation the body goes into a parasympathetic response where heart rate and systolic blood pressure decrease. Studies (da Silva et al., 2023; Slagter et al., 2022) have shown that mindfulness meditation can have numerous benefits for mental and physical well-being, including reducing stress, anxiety and depression; improving focus and attention; enhancing emotional regulation; and promoting overall resilience and well-being. In short, mindfulness meditation has been shown to be effective in reducing stress and anxiety.

Mindfulness meditation can be done while you are sitting quietly, listening to classical music or accomplishing daily routine tasks like cleaning house or working in the garden. Practicing mindfulness meditation involves breathing methods, guided imagery and other practices to relax the body and mind and help reduce stress. Below are general recommendations for incorporating meditation into your everyday schedule.

1. Practice meditation every day, such as ten minutes in the afternoon or 10–20 minutes right before dinner. Do not take any stimulants before meditating because they will keep the body aroused and interfere with the effects of relaxation. Think of meditation as a relaxation exercise that becomes part of your healthy schedule of aerobic exercise, nutritious diet and stress reduction.
2. Select a quiet place to meditate at home or while taking a walk.
3. Meditate in a comfortable chair with your feet on the ground, your hands in your lap and your head in a comfortable position. Do not attempt to fall asleep during meditation. Maintain a passive attitude while you meditate and try to focus on one object, on breathing or on a point in space. If your mind wanders to obsessive thoughts or anxieties, try to distract it by thinking of pleasant scenes that you have experienced in the past or by counting after each breath.
4. Do a body scan to determine if your muscles are tense or relaxed. Massage with a gentle circular movement the muscles that seem tense.
5. Start a meditation program with as little as five minutes and then condition yourself to increase the amount of time to 20 minutes. You will be surprised how long ten minutes is when you are in a state of relaxation.

6. Meditation is helpful in increasing your energy so that it may be beneficial to meditate during the afternoon when most people feel less energetic.
7. Focus on an internal bodily process, such as visualizing your heart pumping nutrients to your body or the warmth of your hands and arms, as you keep your eyes closed.
8. If you want to keep your eyes open during meditation, then focus on an object in the room while letting go of obsessive or anxious thoughts.
9. Use diaphragmatic breathing. This refers to breathing inward through your nose while expanding your abdomen, holding your breath for a moment and then letting go by breathing through your mouth while contracting your abdomen. Practice diaphragmatic breathing before meditating and then incorporate it into the relaxation exercise.
10. Use a relaxing and calm subvocal phrase, or mantra, repeatedly while you are meditating, such as "alert mind calm body," "one," "my arms are warm and heavy," "I feel happy" or "pleasant scenes."

The following specific example of a mindfulness meditation exercise (Building a Dream House) has been used by the first author with individuals with depression, older adults and occupational therapy graduate students.

MINDFULNESS MEDITATION VISUALIZATION EXERCISE: BUILDING A DREAM HOUSE

1. Time for exercise: usually half an hour
2. Steps in completing the procedure:
    a. in a hard-backed chair in an ergonomic position, feet on the ground, eyes closed with hands in one's lap.
    b. The individual is told to become aware of one's abdominal deep breathing: breathing in through the nose and out through the mouth
    c. The individual sitting quietly becomes aware of inner bodily sensations, feelings and thoughts. The individual tries to be objective in filtering these experiences while focusing on breathing and the internal environment and not being distracted by current worries.
    d. The therapist explains the purposes of the exercise to the client by stating, "this exercise is to create a mental state of serenity by building a dream house through visual imagery. The exercise can be used to reduce anxiety, increase relaxation and to be used as an aid to restful sleep as a countermeasure to insomnia."

Specific Directions for Building a Dream House.

a. The therapist reads the following to the client: "Select an area in nature where you would like to build the dream house, such as in a forest, near a lake, along a river or in the mountains or a sunny field or prairie.
b. Now build the structure of the house such as a one-story ranch, a two-story colonial, town house, condominium, log cabin, farmhouse or large mansion.
c. Now build the structure of the house with wood, brick, stone, stucco or a combination of building materials. Visualize the house firmly in your mind so that you can describe it to someone else.
d. Open the door of the house and now start furnishing the house beginning with the living room. Start with comfortable chairs to relax in, chat with friends and family, listen to music you enjoy and read or watch favorite videos. Build large windows so you can enjoy nature outside and watch sunrises and sunsets. To decorate the walls, select your favorite paintings, prints and photographs that make you feel close to nature or remind you of loving family members. Visualize the living room firmly in your mind so that you can return to that scene as a familiar place that makes you feel serene and less stressful.
e. Now invite someone you love to visit your dream house."

g. Handout on Exercise for Alleviating Depression

EXERCISE FOR ALLEVIATING DEPRESSION

"Exercise is an effective treatment for depression, with walking or jogging, yoga, and strength training more effective than other exercises, particularly when intense. Yoga and strength training were well tolerated compared with other treatments" (Noetel et. el., 2024, p. e075847).

In setting up an exercise program for depression, it is important to consider the amount of time for a session (30 or 40 minutes), the intensity of the exercise (moderate or fast walking) and the duration (five times a week). In a meta-analysis of exercise and depression by Li et al. (2024), it was found that the median effective exercise routine for people who have symptoms of depression was 40 minutes of moderate aerobic exercise done three times a week for 6–11 weeks.

1. Purpose of exercise
2. Setting for exercise
3. Furniture and materials needed
4. Approximate time for exercise
5. Steps in completing exercise
6. Adherence and establishing healthy habits

h. Adherence to the Stress Management Program

An important aspect of any stress management program is to help the client comply with the recommendations that were jointly agreed on by the occupational therapist and individual. The model below is an example of operationalizing a stress management program by defining the activity to be engaged in, explaining the therapeutic purpose of the activity and having the individual personalize the activity so that it is feasible and meets the person's unique needs. For example, in the first activity, the therapist and individual agree that talking to a personal friend or relative on an ongoing basis will help the person release feelings and be able to analyze a situation objectively as a means of dealing with the stress of everyday life. In the individual response, the person records the specific plan to meet this objective and how he or she monitors the implementation.

ADHERENCE: INDIVIDUALIZED STRESS MANAGEMENT PROGRAM

1. Activity – Talk to a personal friend or relative on an ongoing basis to discuss the stresses and strains of everyday life.
   Purpose – Release of feelings and opportunity to analyze situations
   Individual Response – "I will telephone a friend twice a week."
2. Activity – Exercise periods of 5–45 minutes every day. For example, I will walk 30 minutes after dinner.
   Purpose – Reduce muscular tension and work out pent-up emotions.
   Individual Response – "Before breakfast I will do stretching exercises for 10 minutes, and at 5 PM. I will take a walk in the neighborhood."
3. Activity – Engage in an ongoing activity that leads to a finished project, such as a home improvement, model or craft project.
   Purpose – Increase self-esteem and feelings of accomplishment.
   Individual Response – "I will crochet 1 hour every day after dinner."
4. Activity – Volunteer in a social service agency, school or library.
   Purpose – Provides opportunity to help others and at the same time creates meaning in one's life. Increases responsibility and commitment.
   Individual Response – "I will volunteer in the library on Saturday mornings."
5. Activity – Active participation in a social support or self-help group such as Recovery Inc., Single People Together, Alcoholics Anonymous (AA) or National Alliance on Mental Illness (NAMI).
   Purpose – Provides for ongoing support, especially during periods of crisis.
   Individual Response – "I will attend a NAMI meeting once a month."
6. Activity – Monitoring diet because of a concern with nutrition.

Purpose – Help the body cope with the physical and psychological effects of stress.
Individual Response – "I will record the daily food I consume and ensure that I eat five fruits and vegetables a day."

7. Activity – Ongoing concern with body appearance.
   Purpose – Increase self-esteem.
   Individual Response – "I will use cleansing cream on my face before going to bed."
8. Activity – Taking responsibility for a plant or an animal.
   Purpose – Increase opportunity to nurture and make a commitment to life.
   Individual Response – "I will care for a cat."
9. Activity – Engage every day in other stress reduction activities, for example, progressive relaxation, yoga, quieting response, visualization, medication and biofeedback.
   Purpose – Inoculate yourself against the negative effects of stress by incorporating the relaxation response.
   Individual Response – "I will take a class in tai chi."
10. Activity – Eliminate or reduce excessive alcohol, reliance on abusive drugs, smoking, excessive caffeine, excessive "junk foods."
    Purpose – Increase the body's resistance to stressors.
    Individual Response – "I will drink only one cup of coffee per day and gradually eliminate smoking."

SUMMARY

Psychoeducation has been used by mental health professionals to increase patients' knowledge of, and insight into, their illness and its treatment. Psychoeducation has been applied effectively with several disabilities and conditions, such as with individuals having symptoms of anxiety and depression, multiple sclerosis and breast cancer. In this chapter, the author discusses how psychoeducation can be applied by occupational therapists in a stress management program. A prototype of a psychoeducational model for individuals diagnosed with depression was described. In this prototype, educational approaches integrating lecture, discussion, handouts, role-playing, behavioral rehearsal, homework and group experiences were described in detail. The main purpose of this psychoeducation experience is to help individuals understand the dynamics of mental illness and to practice and develop stress management techniques. These stress management techniques include mindfulness meditation, sleep hygiene, nutrition, aerobic exercise and humor. For helping individuals incorporate stress management techniques into their everyday lives, a model for operationalizing therapeutic goals was presented.

DISCUSSION QUESTIONS

1. How would occupational therapists define psychoeducation?
2. What are the components of a psychoeducation program for helping individuals manage stress?
3. What skills does an occupational therapist need for coordinating a psychoeducation program?
4. What are the benefits to the individual from engaging in a psychoeducation program?
5. How can occupational therapists help individuals comply with a positive, holistic program that helps them manage stress?

REFERENCES

American Psychological Association. (2018). *Stress effects on the body*. https://www.apa.org/topics/stress/body

Chernata, T. (2024). Personal boundaries: Definition, role, and impact on mental health. *Personality and Environmental Issues, 3*(1), 24–30. https://doi.org/10.31652/2786-6033-2024-3(1)-24-30

Colodro-Conde, L., Couvy-Duchesne, B., Zhu, G., Coventry, W. L., Byrne, E. M., Gordon, S., Wright, M. J., Montgomery, G. W., Madden, P. A. F., Major Depressive Disorder Working Group of the Psychiatric Genomics Consortium, Ripke, S., Eaves, L. J., Heath, A. C., Wray, N. R., Medland, S. E., & Martin, N. G. (2018). A direct test of the diathesis-stress model for depression. *Molecular Psychiatry, 23*(7), 1590–1596. https://doi.org/10.1038/mp.2017.130

Cowls, J., & Hale, S. (2005). It's the activity that counts: What clients value in psycho-educational groups. *Canadian Journal of Occupational Therapy, 72*(3), 176–182. https://doi.org/10.1177/000841740507200305

da Silva, C. C. G., Bolognani, C. V., Amorim, F. F., & Imoto, A. M. (2023) Effectiveness of training programs based on mindfulness in reducing psychological distress and promoting well-being in medical students: A systematic review and meta-analysis. *Systematic Reviews, 12*(1), 79. https://doi.org/ 10.1186/s13643-023-02244-y

Dolan, N., Simmonds-Buckley, M., Kellett, S., Siddell, E., & Delgadillo, J. (2021). Effectiveness of stress control large group psychoeducation for anxiety and depression: Systematic review and meta-analysis. *British Journal of Clinical Psychology, 60*(3), 375–399. https://doi.org/10.1111/bjc.12288

Donker, T., Griffiths, K. M., Cuijpers, P., & Christensen, H. (2009). Psychoeducation for depression, anxiety and psychological distress: A meta-analysis. *BMC Medicine, 7*, 79. https://doi.org/10.1186/1741-7015-7-79

Early, M. B. (2009). *Mental health concepts and techniques for the occupational therapy assistant* (4th ed.). Wolters Kluwer Health/Lippincott Williams & Wilkins.

Finicelli, M., Di Salle, A., Galderisi, U., & Peluso, G. (2022). The Mediterranean diet: An update of the clinical trials. *Nutrients, 14*(14), 2956. https://doi.org/10.3390/nu14142956

Fogarty, C., Hevey, D., & McCarthy, O. (2019). Effectiveness of cognitive behavioural group therapy for social anxiety disorder: Long-term benefits and aftercare. *Behavioural and Cognitive Psychotherapy, 47*(5), 501–513. https://doi.org/10.1017/S1352465819000079

Frankl, V. E. (1975). Paradoxical intention and dereflection. *Psychotherapy: Theory, Research & Practice, 12*(3), 226–237. https://doi.org/10.1037/h0086434

Günaydin, N. (2022). Effect of group psychoeducation on depression, anxiety, stress and coping with stress of nursing students: A randomized controlled study. *Perspectives in Psychiatric Care, 58*(2), 640–650. https://doi.org/10.1111/ppc.12828

Hale, S., & Cowls, J. (2009). Psychoeducational groups. In I. Söderback (Ed.) *International handbook of occupational therapy interventions* (pp. 255–260). Springer. https://doi.org/10.1007/978-0-387-75424-6_24

Herrera, S. N., Sarac, C., Phili, A., Gorman, J., Martin, L., Lyallpuri, R., Dobbs, M. F., DeLuca, J. S., Mueser, K. T., Wyka, K. E., Yang, L. H., Landa, Y., & Corcoran, C. M. (2023). Psychoeducation for individuals at clinical high risk for psychosis: A scoping review. *Schizophrenia Research, 252*, 148–158. https://doi.org/10.1016/j.schres.2023.01.008

Higgins, A., Murphy, R., Downes, C., Barry, J., Monahan, M., Hevey, D., Kroll, T., Doyle, L., & Gibbons, P. (2020). Factors impacting the implementation of a psychoeducation intervention within the mental health system: A multisite study using the consolidation framework for implementation research. *BMC Health Services Research, 20*(1), 1023. https://doi.org/10.1186/s12913-020-05852-9

James, K. A., Stromin, J. I., Steenkamp, N., & Combrinck, M. I. (2023). Understanding the relationships between physiological and psychosocial stress, cortisol and cognition. *Frontiers in Endocrinology, 14*, 1085950. https://doi.org/10.3389/fendo.2023.1085950

Langeveld, J. H., Hatløy, K., Ten Velden Hegelstad, W., Johannessen, J. O., & Joa, I. (2025). The TIPS family psychoeducational group work approach in first episode psychosis and related disorders: 25 years of experiences. *Early Intervention in Psychiatry, 19*(1), e13591. https://doi.org/10.1111/eip.13591

LeMoult, J., Battaglini, A. M., Grocott, B., Jopling, E., Rnic, K., & Yang, L. (2023). Advances in stress and depression research. *Current Opinion in Psychiatry, 36*(1), 8–13. https://doi.org/10.1097/YCO.0000000000000831

Li, W., Liu, Y., Deng, J., & Wang, T. (2024). Influence of aerobic exercise on depression in young people: A meta-analysis. *BMC Psychiatry, 24*(1), 571. https://doi.org/10.1186/s12888-024-06013-6

Mirhosseini, S., Heshmati Nabavi, F., Behnam Vashani, H., & Vaghee, S. (2025). Evaluating the effect of online psychoeducational support group on perceived stress in family caregivers of COVID-19 survivors. *OMEGA - Journal of Death and Dying, 90*(4), 1685–1700. https://doi.org/10.1177/00302228221126219

Noetel, M., Sanders, T., Gallardo-Gómez, D., Taylor, P., Del Pozo Cruz, B., van den Hoek, D., Smith, J. J., Mahoney, J., Spathis, J., Moresi, M., Pagano, R., Pagano, L., Vasconcellos, R., Arnott, H., Varley, B., Parker, P., Biddle, S., & Lonsdale, C. (2024). Effect of exercise for depression: Systematic review and network meta-analysis of randomised controlled trials. *BMJ Clinical Research, 384*, e075847. https://doi.org/10.1136/bmj-2023-075847

O'Brien, M. P., Zinberg, J. L., Bearden, C. E., Daley, M., Niendam, T. A., Kopelowicz, A., & Cannon, T. D. (2007). Psychoeducational multi-family group treatment with adolescents at high risk for developing psychosis. *Early Intervention in Psychiatry, 1*(4), 325–332. https://doi.org/10.1111/j.1751-7893.2007.00046.x

Oz, H. S., & Oz, F. (2020). A psychoeducation program for stress management and psychosocial problems in multiple sclerosis. *Nigerian Journal of Clinical Practice, 23*(11), 1598–1606. https://doi.org/10.4103/njcp.njcp_462_19

Pedersen, P., Søgaard, H. J., Labriola, M., Nohr, E. A., & Jensen, C. (2015). Effectiveness of psychoeducation in reducing sickness absence and improving mental health in individuals at risk of having a mental disorder: A randomised controlled trial. *BMC Public Health, 15*, 763. https://doi.org/10.1186/s12889-015-2087-5

Pekkala, E., & Merinder, L. (2002). Psychoeducation for schizophrenia. *The Cochrane Database of Systematic Reviews, 2002*(4), CD002831. https://doi.org/10.1002/14651858.CD002831

Riachi, E., Holma, J., & Laitila, A. (2022). Psychotherapists' views on triggering factors for psychological disorders. *Discover Psychology, 2*(1), 44. https://doi.org/10.1007/s44202-022-00058-y

Rocamora-Montenegro, M., Compañ-Gabucio, L. M., & Garcia de la Hera, M. (2021). Occupational therapy interventions for adults with severe mental illness: A scoping review. *BMJ Open, 11*(10), e047467. https://doi.org/10.1136/bmjopen-2020-047467

Salonen, K., Hyvönen, K., Paakkolanvaara, J. V., & Korpela, K. (2022). Flow with nature treatment for depression: Participants' experiences. *Frontiers in Psychology, 12*, 768372. https://doi.org/10.3389/fpsyg.2021.768372

Setyowibowo, H., Yudiana, W., Hunfeld, J. A. M., Iskandarsyah, A., Passchier, J., Arzomand, H., Sadarjoen, S. S., de Vries, R., & Sijbrandij, M. (2022). Psychoeducation for breast cancer: A systematic review and meta-analysis. *Breast, 62*, 36–51. https://doi.org/10.1016/j.breast.2022.01.005

Slagter, L., Demyttenaere, K., Verschueren, P., & De Cock, D. (2022). The effect of meditation, mindfulness, and yoga in patients with rheumatoid arthritis. *Journal of Personalized Medicine, 12*(11), 1905. https://doi.org/10.3390/jpm12111905

Smith, P. J., & Merwin, R. M. (2021). The role of exercise in management of mental health disorders: An integrative review. *Annual Review of Medicine, 72*, 45–62. https://doi.org/10.1146/annurev-med-060619-022943

Steed, R. (2014). A client-centered model of instructional design for psychoeducation interventions. *Occupational Therapy in Mental Health, 30*(2), 126–143. https://doi.org/10.1080/0164212X.2014.878536

Stein, F., & Cutler, S. K. (2002). *Psychosocial occupational therapy: A holistic approach* (2nd ed.). Delmar Thomson Learning.

Thimm, J. C., & Antonsen, L. (2014). Effectiveness of cognitive behavioral group therapy for depression in routine practice. *BMC Psychiatry, 14*(1), 292. https://doi.org/10.1186/s12888-014-0292-x

Tucker, R. M., Contreras, D. A., Carlson, B. R., Carter, A., Drake, C. L. (2021). Sleep education for elders program (SLEEP): Promising pilot results of a virtual, health educator-led, community-delivered sleep behavior change intervention. *Nature and Science of Sleep, 13*, 625–633. https://doi.org/10.2147/NSS.S304035

Tursi, M. F., Baes, C. v. W., Camacho, F. R., Tofoli, S. M., & Juruena, M. F. (2013). Effectiveness of psychoeducation for depression: A systematic review. *Australian and New Zealand Journal of Psychiatry, 47*(11), 1019–1031. https://doi.org/10.1177/0004867413491154

Wirz-Justice, A. (2018). Seasonality in affective disorders. *General and Comparative Endocrinology, 258*, 244–249. https://doi.org/10.1016/j.ygcen.2017.07.010

Xia, J., Merinder, L. B., & Belgamwar, M. R. (2011). Psychoeducation for schizophrenia. *Cochrane Database of Systematic Reviews, 2011*(6), CD002831. https://doi.org/10.1002/14651858.CD002831.pub2

Epilouge

Authors' Personal Responses to Stress in Their Lives

Franklin Stein

Madison, Wisconsin, USA

I was born into a Jewish working-class family in Brooklyn, New York. Both my grandparents immigrated to New York City from Romania around 1890. They fled Romania because of religious persecution. They settled in the Lower East Side in New York City in tenement housing with little resources as well as not being able to speak English. They were Orthodox Jewish families who did not work on the Sabbath (Saturday), and they observed all the Jewish holidays of Rosh Hashanah, Yom Kippur, Sukkot, Passover and Hanukkah. My maternal grandfather worked as a peddler with a pushcart in the streets selling fruits and vegetables, while my paternal grandfather was a tailor. My grandmothers were homemakers and raised the children in their large families. As children of immigrant families, my parents had a limited education. They married in 1927 and moved to a one-bedroom apartment in a Jewish neighborhood in Brooklyn. I had an older brother who was six years older than me. My father worked as a gas station attendant most of his adult life. He frequently changed jobs and was unemployed multiple times. My mother was primarily a homemaker and enjoyed cooking, baking, socializing with the family and neighbors and taking care of the apartment. In general, our family lived from paycheck to paycheck, and money was always scarce. As a family, we spent much of our spare time with our relatives and celebrating the Jewish holidays. I had a public education and enjoyed all of the street games that we played as kids growing up in the 1940s. We organized our own sports, such as stickball, punchball, sandlot football and schoolyard softball. I had a good childhood with loving parents and an older brother whom I admired. Sports and street games were a priority during my childhood. I formed a club called the Cheyennes with my neighborhood friends. I later played football in high school. Growing up in a Jewish

DOI: 10.4324/9781003671084-13

household meant that I went to Hebrew School in the afternoon, preparing for my Bar Mitzvah when I was 13 years old. I was an active child engaging in all the group sports, and I was self-directed and developed a strong sense of confidence in my ability to cope with new situations. I became very adaptable working in the many part-time jobs that I had during high school and college, such as salesman in a department store, bus boy, waiter, bellhop and Playstreet director. I handled major life transitions well, such as starting high school, college, graduate school, marriage, numerous professional positions and being a parent to three children, all of whom have graduated from a university. I am very goal-directed and motivated to succeed in education and work. I am also very disciplined in my daily life in exercising, eating a healthy diet and managing all the time commitments I have, combining my scholarly pursuits as well as my interests in reading, classical music, art, theater, opera, international travel and sports.

What have been major stresses in my life, and how have I handled them? The biggest stressor in my life was the death of my brother in 1955 when I was 21 years old and a senior at Brooklyn College. My brother had been a draftee into the Army during the Korean War. He suffered an emotional breakdown, which now we would identify as post-traumatic stress disorder. He was hospitalized in a military hospital. His breakdown was a shock to my parents and to me. My brother, prior to his Army experience, was a stalwart in the family, contributing financial support. He was an excellent student in high school, good at sports and he had many friends. In the Army he had been promoted and successfully completed leadership school while being in the Signal Corps. After he was honorably discharged from an Army hospital in Fayetteville, North Carolina, he did not return home but became a missing person for almost three years, traveling the country as a homeless person. He did finally return home and seemed a completely different person than he had been prior to his army experience. He felt ashamed for becoming ill, a disappointment to the family and a failure in life. After being home for a week, he was unable to find a job as a clothing salesman that he had worked at after he graduated from high school. Then the worst happened. During the night he left the apartment and committed suicide by jumping off a bridge in the East River in Manhattan. This was a devastating blow to my parents and me. It was heartbreaking for my mother who had such high hopes for my brother's future. My father tried to console my mother and to continue his life.
Nothing could bring back my brother. I was shocked. How did my brother break down from being a strong, supportive person? It was depressing for me and sent me into an emotional tailspin. My close friends in college were supportive of me. Even though I was emotionally hurt I decided to "pick up the pieces" and continue my life. I graduated from Brooklyn College with a major in psychology and a minor in philosophy. I decided at that time to devote myself to a social service profession.

My first job after graduation was as a social worker for the New York City Department of Welfare. I then discovered the field of occupational therapy and received a full scholarship from the New York State Department of Mental Hygiene. After my professional education, I worked at the New York Psychiatric Institute and later became the Director of Occupational Therapy at the Brooklyn Day Hospital. I then received a full scholarship from New York University toward a doctorate in counseling psychology. I completed a two-year doctoral internship in psychology at Queens College in New York City. After receiving my doctorate, I was offered an Assistant Professor position at Boston University in the graduate program in occupational therapy. After a ten-year tenure, I became Director of the Occupational Therapy Program at UW-Milwaukee, then Director of the School of Medical Rehabilitation in Winnipeg, Canada, and Professor at the University of South Dakota. I have been fortunate in my life to have a successful career, marriage and full life with extensive foreign travel. I have been able to publish a number of books and to have visiting professorships at Cambridge University in England, McGill University, Alberta University in Canada, the University of Uppsala in Sweden and Dorset House on Oxford, England. In general, I have coped with the stressors in my life by being disciplined in my everyday activities, emphasizing positive health. I use breathing, aerobic exercise, walks in the woods, music and reading to reduce my everyday stress. My wife and family have been anchors in my life. I have also had mentors who have been encouraging and supportive. A strong commitment to a career in occupational therapy that is self-fulfilling while helping others has given my life purpose and meaning. My love of the arts, music, literature and an intellectual life has balanced my strong involvement in my professional life.

Khader A. Almhdawi

Irbid, Jordan

Success might be the best cure for many stressful situations. However, it is all about perception! I truly believe that your own perception plays much more important roles in your life consequences than the events or situations themselves. Your perception about any achievement or event, its importance and its consequences is the fundamental component of the potential stress level it may evoke.

Stress, this amazing but yet terrifying monster, might be utilized as a job facilitator if well and deeply understood. It took me about 30 years to develop and adopt my current analogy that helped me to initially understand stress and then overcome its potential negative impact on my achievements and well-being. For me, stress acts like "salt." Unless prohibited for medical reasons, you almost cannot cook anything without "salt." However, you need to carefully titrate the "salt" amount used. Underusing or overusing "salt" might jeopardize the meal regardless of how nice the ingredients or how skillful the chef. Individuals who either have excessive or negligible levels of stress might lose the success pathway.

I was born to a Muslim Arabic family in Jordan early in the eighties of the last century. Jordan is a relatively poor country with limited economic and natural resources. The Middle East is an unstable area of the world with excessive political, environmental, economic, and demographic stressors. My parents were Palestinian refugees who worked very hard and managed to offer a nice living standard for our eight-member family. Despite my father not being formally educated, he was highly cultured and knowledgeable. My father's life was very tough, and this was reflected onto the entire family. That led me to believe that stress is contagious or can be inherited. My father had tons of love in his heart but most of the time omitted expressing love as a priority. Often client-centered parenting (taking care of each individual's needs and emotions) was not available from him for each child. On the other hand, my late mother's personality was much more expressive. She used to talk with each family member and tailor her care to fit each one's needs. She had an extensive social network, was an amazing elementary school teacher and was great at managing the household. Truly, my mother was a warm nest filled with love.

Stress started to build up in me consciously and subconsciously early in life. During my childhood, I learned the hard way that I couldn't always get what I wanted. I used to compare myself with others all the time. The method I used to fight stress in my childhood was to be distinguished in as many fields as possible. I was one of the top students in the school, played sports, practiced some handcrafts and memorized parts of the Islamic holy book "Quran." I have always expected to be the first ranked in all of these activities and never accepted compromises. Truly, I had a pure type A personality. In most cases I was the elite among my colleagues, whom I used to see as opponents or competitors. Often my heart was broken when someone exceeded my achievements. The situation was made worse, given that my family's and friends' expectations of me were not less than my own. Clearly, I had far more "salt" than needed in my recipe! Stress had been accumulating in my childhood due to my distorted perception of achievements and satisfaction.

In high school my distorted self-perception continued. I had very high expectations regarding my potential academic achievements. My school teachers also contributed with very high expectations. Having a much lower GPA than expected, and consequently getting into a university major that did not meet my ambitions at that time, was my first serious psychological trauma in life. My father refused to allow me to travel to study abroad due to his past negative experience, leaving me having to love the best major available for me, occupational therapy (OT). Tons of "salt" were deployed into my recipe! To fight the accumulated stress, I used many subconscious self-defense mechanisms. Although faith and religion and believing in destiny helped me reduce stress, I was stuck for many years in denial and rationalization. I was right about one thing: in every catastrophe lies an opportunity. OT was a new major in Jordan with a lot of opportunities at that time. This helped me later get a scholarship from the government to earn a PhD. During my college life, I learned that talent is not enough to achieve what someone wants. I realized that I needed to plan and work by deadlines to complete achievements, to avoid running out of time as happened before my high school examinations. I also started to regard the filled half of the glass. No, I did not get the major I loved, but I could come to love the major I got and one day be distinguished. Learning from past mistakes and being optimistic helped me adjust the amount of "salt" in my recipe!

My most severe life psychological trauma happened in the middle of my college years. Although I took the event as a grown man who assumed the care of the family, losing my late beloved mother was something I have never gotten over. My mother was the sweet buffer in my life. She used to absorb tons of my stress and spread nice breezes of optimism and love throughout. The old saying is, "what does not kill you makes you stronger." I will never forget my mother, but I had to quickly get over the shock and manage the deep sadness, as my more fragile siblings needed my support. The instinct for survival shaped my personality to be stronger and more independent. I began to face stress, believing that I should never lose a battle without fighting. If you can change things, why panic? If not, why panic? I started to play a key role in managing the household after my mother's death. I also took my academic future more seriously. I managed to become the top-ranked student in my class, which guaranteed receiving a full PhD scholarship a few years later. I believe that the amount of "salt" started to reach the optimal level at this stage of my life. I became more realistic, braver and task-oriented.

In the PhD stage of my life, I had extensive success in gaining admissions and scholarships. Stress kept building up, though, through many transitions. First was going from the undergraduate linear scientific world to the scholarly-based thinking and critiquing world. Second, I had to secure a huge financial guarantee to fulfill my Jordanian government PhD scholarship requirements. Finally, during my studies in the USA, I had to survive living in a new society with a totally different culture, language and values. Particularly in the first two years of my five-year graduate studies journey, I had many moments where I lost belief in myself and my abilities. I had nightmares about academic failure. "Salt" almost contaminated my meal! I wanted to conduct a meaningful clinical rehabilitation study in stroke rehabilitation, which would cause me to shed sweat and tears. Here is when I truly learned to work with my resources and make my goals "SMART": *Specific, Measurable, Achievable, Realistic and Timely*, as we do in OT. I started to believe that "it is totally perfect not to be perfect" and that plans and consistency are as important as talent in achieving what you want. To this point, I remember three of my academic mentor's statements, which I consider to be good life lessons:

A. "When you get your PhD, you become smarter in a small area and dumber in the rest!"
B. "PhD study is more about persistence than being smart."
C. "Khader, always take a bite that you can swallow."

I have generalized these lessons into many aspects of my life, including social, personal, professional and financial goals. This way, the amount of "salt" became more optimal.

After a successful PhD experience, I decided to return to my country to serve the growing rehabilitation profession. At this stage, "salt" started to accumulate again. But luckily, I was not a student anymore. As a great teacher of mine foretold, "I was on the right side of the pen!" I learned that stress can be due to a lack of choices or when you have more than one good choice! I learned to compare choices objectively and decide in a timely way what is the best fit for my own needs and situation. I think that 70% right but timely decision is far better than 100% right but late. Here I started to realize that I am as unique as my own fingerprint. What works for others might not necessarily fit me. I got back to Jordan after living a nice, steady, and relatively modern life in the USA. I had to adjust back to my original community. Starting my own family dictated going through a stressful dilemma between finding someone you love and the commonly available arranged marriage process, not mentioning marriage's high social and financial demands. Furthermore, I had to manage my growing career as an assistant professor who needed to teach many courses for the first time and publish frequently to get tenured. "Salt" amounts started to hit critically high levels again!

Managing the balance between my social and professional life was a major source of stress at this stage. Here is another time when I leaned on my OT skills: dividing the world into "work, leisure and self-care." In this "royal" stage of my life, I have made many decisive choices to optimize the amount of "salt" in my recipe. I stopped work at 4 PM and on weekends. I also revived many of my old beloved hobbies, including crafts, soft music, home maintenance and playing sports.

Furthermore, I designated time for my family's and friends' activities. I quit smoking after more than 20 years of addiction, when I used to deceive myself that smoking relieved stress. I developed enough courage to say "no" when I needed to. Now, my life is filled with things I really want and truly enjoy, and I only keep positive, helpful individuals in my social and professional networks. Nowadays, I live for myself and the ones I truly love and for the causes I truly believe in. I started to compete with myself, working on my own timely goals, and entirely stopped comparing myself to colleagues. This way, I experienced a significant boost in my social and professional lives. I have also encountered numerous new personal and professional life-changing stressors. Such challenges, however, are an inevitable part of life, and I have managed to navigate through them successfully. Finally, I would like to express my deepest appreciation to my stress-relief heroes – my invaluable circle of friends, my beloved family and my extended family.

I have been told recently that I resemble an inspiring stress management role model for others. I still believe that success is the best stress reliever; however, success is subjective. It is all about perception! I truly believe that your own perception plays a much more important role in your life than the events themselves.

Ryan Thomure

Chicago, Illinois, USA

I'm a clinical social worker and occupational therapist currently serving as a faculty member and academic fieldwork coordinator in a graduate occupational therapy program. My professional roles have always focused on supporting others – whether through direct care or teaching. That work is meaningful to me, and I consider myself very lucky to get to do it. But like many people, I've also had periods in my life when stress has impacted me, sometimes to the point where it barely feels manageable.

While I don't claim to be an expert at managing stress (or any other difficulties, really) in my own life, I've developed a set of strategies that help me manage stress more effectively. That process hasn't been linear, and I haven't always been consistent or successful in implementing the kinds of strategies I'd suggest to others. I've engaged in therapy at various points and have taken prescribed medications that supported my well-being. In moments of acute stress, I often turn to cognitive-behavioral techniques – pausing to ask whether my concerns are reasonable or shaped by distorted assumptions or worst-case thinking. That habit, when I'm able to successfully implement it, has helped me regulate my "gut" reactions and stay focused on what's actually within my control.

That said, much of the stress I experience isn't necessarily that "acute" stress – it's cumulative. It builds gradually through the intersection of too many demands, too little time, and an internal sense that more could or should be done. I don't think such stress is unique to me, but recognizing how it shows up in my life has helped me design routines that support my mental health. The strategies I use might not work for everyone, but they work for me. I bike frequently as a means of both commuting and relaxation, which serves both as physical activity and a mental reset. I walk my dog, which gives me a reason to get outside and take a break. I read regularly to broaden my horizons beyond my personal struggles. I spend time with my family to reorient my priorities and remind myself of what matters.

Working as an academic fieldwork coordinator means that work-related stress isn't always confined to "business hours." Students encounter challenges on fieldwork, and oftentimes the only times that we can collaborate on solutions to those challenges are in the evenings, after their fieldwork day ends. I accept a degree of ongoing availability as part of the job. At the same time, I've become much more deliberate about protecting key parts of my schedule. I do my best not to work on weekends. I avoid email in the hours when my daughter expects my attention. And when I do need to be available outside traditional hours, I try to respond efficiently and then step back. I don't pretend to have perfect boundaries, but I've gotten clearer about which parts of the day or week need to be reserved – because they're restorative, or because someone else is counting on me to be present.

My professional background in both occupational therapy and social work informs how I think about stress. In my teaching and in my clinical work, I try to reinforce that managing stress doesn't mean avoiding it entirely – that's impossible. It means being proactive about the steps you can take that make the hard parts more sustainable.

Farrukh A. Chishtie

Vancouver, British Columbia, Canada

When I reflect on my journey from theoretical physics to climate science to humanitarian service and occupational therapy research, I realize that what might appear as a scattered path has actually been a continuous flow experience, one where my deepest character strengths have served as both compass and anchor through periods of intense stress and uncertainty. With humble beginnings from Karachi, Pakistan, where I was born, it has been an enriching journey for which I am grateful to all.

My transition from studying quantum field theory to investigating long COVID experiences might seem like an impossible leap, but it represents the essence of what Mihaly Csikszentmihalyi describes as flow: that optimal experience where challenge meets skill in perfect balance. Each career pivot has required me to stretch beyond my comfort zone while building upon existing capacities, creating what I now recognize as a sustained state of growth-oriented engagement with life's complexities.

SPIRITUALITY: FINDING SACRED PURPOSE IN SERVICE

My Islamic spiritual foundation has been the bedrock of my stress management approach, though it manifests not through traditional religious practices alone but through a deep sense of connection to something larger than myself. Whether responding to the 2005 northern Pakistan earthquake, developing climate resilience services for vulnerable populations, or researching long COVID experiences, I have found that viewing my work as service to humanity transforms stress from burden into sacred calling.

During the most challenging periods, establishing SERVIR-Mekong in Thailand while managing complex international partnerships or founding the Peaceful Society Science and Innovation Foundation while completing my PhD, my spiritual practice centers on recognizing that each challenge is an opportunity to contribute to human flourishing. This perspective, deeply aligned with Islamic principles of service and stewardship, has consistently transformed what could be overwhelming stress into meaningful engagement.

The spirituality dimension of my stress management integrates beautifully with post-traumatic growth principles from our framework. Working with earthquake survivors in Muzaffarabad revealed how adversity can deepen spiritual connection and life purpose. That experience taught me that stress, when approached with spiritual openness, becomes a pathway to greater meaning and service capacity.

LOVE: RELATIONSHIPS AS STRESS RESILIENCE

Love, in its broadest sense of deep care for others and genuine connection, has been my most powerful stress-buffering resource. Whether it's love for family that grounds me during intense travel periods, love for students that energizes my teaching despite academic pressures or love for communities affected by climate change that drives my research, this character strength transforms stress from a solitary burden into shared purpose.

My work across multiple countries and cultures has taught me that love transcends linguistic and cultural boundaries. Developing flood forecasting systems for Lower Mekong communities wasn't just technical work; it was an expression of love for vulnerable populations facing climate risks. This emotional investment, rather than increasing stress, actually created flow states where technical challenges became opportunities for meaningful impact.

The collaborative nature of my research, from NASA partnerships to community-based rehabilitation projects, reflects how love manifests as genuine care for colleague well-being and shared success. When stress arises from deadline pressures or complex negotiations, returning to the underlying love that motivates the work consistently restores both energy and perspective.

HONESTY: INTEGRITY FOR STRESS NAVIGATION

Integrity and scientific honesty have been crucial in managing the stress that comes with working across disciplines where I'm not always the expert. Moving from physics to climate science to occupational therapy required me to honestly acknowledge knowledge gaps while confidently contributing unique perspectives. This intellectual humility, rather than creating impostor syndrome stress, has actually facilitated rapid learning and meaningful collaboration.

When developing the integrated SMQ-positive psychology framework, honesty about the limitations of traditional stress assessment approaches opened space for innovative solutions. Rather than defending existing paradigms, acknowledging what was not working created opportunities for breakthrough thinking. This honest engagement with complexity has consistently transformed potentially stressful uncertainty into exciting discovery opportunities.

Honesty also manifests in transparent communication with collaborators about capacity limitations and competing priorities. Rather than overcommitting and creating stress, honest boundary-setting has enabled sustainable engagement with multiple high-impact projects simultaneously.

LOVE OF LEARNING: STRESS AS A GROWTH CATALYST

Perhaps no character strength has been more central to my stress management than love of learning. Each career transition, from mathematical physics to environmental science to rehabilitation research, required mastering entirely new knowledge domains under significant time pressure. Rather than experiencing this as a stressful burden, my deep love of learning transformed these transitions into exhilarating flow experiences.

Learning Google Earth Engine programming to develop flood monitoring systems in Southeast Asia exemplifies this process. The technical complexity could have been overwhelming stress, but genuine curiosity about satellite data applications to disaster preparedness created sustained engagement that felt more like play than work. This aligns perfectly with Dweck's growth mindset research – viewing challenges as learning opportunities rather than threats to competence.

My approach to stress management increasingly involves asking, "What is this situation teaching me?" Whether navigating complex international partnerships, managing competing deadlines, or addressing reviewer critiques, reframing stress as a learning opportunity consistently restores both energy and optimism. The 100+ peer-reviewed publications in my career represent not just academic output, but evidence of how love of learning can transform research stress into sustained intellectual flow.

COURAGE: TRANSFORMING FEAR INTO FORWARD MOVEMENT

Courage has been essential for managing the stress that accompanies meaningful innovation. Proposing the integration of positive psychology with traditional stress assessment required courage to challenge established approaches. Moving from tenured positions to entrepreneurial ventures required courage to embrace uncertainty. Each major career decision has involved courageously choosing growth over security.

But I've learned that courage isn't the absence of fear – it's the willingness to move forward despite fear. When establishing research collaborations across 15+ countries, or when proposing novel intervention frameworks, the initial stress of potential failure transforms into excitement about potential impact when approached with courage.

Courage also manifests in vulnerability – the willingness to admit uncertainty, ask for help and acknowledge mistakes. This emotional courage has been crucial for maintaining authentic relationships across cultural and professional boundaries, creating the social support networks that buffer stress most effectively.

GROWTH MINDSET: STRESS AS DEVELOPMENT OPPORTUNITY

Carol Dweck's growth mindset concept has been transformational for my stress management approach. Rather than viewing challenging situations as threats to my competence or identity, I have learned to see them as opportunities for development. This shift, from fixed mindset stress about "being good enough" to growth mindset excitement about "getting better," has been liberating.

When peer reviewers initially rejected our occupational security framework manuscript, growth mindset thinking transformed potential stress into an improvement opportunity. Rather than viewing criticism as a personal attack, I approached feedback as collaborative input for strengthening our contribution. This perspective has consistently enabled productive engagement with academic challenges that might otherwise create defensive stress.

The growth mindset also applies to failure management. When early flood forecasting models showed poor accuracy, rather than experiencing this as professional stress, growth mindset framing enabled rapid iteration toward improved solutions. Each setback became data for better approaches rather than evidence of inadequacy.

INTEGRATION

These character strengths do not operate in isolation; they create synergistic effects that transform the stress experience entirely. Spirituality provides ultimate meaning and context, love creates motivation and connection, honesty enables authentic engagement, love of learning transforms challenge into opportunity and courage enables forward movement despite uncertainty.

When these strengths operate together within a growth mindset framework, stress becomes less about threat management and more about optimization for flow states. Rather than asking, "How do I avoid stress?" I've learned to ask, "How do I engage with this challenge in ways that honor my values and facilitate growth?"

This integrated approach aligns perfectly with the positive psychology framework we've developed in this book. Rather than merely managing stress symptoms, we can cultivate the character strengths and mindset approaches that transform stress into flourishing. My personal experience suggests that this is not just a theoretical possibility; it is a practical pathway accessible to anyone willing to develop these capacities systematically.

DAILY PRACTICES AND SUSTAINED TRANSFORMATION

The integration of these insights into daily practice has required systematic attention to both micro-moments and macro-patterns. Morning reflection on spiritual purpose sets intention for engaging challenges as service opportunities.

Regular check-ins with loved ones maintain the relationship infrastructure that buffers stress. An honest assessment of energy and capacity guides sustainable project engagement.

Perhaps most importantly, I've learned to recognize when I'm in flow states and create conditions that support them. Whether writing research papers, developing community partnerships or analyzing earth science data, optimal engagement occurs when challenge-skill balance is maintained and intrinsic motivation is activated.

The positive psychology interventions we describe in our framework, gratitude practices, character strengths usage, benefit finding, have become integrated into my daily stress management approach. But they work not as isolated techniques, but as expressions of deeper character development that transforms how stress is experienced and utilized.

MOVING FORWARD: STRESS AS A TEACHER AND ALLY

As I continue navigating the complex landscape of interdisciplinary research and international collaboration, my relationship with stress continues evolving. Rather than something to be eliminated, stress has become a trusted signal system, indicating when growth opportunities are present, when values alignment needs attention, or when capacity limits require respect.

The framework we have developed for integrating positive psychology with stress management reflects not just academic synthesis but lived experience of how human beings can thrive in the face of adversity. By cultivating character strengths, maintaining growth mindset and creating conditions for flow states, we can transform stress from enemy into ally, a teacher that guides us toward our highest potential for service, growth and contribution.

This personal journey from quantum physics to community resilience has taught me that our deepest challenges often become our greatest gifts. When approached with the right character strengths and mindset, stress does not diminish us, it reveals who we can also potentially become.

George S. Tomlin

Tacoma, Washington, USA

As the middle child of five in a U.S. middle class family of the 1950s, I had the advantage of my older brother taking the blame when I managed to mess things up around our home, but the disadvantage of my younger sister and brother receiving what attention our parents, after their considerable daily tasks were done, could devote to us. The coping skills to life's challenges/stressors that I was taught non-verbally consisted of stuffing one's own feelings and throwing oneself into whatever was coming along next. It took the accumulated effects of the 1960s, 1970s and OT school in the early 1980s, and several years of living overseas, to undo the effects of my childhood stress response training. What works in one stage of one's life will not necessarily be sufficient for the next stage.

In this transition from protected childhood to becoming an adult was the most stressful period of my life: my first semester of college. In high school I had been among the best in my class in mathematics and science. Suddenly I was one of a thousand first year students who had all been among the best in their high schools. My plummet from the top to the bottom of the class precipitated a demolition and reconstruction of my intellectual identity. This dangerous and potentially unhealthy process entailed a reorganization of my daily thoughts and a decade-long reordering of my life's career goals. From math to philosophy to public health (my first serious job after college), unbeknownst to me I was walking a path to occupational therapy. When I first encountered the field, through my wife Sybille, I recognized it as the perfect blend of public health (with its emphasis on protecting society by protecting individuals) and existential philosophy (which emphasizes the instinctive pursuit of meaning in one's own life).

In high school my two coping mechanisms had been active sports and adopting somewhat unfashionable hobbies (chess and Boy Scouts). With the exponentially greater stressors of a math/science college these two approaches were woefully inadequate. Despite the dissolution of my academic identity, I kept one image tenaciously in mind: in my life plot throughline I retained the belief that it was worth fighting for society-wide justice. That pushed me to explore new ways of contributing to this historical campaign: through community organizing, political activity and eventually through occupational therapy and being an OT educator- all aim to empower others. In college I also tried to maintain a strong affiliation with just a very few friends and family members. I cultivated a proactive stance toward my younger sister and brother, initiating outdoor activities with them to give them a stronger sense of place in the world. In my younger brother this engendered a lifelong avocation of trail maintenance, conservation, and trail GPS mapping. (I am so proud of him!) In my second year of college, I resolved to spend my junior year abroad. This flight had the liberating effect of getting me out of the pressure cooker atmosphere of an elite college for 12 months. It afforded me opportunities to experience different languages, cultures, and approaches to life. Piece by piece I built back my identity.

Throughout this time one specific goal endured. When I was nine years old, my maternal grandmother consented to listen to me give a talk about my penny collection. At the end of it she resolutely announced, "You should be a teacher." It was the one identity integrity thread I was able to maintain through all the unsettling early education and career transitions. I leaped at the chance in 1984 to teach in the occupational therapy program at the University of Puget Sound. As my responsibilities grew over the years, both on campus and in my own growing family, I discovered that the stress management techniques of the past would no longer suffice. Intramural sports and reminding myself that there were bigger problems in the world than my own were no longer enough to keep me healthy. A beginning stomach ulcer shook me to the realization that I needed to pay stricter attention to diet, rest and incorporating reflective, calming moments into my daily life. The breakthrough, however, came when a graduate OT student of mine, having accurately diagnosed my condition of hyperstress and sleep deprivation, loaned me his copy of a book on the new science of sleep. Suddenly I understood why I was waking up in the middle of the night (usually after three hours of sleep), getting stressed about being awake and tossing and turning for hours. Understanding that there are 90-minute sleep cycles allowed me to stop stressing over waking up at 2 AM after getting to sleep at 11! I began to make much better use of the time allotted to rest each night.

In retirement I have maintained a strict sleep hygiene: relaxing by reading a book (an actual, paper-based book) just before turning off the light. Not watching or reading any "news" (fake or otherwise). Only watching the season finale of a detective series in the evening when I could allow myself an additional 90 minutes in bed the next morning. Diet is a wide variety of vegetables and fruits (much of it home-grown or direct from the farm), grains and cheeses, seafood and very little meat, and virtually all meals made from scratch. Sports have been replaced by hiking, folk dancing, tai chi and gardening. Listening to music has become an important part of many days. Flute pieces in summer, jazz in autumn, piano concertos and classical symphonies in winter and big band sound in spring, resonate seasonally, lift my mood and make me feel optimistic. Being able to allot more time to talk with family, friends and neighbors is another stress-busting luxury of retirement.

Transitions in life have called for transitions in stress management plans. These have actually been somewhat effective at keeping the effects of aging at bay, and at helping me preserve an attitude of growth toward life.

Appendix
Stein's Stress Management Questionnaire

For the purpose of this questionnaire, distress refers to the personal responses or symptoms that are the result of daily personal interactions, events or thoughts that make life difficult and/or create discomfort.

I. When I feel stressful at work, I experience the following symptoms, feelings or problems.

(Circle yes [Y] or no [N] for each item.)

Y N 101. Bleeding ulcer

Y N 102. Blushing

Y N 103. Chest pains

Y N 104. Cold hands/feet

Y N 105. Constipation

Y N 106. Diarrhea

Y N 107. Difficulty swallowing

Y N 108. Dizziness

Y N 109. Dryness of mouth

Y N 110. Fatigue

Y N 111. Frequent urination

Y N 112. Grinding teeth

Y N 113. Headaches

Y N 114. Heartburn

Y N 115. High blood pressure

Y N 116. Hot flashes

Y N 117. Indigestion

Y N 118. Menstrual changes

Y N 119. Muscle tension

Y N 120. Nausea

Y N 121. Neck/low back pain

Y N 122. Rapid heart rate

Y N 123. Skin disorder

Y N 124. Stomach pain

Y N 125. Sweaty palms

Y N 126. Tremors

Y N 127. Trouble breathing

DIFFICULTY:

Y N 128. Concentrating

Y N 129. Reacting

Y N 130. Decision making

Y N 131. Reasoning

Y N 132. Listening

Y N 133. Remembering

Y N 134. Problem solving

Y N 135. Thinking

FEELING:

Y N 136. Angry

Y N 137. Anxious

Y N 138. Apathetic

Y N 139. Defensive

Y N 140. Fearful

Y N 141. Guilty

Y N 142. Hopeless

Y N 143. Irritable

Y N 144. A loss of control

Y N 145. Low tolerance/others

Y N 146. Moody

Y N 147. Nervous

Y N 148. Panicky

Y N 149. Resentful

Y N 150. Restless

Y N 151. Sad

Y N 152. Tense

Y N 153. Upset

PROBLEMS WITH:

Y N 154. Being lazy

Y N 155. Biting nails

Y N 156. Being obnoxious

Y N 157. Being sarcastic

Y N 158. Changing tone of voice

Y N 159. Complaining

Y N 160. Compulsiveness

Y N 161. Drinking

Y N 162. Eating

Y N 163. Giving compliments

Y N 164. Keeping eye contact

Y N 165. Relating to others

Y N 166. Sitting still

Y N 167. Sleeping

Y N 168. Smoking

Y N 169. Speaking

Y N 170. Spending money

Y N 171. Talking excessively

Y N 172. Twisting hair

Y N 173. Other: ____________

After you have checked all the items you experience, go back to your responses and rank-order them below from 1 to 10* with the rank of 1 being the item experienced most often and being the most troublesome.

SYMPTOMS EXPERIENCED

1. ______________________________
2. ______________________________
3. ______________________________
4. ______________________________
5. ______________________________
6. ______________________________
7. ______________________________
8. ______________________________
9. ______________________________
10. ______________________________

*Not everyone will have as many as ten symptoms or problems.

II. What are the everyday work situations or thoughts that cause stress for you?

(Circle yes [Y] or no [N] for each item.)

Y N 201. Arguments with family members, co-workers or others

Y N 202. Being evaluated for performance

Y N 203. Being in crowds

Y N 204. Criticism by others

Y N 205. Doing new things for the first time

Y N 206. Driving in traffic to work

Y N 207. Excessive noise at work

Y N 208. Feeling too much pressure at work

Y N 209. Financial situations at work

Y N 210. Having problems in relationship with Family members, friends or co-workers

Y N 211. Hearing sad or depressing news at work

Y N 212. Mechanical breakdown at home or work

Y N 213. Being overwhelmed by documentation and paperwork

Y N 214. Speaking in front of groups at work

Y N 216. Being alone at work

Y N 217. Being bored

Y N 219. Being unprepared

Y N 220. Being watched by others

Y N 221. Failure to meet goals (expected of you)

Y N 222. Feeling guilty for inadequate behavior

Y N 223. Feeling frustrated

Y N 224. Having no control over a situation

Y N 225. Having too many things to do with not enough time

Y N 226. Lack of confidence in oneself

Y N 227. Misplacing something at work

Y N 228. Meeting deadlines

Y N 229. Not having any free time for oneself or friends

Y N 230. Not knowing what is expected of you

Y N 231. Poor performance at work

Y N 232. Trying to please people at work ____________________

____

Y N 233. Waiting for expected letter or decision from superiors ____________________

Y N 234. Other (please list): ____________________

Stress Management Questionnaire 3

After you have checked all the items you experience, go back to your responses and rank-order them below from 1 to 10* with the rank of 1 being the most stressful situation or thought.

SITUATIONS OR THOUGHTS CAUSING STRESS

1. ____________________
2. ____________________
3. ____________________
4. ____________________
5. ____________________
6. ____________________
7. ____________________
8. ____________________
9. ____________________
10. ____________________

*Rank-order only those situations or thoughts that apply to you. Not everyone will have ten items.

III. List the following activities that help you relieve stress by circling yes [Y] or no [N] for each item

Y N 301. Analyze situation

Y N 302. Avoid situation

Y N 303. Be active in social club

Y N 304. Baking

Y N 305. Being by myself

Y N 306. Being busy

Y N 307. Bicycling

Y N 308. Cleaning house

Y N 309. Cooking

Y N 310. Crocheting

Y N 311. Crying

Y N 312. Dancing

Y N 313. Deep breathing

Y N 314. Drawing

Y N 315. Eating

Y N 316. Exercising

Y N 317. Gardening

Y N 318. Go shopping

Y N 319. Go to dinner

Y N 320. Go to movie

Y N 321. Hot shower/bath

Y N 322. Jogging

Y N 323. Listen to music

Y N 324. Meditate or pray

Y N 325. Needlecraft

Y N 326. Painting

Y N 327. Play musical instrument

Y N 328. Prepare for school/work

Y N 329. Read for pleasure

Y N 330. Relax (lie down)

Y N 331. Running long distance

Y N 332. Screaming

Y N 333. Sex

Y N 334. Singing

Y N 335. Sleeping

Y N 336. Stretching muscles

Y N 337. Swimming

Y N 338. Take a drive in a car

Y N 339. Take care of a pet

Y N 340. Talk to a friend

Y N 341. Throw something

Y N 342. Visit friends

Y N 343. Watch TV

Y N 344. Walking

Y N 345. Writing letters

Y N 346. Writing poetry

Y N 347. Writing short stories

Y N 348. Yoga

Please list any other activities that help you relieve stress.

Y N 349. Other ______________________________

SUPPORT MATERIAL

Again rank-order your responses 1–10* with the rank of 1 being the activity that most relieves your stress.

ACTIVITIES THAT RELIEVE STRESS

1. ______________________	6. ______________________
2. ______________________	7. ______________________
3. ______________________	8. ______________________
4. ______________________	9. ______________________
5. ______________________	10. ______________________

*Rank as many items up to 10 that are appropriate to you.

Glossary

Acetylcholine (ACh) Neurotransmitter released by cholinergic neurons, responsible for transmitting nerve impulses in the parasympathetic nervous system and influencing muscle contraction, heart rate, and digestion.

Activity based groups Groups that emphasize learning through doing, engaging participants in meaningful activities that build coping skills and promote stress management. These groups focus on participation and skill practice rather than discussion alone.

Adrenal cortex Outer portion of the adrenal glands that secretes cortisol and other steroid hormones during stress.

Adrenal medulla Inner region of the adrenal glands that releases adrenaline (epinephrine) and norepinephrine during the fight-or-flight response.

Adrenocorticotropic hormone (ACTH) Hormone secreted by the pituitary gland that stimulates the adrenal cortex to produce cortisol.

Adjustment disorder Condition triggered by undesirable life events, marked by excessive worry or rumination and significant functional impairment.

Aerobic exercise Cardiovascular activity that increases heart rate, breathing, and oxygen uptake. It includes activities such as running, swimming, bicycling, and sports such as tennis, basketball, and soccer.

Allostasis Process of achieving stability through physiological or behavioral change in response to stressors, involving active adjustment rather than simple maintenance of equilibrium (McEwen & Stellar, 1993).

Allostatic load Cumulative physiological wear and tear resulting from chronic overactivity or inactivity of systems involved in adaptation to environmental challenges, potentially leading to disease.

Amygdala Brain region in the limbic system that detects threats and triggers emotional and physiological responses to stress.

Anxiety Feeling of fear about an impending or stressful event such as driving in a snowstorm or taking an examination when unprepared. Anxiety can be linked to phobias (e.g., fear of heights or flying). It may be accompanied by physiological reactions such as sweating, rapid heart rate, and tremors.

Autonomic nervous system (ANS) Division of the peripheral nervous system that regulates involuntary physiological processes including heart rate, blood pressure, respiration, digestion and sexual arousal. It contains three anatomically distinct divisions: sympathetic, parasympathetic and enteric (Waxenbaum et al., 2024).

Biopsychosocial perspective Framework that systematically considers biological, psychological and social factors and their complex interactions in explaining health, illness and health care delivery.

Breathing exercise Conscious practice to improve breathing patterns, enhance lung efficiency and reduce stress.

Burnout State of emotional, mental and physical exhaustion caused by prolonged and excessive workplace stress, characterized by emotional exhaustion and reduced personal accomplishment.

Catecholamines Group of hormones (including adrenaline and noradrenaline) released during stress that stimulate the sympathetic nervous system.

Central nervous system (CNS) Comprises the brain and spinal cord; processes information and coordinates responses to stimuli.

Challenge appraisal Cognitive evaluation of a stressor as an opportunity for growth, mastery or gain that can be met with available resources, typically leading to salutogenic responses and positive adaptation.

Chronic diseases Long-lasting conditions (one year or more) that require ongoing medical attention or limit daily activities. Examples include heart disease, cancer, diabetes, arthritis and chronic obstructive pulmonary disease (Centers for Disease Control and Prevention, n.d.).

Cognitive appraisal Mental process by which individuals evaluate and interpret the personal significance of events, determining whether situations represent threats, challenges or benign circumstances (Lazarus & Folkman, 1984).

Cole's Seven Steps of Group Leadership Structured process for leading OT groups that includes introduction, activity, sharing, processing, generalizing, application and summary. The model keeps sessions goal-directed, predictable and connected to real-life application

Compassion fatigue Emotional and physical exhaustion leading to a diminished ability to empathize or feel compassion for others, often experienced by healthcare providers.

Complex post-traumatic stress disorder (CPTSD) Mental health condition resulting from repeated exposure to traumatic events, characterized by difficulties in emotional regulation, self-perception, and relationships.

Constellation metaphor Bernstein's framework for understanding how diverse theories and concepts, while separated by time or academic discipline, can illuminate each other when viewed as interconnected elements forming meaningful patterns of knowledge.

Coping resources Personal, social and material assets available to individuals for managing stressful situations, including psychological capital, social support networks and tangible resources.

Corticotropin-Releasing Hormone (CRH) Hormone secreted by the hypothalamus that stimulates the pituitary gland to release ACTH during stress.

Cortisol Glucocorticoid hormone produced by the adrenal cortex that helps the body respond to long-term stress by regulating metabolism, blood pressure and immune function.

Critical life skills Abilities for adaptive and positive behavior that enable individuals to effectively manage stresses, demands, and challenges of daily life.

Cyberbullying Harassment or bullying that occurs through digital devices such as smartphones or computers, often via social media or messaging platforms.

Diathesis–stress approach Psychological theory explaining the interaction between genetic vulnerability and predisposition to a disorder and the effects of stress in precipitating onset of symptoms (Fauver et al., 2024).

Digital detox Period of refraining from using digital devices to reduce mental fatigue.

Digital minimalism Practice of reducing digital clutter by minimizing app usage and focusing only on essential digital interactions.

Distress Negative or harmful stress resulting from circumstances perceived as threatening, overwhelming or beyond one's coping capacity, potentially leading to adverse psychological and physiological outcomes (Selye, 1974).

Dopamine Neurotransmitter released during pleasurable activities.

Endocrine system Network of glands that secrete hormones into the bloodstream to regulate metabolism, growth and stress responses.

Endorphin Hormones with an analgesic (pain reduction) effect.

Epinephrine (adrenaline) Hormone and neurotransmitter released during acute stress that increases heart rate, blood pressure, and energy supply.

Eustress Positive or beneficial stress associated with optimal challenge, motivation and performance enhancement; stress that promotes growth and adaptation rather than harm (Selye, 1974).

Fear of missing out (FOMO) Anxiety that others are having rewarding experiences without you, often exacerbated by social media.

Fight-or-flight response Acute physiological reaction to perceived threats involving sympathetic nervous system activation, preparing the body for confrontation or escape through increased heart rate, respiration, and energy mobilization (Cannon, 1932).

Flow "Psychological flow is a state of mind where an individual is fully absorbed, and engaged in an activity, deriving immense pleasure from it." (Burke et al., 2025, pp. 44–45).

Formal strategies Structured methods for managing stress, such as consulting with supervisors, seeking professional services or using institutional resources.

General adaptation syndrome (GAS) Selye's (1956) three-stage model of stress response comprising alarm (initial reaction), resistance (adaptation), and exhaustion (depletion of adaptive resources) phases.

Guided imagery Relaxation technique that involves visualizing positive images or scenarios to enhance well-being and reduce stress, pain, anxiety and depression (National Cancer Institute, n.d.).

Hardiness Personality characteristic involving commitment, control and challenge orientation that enhances resilience and protects against stress-related illness (Kobasa, 1979).

Hassles and Uplifts Scale Assessment tool developed by Lazarus and Folkman (1989) to measure daily positive and negative experiences, recognizing that minor daily events significantly influence stress and well-being.

Homeostasis Tendency of biological systems to maintain stable internal conditions despite external fluctuations through self-regulating mechanisms, termed "the wisdom of the body" by Cannon (1932).

Hormesis Biological theory in which an exposure that in high doses is harmful can, in low doses, have the effect of challenging and strengthening the individual.

Horticulture therapy Growing of plants and gardening as stress reduction activities.

Hyperstress Extreme psychological strain caused by overwhelming stressors in work, school, social or financial contexts (Selye, 1976).

Hypofrontality In a flow state, the transient temporary downregulation of prefrontal cortex activity that reduces self-criticism and overthinking (Dietrich, 2004)

Hypostress Apathy, boredom or lack of motivation when under-stimulated, which can lead to disengagement from activities.

Hypothalamic-Pituitary-Adrenal (HPA) Axis Major neuroendocrine system controlling reactions to stress through the release of CRH, ACTH and cortisol.

Hypothalamus Brain region that regulates homeostasis and coordinates the body's response to stress via the ANS and endocrine systems.

Immune System Body's defense mechanism against pathogens that can be suppressed by chronic stress and cortisol overexposure.

Information overload Stress and difficulty of processing overwhelming amounts of information, often linked to digital connectivity.

Informal strategies Unstructured personal methods for coping with stress, such as hobbies, socializing or mindfulness.

Integrated-pathway model Comprehensive framework recognizing that stress responses involve dynamic interactions between pathogenic and salutogenic pathways, with cognitive appraisal serving as a bifurcation point determining responses.

International Classification of Diseases (ICD-11) 11th revision of the World Health Organization's classification of diseases, including stress-related disorders.

Job stress Harmful physical and emotional responses that occur when job demands do not match worker resources or needs, potentially leading to poor health and injury (National Institute for Occupational Safety and Health, n.d.).

Meta-analysis Statistical technique that synthesizes findings from multiple research studies to identify trends and draw conclusions.

Milieu intérieur Bernard's (1865) concept of the internal environment that organisms actively maintain in stable conditions despite external variations established the foundation for understanding physiological adaptation.

Mindfulness-based cognitive therapy (MBCT) Therapeutic intervention that combines mindfulness-based stress reduction (MBSR) with cognitive behavioral therapy to treat conditions such as depression (APA, n.d.-b).

Mindfulness-based stress reduction (MBSR) Structured program combining mindfulness meditation and yoga to reduce distress.

Mindfulness meditation Attending to the present moment with awareness of breath, thoughts, bodily sensations and feelings without judgment.

Music therapy Evidence-based use of music interventions to achieve individualized goals in health and education settings (American Music Therapy Association, n.d.).

Norepinephrine (noradrenaline) Neurotransmitter and hormone involved in alertness and the body's response to stress; released from sympathetic nerve endings and the adrenal medulla.

Oxytocin Hormone and neurotransmitter playing a role in bonding and emotional regulation.

Parasympathetic nervous system (PSNS) Division of the autonomic nervous system responsible for "rest and digest" functions, slowing heart rate, promoting digestion, and conserving energy (National Cancer Institute, n.d.).

Pathogenic approach Traditional medical model focusing on disease etiology, risk factors, and pathology; asking "What causes illness?" rather than "What creates health?" (Antonovsky, 1979).

Pathogenic pathway Stress response trajectory characterized by threat appraisal, dysregulated physiological activation, and potential progression toward disease, reduced functioning and decreased well-being.

Pathological stress Overwhelming stress contributing to physiological and psychological problems in vulnerable individuals.

Peripheral nervous system (PNS) Body's nervous system outside the brain and spinal cord.

Pituitary Gland Endocrine gland at the base of the brain that secretes hormones influencing growth, metabolism and stress responses (e.g., ACTH).

Post-traumatic growth (PTG) Positive psychological change experienced following struggle with highly challenging life circumstances, encompassing enhanced relationships, personal strength, new possibilities, spiritual development and life appreciation (Tedeschi & Calhoun, 2004).

Post-traumatic stress disorder (PTSD) Mental health condition triggered by experiencing or witnessing trauma, with symptoms such as flashbacks, nightmares and hyperarousal (Mayo Clinic, n.d.)

Prescriptive exercise Specific fitness plan developed for health or rehabilitation purposes, including exercise type, intensity, duration and frequency.

Progressive relaxation Relaxation technique involving sequential tensing and relaxation of muscle groups, also known as the Jacobson method.

Prolactin Hormone produced in the pituitary gland normally to enhance breastmilk production; released after sexual activity, it promotes sleep and better sleep quality, thus its presumed role in stress reduction.

Prolonged grief disorder Persistent and intense grief that exceeds cultural, social, or religious norms.

Psychological capital Positive psychological resources, including self-efficacy, optimism, hope and resilience, that individuals can develop and deploy to enhance performance and well-being.

Psychological well-being State of mind enabling individuals to realize potential, cope with stress, work productively and contribute to their community (World Health Organization, n.d.).

Psychoeducation Therapeutic approach that provides education about mental health conditions, coping strategies and recovery processes incorporating meaningful activities.

Psychoneuroimmunology Study of interactions between behavior, neural and endocrine functions and immune processes (Ader et al., 1995).

Relaxation response Stress reduction technique introduced by Benson (1975), involving meditation steps to elicit relaxation.

Salutogenic approach Antonovsky's (1979) health-promotion model focusing on factors that create and maintain health rather than those that cause disease.

Salutogenic pathway Stress response trajectory characterized by challenge appraisal, optimal physiological activation and potential progression toward growth, enhanced resilience and flourishing.

Salutogenesis Approach to health that emphasizes factors promoting well-being rather than disease (Antonovsky, 1979).

Self-care Activities undertaken to maintain physical, mental, and emotional health.

Self-defeating behavior Repetitive actions that hinder goal achievement, such as procrastination or poor health habits.

Self-regulation Ability to control emotions, set goals and maintain health.

Sense of coherence (SOC) Antonovsky's (1987) construct comprising three components – comprehensibility (understanding events), manageability (accessing resources), and meaningfulness (finding purpose) – that determines how individuals respond to stressors.

Sentics Field of study exploring the biological basis of emotional communication (Clynes, 1973).

Serotonin Hormone and neurotransmitter that regulates mood ("feel-good" hormone).

Sleep hygiene Practices designed to promote healthy sleep, including routines, environment adjustments and avoidance of naps.

Social comparison Process of comparing oneself to others, often based on idealized portrayals on social media, which can create feelings of inadequacy.

Social isolation Withdrawal from social interaction, resulting in loneliness and lack of support.

Social Learning Theory Theory that explains how people learn by observing and interacting with others. In groups, members model, practice and reinforce adaptive coping behaviors.

Social media Online platforms that facilitate communication, information sharing and social interaction.

Social stress Stress resulting from social threats to relationships, belonging or esteem (Kiecolt-Glaser et al., 2010).

Social stressors Negative social interactions such as bullying, conflict or unfair treatment that contribute to stress.

Stress Non-specific internal or external demand disrupting physiological and psychological balance.

Stress diary Recording of stressors, symptoms and coping activities used to monitor stress.

Stress inoculation training (SIT) Cognitive behavioral intervention that builds stress resilience through graduated exposure to manageable stressors combined with coping skills training; analogous to biological immunization (Meichenbaum, 1993).

Stress management Coping strategies including exercise, meditation and relaxation, used to reduce stress.

Stress mindset Individual's belief system about the nature and effects of stress; either stress-is-enhancing (stress as potentially beneficial) or stress-is-debilitating (stress as inherently harmful; Crum et al., 2013).

Stress response Physiological or psychological reaction to a stressor.

Stressor Any external environmental demand or internal perception that requires adaptation or coping, potentially triggering physiological and psychological stress responses.

Sympathetic nervous system (SNS) Division of the autonomic nervous system responsible for "fight-or-flight" responses, activating physiological arousal through increased heart rate, respiration, and energy mobilization.

Tai chi Originally a martial art, now involving gentle movements, breathing and meditation for health promotion or rehabilitation (National Center for Complementary and Integrative Health, n.d.).

Threat appraisal Cognitive evaluation of a stressor as dangerous, harmful or exceeding available coping resources, typically leading to pathogenic responses and negative adaptation.

Transactional model of stress Folkman and Lazarus' (1984) framework conceptualizing stress as a dynamic interaction between person and environment mediated by cognitive appraisal and coping processes rather than a simple stimulus-response phenomenon.

Traumatic event Event threatening death, injury, or violence, often linked to PTSD.

Universality Shared realization that others experience similar struggles. Recognizing this commonality reduces isolation and fosters connection within a group.

Upward spirals Self-reinforcing positive cycles wherein positive emotions broaden thinking and build resources, generating further positive emotions and continued psychological growth (Fredrickson & Joiner, 2002).

Walking meditation Mindfulness practice of walking slowly and attentively, often in nature (Hanh, n.d.).

Well-being Holistic state encompassing physical, mental and emotional health, life satisfaction and fulfillment.

REFERENCES

Ader, R., Felten, D. L., & Cohen, N. (1995). *Psychoneuroimmunology* (2nd ed.). Academic Press.

American Music Therapy Association. (n.d.). Definition and quotes about music therapy. https://www.musictherapy.org/about/quotes/

American Psychological Association. (2014). The road to resilience. https://www.apa.org/topics/resilience

American Psychological Association. (n.d.-a). APA dictionary of psychology: Hardiness. https://dictionary.apa.org/hardiness

American Psychological Association. (n.d.-b). APA dictionary of psychology: Mindfulness-based cognitive therapy (MBCT). https://dictionary.apa.org/mindfulness-based-cognitive-therapy

Antonovsky, A. (1979). *Health, stress and coping*. Jossey-Bass.

Antonovsky, A. (1987). *Unraveling the mystery of health: How people manage stress and stay well*. Jossey-Bass.

Benson, H. (1975). *The relaxation response*. HarperCollins.

Bernard, C. (1865). *An introduction to the study of experimental medicine*. Dover Publications.

Bienertova-Vasku, J., Lenart, P., & Schering, A. (2020). Eustress and distress: Neither good nor bad, but rather the same? *Stress and Health*, *36*(1), 1–10. https://doi.org/10.1002/smi.2923

Burke, J., Dunne, P. J., Byrne, E., & O'Boyle, C. (2025). *Positive health: The basics*. Routledge.

Cannon, W. B. (1932). *The wisdom of the body*. W. W. Norton.

Centers for Disease Control and Prevention. (n.d.). Chronic diseases in America. U.S. Department of Health and Human Services. https://www.cdc.gov/chronicdisease/

Clynes, M. (1973). Sentics: Biocybernetics of emotion communication. *Annals of the New York Academy of Sciences*, *220*(3), 55–131. https://doi.org/10.1111/j.1749-6632.1973.tb40248.x

Crum, A. J., Salovey, P., & Achor, S. (2013). Rethinking stress: The role of mindsets in determining the stress response. *Journal of Personality and Social Psychology*, *104*(4), 716–733. https://doi.org/10.1037/a0031201

Dietrich, A. (2004). Neurocognitive mechanisms underlying the experience of flow. *Consciousness and Cognition*, *13*(4), 746–761. https://doi.org/10.1016/j.concog.2004.07.002

Fauver, C., Maier, S. F., & Watkins, L. R. (2024). The diathesis–stress model revisited: Epigenetics and stress sensitivity. *Annual Review of Clinical Psychology*, *20*, 421–446. https://doi.org/10.1146/annurev-clinpsy-032423-104356

Folkman, S., & Lazarus, R. S. (1984). *Stress, appraisal, and coping*. Springer.

Fredrickson, B. L., & Joiner, T. (2002). Positive emotions trigger upward spirals toward emotional well-being. *Psychological Science*, *13*(2), 172–175. https://doi.org/10.1111/1467-9280.00431

Hanh, T. N. (n.d.). *Walking meditation*. Plum Village. https://plumvillage.org/library/books/walking-meditation

Kiecolt-Glaser, J. K., Gouin, J. P., & Hantsoo, L. (2010). Close relationships, inflammation, and health. *Neuroscience & Biobehavioral Reviews*, *35*(1), 33–38. https://doi.org/10.1016/j.neubiorev.2009.09.003

Kobasa, S. C. (1979). Stressful life events, personality, and health: An inquiry into hardiness. *Journal of Personality and Social Psychology*, *37*(1), 1–11. https://doi.org/10.1037//0022-3514.37.1.1

Lazarus, R. S., & Folkman, S. (1989). *Hassles and Uplifts Scales (HSUP)*. APA PsycTests. https://doi.org/10.1037/t06473-000

Maslach, C., & Leiter, M. P. (2016). Burnout. In G. Fink (Ed.), *Stress: Concepts, cognition, emotion, and behavior* (pp. 351–357). Elsevier.

Mayo Clinic. (n.d.). Post-traumatic stress disorder (PTSD). https://www.mayoclinic.org/diseases-conditions/post-traumatic-stress-disorder

McEwen, B. S., & Stellar, E. (1993). Stress and the individual: Mechanisms leading to disease. *Archives of Internal Medicine*, *153*(18), 2093–2101. https://doi.org/10.1001/archinte.1993.00410180039004

Meichenbaum, D. (1993). Stress inoculation training: A 20-year update. In P. M. Lehrer & R. L. Woolfolk (Eds.), *Principles and practice of stress management* (2nd ed., pp. 373–406). Guilford Press.

National Cancer Institute. (n.d.). NCI dictionary of cancer terms. https://www.cancer.gov/publications/dictionaries/cancer-terms

National Center for Complementary and Integrative Health. (n.d.). Tai chi: What you need to know. https://www.nccih.nih.gov/health/tai-chi-what-you-need-to-know

National Institute for Occupational Safety and Health. (n.d.). Stress at work. Centers for Disease Control and Prevention. https://www.cdc.gov/niosh/topics/stress/

Seligman, M. E. P. (1975). *Helplessness: On depression, development, and death*. W. H. Freeman.

Selye, H. (1956). *The stress of life*. McGraw-Hill.

Selye, H. (1974). *Stress without distress*. Lippincott.

Selye, H. (1976). *Stress in health and disease*. Butterworth-Heinemann.

Stern, R. M., Ray, W. J., & Quigley, K. S. (2014). *Psychophysiological recording* (2nd ed.). Oxford University Press.

Tedeschi, R. G., & Calhoun, L. G. (2004). Posttraumatic growth: Conceptual foundations and empirical evidence. *Psychological Inquiry*, *15*(1), 1–18. https://doi.org/10.1207/s15327965pli1501_01

Waxenbaum, J. A., Varacallo, M., & Jialal, I. (2024). Autonomic nervous system. In *StatPearls*. StatPearls Publishing. https://www.ncbi.nlm.nih.gov/books/NBK539845/

World Health Organization. (n.d.). Mental health: Strengthening our response. https://www.who.int/news-room/fact-sheets/detail/mental-health-strengthening-our-response

Index

For Product Safety Concerns and Information please contact our EU representative GPSR@taylorandfrancis.com Taylor & Francis Verlag GmbH, Kaufingerstraße 24, 80331 München, Germany